# The Psychoimmunology of Cancer

# The Psychoimmunology of Cancer
## Mind and Body in the Fight for Survival?

*Edited by*

C. E. Lewis,
C. O'Sullivan,
and
J. Barraclough

Oxford   New York   Tokyo
OXFORD UNIVERSITY PRESS
1994

Oxford University Press, Walton Street, Oxford OX2 6DP

Oxford   New York
Athens   Auckland   Bangkok   Bombay
Calcutta   Cape Town   Dar es Salaam   Delhi
Florence   Hong Kong   Istanbul   Karachi
Kuala Lumpur   Madras   Madrid   Melbourne
Mexico City   Nairobi   Paris   Singapore
Taipei   Tokyo   Toronto
and associated companies in
Berlin   Ibadan

Oxford is a trade mark of Oxford University Press

Published in the United States
by Oxford University Press Inc., New York

A catalogue record for this book is available from the British Library

Library of Congress Cataloging in Publication Data
The psychoimmunology of cancer : mind and body in the fight for
survival? / edited by C. E. Lewis, C. O'Sullivan, and J. Barraclough.
Includes bibliographical references and index.
1. Cancer—Immunological aspects.   2. Cancer—Psychological
aspects.   3. Psychoneuroimmunology.   4. Mind and body.   I. Lewis,
Claire E.   II. O'Sullivan, C.   III. Barraclough, Jennifer.
[DNLM: 1. Neoplasms—psychology.   2. Neoplasms—immunology.
3. Psychoneuroimmunology.   QZ 200 P9725 1994]
RC267.3.P79      1994      616.99′4′0019—dc20      94-8027
ISBN 0 19 262365 6

Typeset by Colset Pte Ltd, Singapore
Printed in Great Britain on acid-free paper by
Bookcraft (Bath) Ltd, Midsomer Norton

# Preface

For many years, physicians, psychologists, and psychiatrists have reported signs of an interrelationship between the mind and body in the fight against cancer. Whether emotional stress and/or personality type play an important role in the onset and progression of this disease is a question of relevance to scientists and clinicians, of concern to patients and their families, and of interest to the general public. Various psychological intervention methods have been developed to help patients cope with the emotional impact of their diagnosis. The importance of these methods, however, may be double-edged. Evidence has now emerged that they may also, in some instances, affect prognosis and the course of the disease.

This book presents the findings of leading specialists working in this rapidly expanding field. Their contributions are divided into three broad categories detailing the most recent evidence for and against:

(1) the presence of various physiological pathways linking brain function with immune cell activity (Part I);
(2) the influence of psychosocial factors on cancer survival (Part II); and
(3) the involvement of immune mechanisms in the effect of emotional status on cancer progression (Part III).

Such a multidisciplinary approach is likely to appeal not only to immunologists, oncologists, surgeons, psychologists, and psychiatrists, but also to medical students aware of the growing need to explore both the psychological and the physiological aspects of a given disease in clinical practice.

C.E.L.
*Oxford*                                                                 C.O'S.
August 1994                                                              J.B.

# Contents

# Contributors

**J. Barraclough**  Sir Michael Sobell House, Churchill Hospital, Headington, Oxford, UK

**D. L. Bellinger**  Department of Neurobiology and Anatomy, University of Rochester School of Medicine, 601 Elmwood Avenue, Box 603, Rochester, New York 14642, USA

**C. Bemis**  Department of Psychiatry, Yale School of Medicine, New Haven, Connecticut, USA

**M. Biondi**  III Clinica Psichiatrica, Universita di Roma, 'La Sapienza', Roma, Italy

**D. H. Bovbjerg**  Department of Neurology, Memorial Sloan Kettering Cancer Center, 1275 York Avenue, New York 10021, USA

**C. Classen**  Department of Psychiatry and Behavioral Sciences, Stanford University School of Medicine, Stanford, California 94305, USA

**A. Dalgleish**  Department of Medical Oncology, St George's Hospital, London, UK

**H. J. Eysenck**  Institute of Psychiatry, 16 De Crespigny Park, Denmark Hill, London, SE5 8AF, UK

**R. E. Faith**  College of Pharmacy, University of Illinois, 833 S. Wood St, Chicago, Illinois 60612, USA

**F. I. Fawzy**  Department of Psychiatry and Biobehavioral Sciences, UCLA School of Medicine, 760 Westwood Place, Los Angeles, California 90024–175919, USA

**N. W. Fawzy**  Department of Psychiatry and Biobehavioral Sciences, UCLA School of Medicine, 760 Westwood Place, Los Angeles, California 90024–175919, USA

**D. L. Felten**  Department of Neurobiology and Anatomy, University of Rochester School of Medicine, 601 Elmwood Avenue, Box 603, Rochester, New York 14642, USA

**S. Y. Felten**  Department of Neurobiology and Anatomy, University of Rochester School of Medicine, 601 Elmwood Avenue, Box 603, Rochester, New York 14642, USA

**P. J. Guillou**  Department of Surgery, St Mary's Hospital, Paddington, London, UK

**K. S. Hermanson**  Department of Psychiatry and Behavioral Sciences, Stanford University School of Medicine, Stanford, California, 94305, USA

**S. P. Hersh**   Medical Illness Counseling Center, Chevy Chase, Maryland 20815, USA

**M. Holden**   Cellular Nutrition Group, Dept of Biochemistry, University of Oxford, South Parks Road, Oxford, OX1 3QU, UK

**C. S. Hynn**   Department of Psychiatry and Biobehavioral Sciences, UCLA School of Medicine, 760 Westwood Place, Los Angeles, California 90024–175919, USA

**G. D. Kotzalidis**   III Clinica Psichiatrica, Universita di Roma, 'La Sapienza', Roma, Italy

**J. F. Kunz**   Medical Illness Counseling Center, Chevy Chase, Maryland 20815, USA

**H. Landrine**   Department of Preventive Medicine, USC School of Medicine, 1420 San Pablo Street, PMB A-301, Los Angeles, California 90033, USA

**J. L. Levensen**   Department of Psychiatry, Virginia Commonwealth University, Medical College of Virginia, Richmond, Virginia 23298–0268, USA

**K. S. Madden**   Department of Neurobiology and Anatomy, Rochester University, Rochester, New York 14642, USA

**G. Marks**   Department of Preventive Medicine, USC School of Medicine, 1420 San Pablo Street, PMB A-301, Los Angeles, California 90033, USA

**E. A. Newsholme**   Cellular Nutrition Group, Department of Biochemistry, University of Oxford, South Parks Road, Oxford, OX1 3QU, UK

**B. A. Presberg**   Department of Psychiatry, Virginia Commonwealth University, Medical College of Virginia, Richmond Virginia 23298–0268, USA

**N. P. Plotnikoff**   College of Pharmacy, University of Illinois, 833 S. Wood Street, Chicago, Illinois 60612, USA

**J. L. Richardson**   Department of Preventive Medicine, USC School of Medicine, 1420 San Pablo Street, PMB A-301, Los Angeles, California 90033, USA

**M. Schedlowski**   Department of Medical Psychology, Hannover Medical School, Hannover, Germany

**H.-J. Schmoll**   Department of Medical Psychology, Hannover Medical School, Hannover, Germany

**T. A. B. Sheard**   CRC Psychological Medicine Group, Christie Hospital NHS Trust, Stanley House, Wilmslow Road, Withington, Manchester, M20 9BX, UK

**S. Somers**   Department of Surgery, St Mary's Hospital, Paddington, London, UK

**B. Souberbielle**   Department of Medical Oncology, St George's Hospital, London, UK

**D. Spiegel**  Department of Psychiatry and Behavioral Sciences, Stanford University School of Medicine, Stanford, California 94305, USA

**U. Tewes**  Department of Medical Psychology, Hannover Medical School, Hannover, Germany

**K. S. Zanker**  Institute of Immunology, University of Witten, Herdecke, 10 Stockumerstrasse, 5810 Witten, Germany

PART I

# Psychoneuroimmunology:
# the interplay between the brain and
# the immune system

# 1

# Psychoneuroimmunology today: current concepts and relevance to human disease

## M. BIONDI AND G. D. KOTZALIDIS

## 1   Introduction

The term 'psychoimmunology' refers to a relatively recently acknowledged discipline, which deals with the interaction between the psyche and the immune system. It was not first coined by Solomon and Moos in their seminal paper in 1964 (1) as has often been claimed, although it is a term usually associated with Solomon. It remained fairly unused in the literature until it was reintroduced to abbreviate and circumscribe the term 'psychoneuro-immunology'. The latter is commonly associated with the work of Ader and colleagues (2, 3), who have pioneered studies in this multidisciplinary field since the mid-1970s.

Obviously, any term involving the word psyche is likely to create confusion since there is no universal consensus on the definition of this aspect of human function. Both psychoimmunology and psychoneuroimmunology are broadly used as synonyms to define a field that considers analogies and mutual interactions between the central nervous system (including all aspects of behaviour and mental activity) and immune function. These interactions may be either direct or indirect (through other systems that are linked to both the immune or the central nervous system). At its broadest definition, therefore, psychoimmunology could be seen to encompass virtually anything within an organism, since most immune cells have access to all organs and tissues of the body, including the central nervous system. This, in turn, influences the peripheral nervous system which then modulates the function of bodily organs.

All those who are acquainted with psychotherapy know that too deep an interpretation, too early in the course of therapy, is likely to be rejected by the patient. Psychoanalysts speak of *resistance* (a term familiar to immunologists as well). It is a kind of 'anaphylactic' reaction that could harm rather than benefit the patient. What happens to the patient is that, should the interpretation be correct, he or she would then re-discuss and re-adapt a host of inner things, to allow 'foreign', non-self elements to be embodied. This, in his/her mind, would cause a loss of personal identity. To preserve the latter, the patient overreacts (the immune system behaves much the same way during hypersensitivity reactions).

Similarly, the medical establishment could overreact to a newly established discipline if the scope of the discipline allows people who have little to do with science to proclaim themselves as psychoimmunologists. Unfortunately, this is what happened in two of the leading nations of psychoneuroimmunological research. During the mid-1980s, a passionate debate took place in the *New England Journal of Medicine*. In an editorial entitled *Disease as a Reflection of the Psyche* (4), the very influential pathologist, Marcia Angell, attacked psychoimmunology (and other aspects of psychosomatics, although she did not mention these new disciplines by name), on the grounds of some negative findings regarding survival of cancer patients (5). She went on to compare cancer in the twentieth century with tuberculosis in the nineteenth, stating that 'the elaborate construct of a tuberculosis-prone personality evaporated when tuberculosis was found to be caused by the tubercle bacillus'. She failed, however, to explain why only some people exposed to the microbe actually get tuberculosis; could personality, redefined by today's standards, have something to do with resistance to infection? Although we, the authors, believe that this is, indeed, the case, we do not yet understand fully the physiological mechanisms responsible for such phenomena. Hence, we believe that much research has still to be done in this exciting new field. By contrast, people who endorse Dr Angell's views would, no doubt, propose that it is a waste of time (and of research funding) to even try.

Both the above editorial, and the research paper that triggered it, caused a heart-felt reaction (6–14). Defendants of psychoimmunology rightly stressed that simply because the links between the psyche and the immune function had not been discovered at that time, this was not proof that such links did not exist. Furthermore, the lack of positive findings of psychoimmune links in a given area could simply reflect inadequate methodology.

Another major debate took place in the early 1990s in the United Kingdom. The trigger was very similar. A group of researchers found the survival of women with breast cancer to be negatively affected when they participated in a treatment programme involving help with psychological aspects of their disease. These research workers presented results first on television, where they took an explicit position against psychoimmunology (although again, the word psychoimmunology was not cited, as such). Thereafter, they published their work in the *Lancet*, where they were increasingly cautious (15, 16). Again, the reaction was marked (17–21) and the arguments in favour of the existence of a mind–immunity connection were similar. It could be argued that even if the results of this study were not biased by the design of the study (something that the authors themselves later implicitly admitted (16)), they would still point to the existence of psychological factors which can influence cancer survival. It is rational to believe, therefore, that some different approach could yield opposite results; hence the need for further research.

The heat of the debate demonstrated that psychoimmunological issues were becomingly increasingly important to clinicians in their understanding and treatment of disease. Physicians, psychologists, and social workers were eager to integrate these into their treatment programmes based on the findings of psychoimmunological research. The ongoing negative reactions of some clinicians could reflect their frustration with the lack of solid, irrefutable data that could be translated into bold new clinical guidelines. Moreover, scientifically based professionals are prone to seeing psychoimmunology as being invaded by people who propose untestable models, over-extrapolate from data, and draw unsubstantiated conclusions. It is clear that some of the so-called psychoimmunological methods of healing have yet to be fully grounded in scientific knowledge; one example is guided imagery. Although a positive effect of imagery has been shown on lymphocyte differentiation and thymic hormone levels (22), this cannot be linked directly (or otherwise), at present, to specific anti-tumour effects or cancer progression.

We should limit ourselves, therefore, to accepting as psychoimmunologically relevant only that which can be scientifically tested, reproduced, or refuted, and concerns changes in behaviour that can be correlated with changes in immune measures and vice versa. It is too early to propose psychoimmunology as a scientific discipline that enables us to fight or avoid cancer or other immunological (or even mental) disorders. One of the aims of psychoimmunology, however, is to study how the fight against, or prevention of, such an illness could be pursued. Hence, to avoid the misuse of psychoimmune principles, such as blame being attributed to patients for their disease (23), a psychoimmunological hypothesis should at least offer a scientifically plausible chain of physiological events to link the immune system with behaviour and/or psychological status. For example, no matter how simplistic or incomplete it may be, the chain linking mental depression with altered hypothalamic–pituitary–adrenal axis, increased corticosteroid secretion, decreased immunity, and finally to increased cancer susceptibility, should be accepted as a scientifically testable hypothesis, and every single link in this chain rigorously investigated. On the other hand, telling cancer patients there is a brand new 'psychoimmune treatment' approach, which involves one or a number of psyche-based ways of boosting the activity of immune cells to destroy their cancer cells and improve survival, is unethical and scientifically incorrect. Rather, patients should be told that there is evidence that cancer usually involves immunological impairment, and that some methods, such as imagery, show positive immunological effects. That their condition is such that they have nothing to lose if they participate in such a novel programme, and that with the committed approach of the patient, it may just help (in a variety of ways). However, clinicians are duty-bound to also explain that it is not fully known how or why this might be the case for *some* patients and not others, and that absence of a beneficial effect is not their fault and will probably not negatively influence the progression of their disease.

Here, we briefly review the evidence for mind–immune interactions in lower species and humans, and assess their relevance to various forms of human disease. The relevance of psychoimmunology to human disease is likely to increase as our knowledge of the molecular mechanisms of physiological and pathological processes expands, and as the concept of a link between the psyche and disease evolves.

Here, the evidence for the influence of psychological stress on the immune system will be reviewed with special emphasis on human studies. The impact of psychoneuroimmunological studies on the development of various human diseases will then be tackled, as well as the problems arising from the use of imperfect experimental designs and confounding variables. Finally, we will discuss the interaction between environmental factors and the biological constitution of an individual in determining susceptibility to disease.

## 2 Stressors as mediators of immune changes

'Stress research' is an area of psychoimmunology for which it was relatively easy to prove a scientific basis. Stress mechanisms are thought to be centrally involved in the relationship between behaviour and immunity. Briefly, stress is the response of a system to environmental influences which tend to push the system's function off-range. A stressor is a stimulus that evokes an abnormal physiological response. In the case of biological organisms, the stressor need not be truly 'external' to the system, but may originate from past material stored in the organism.

The link between stress and changes in immune function was first proposed by Hans Selye, who observed lymphatic involution and increased susceptibility to infection in animals subjected to certain stressful procedures (24, 25). Various stressors were subsequently found to affect almost all aspects of immunity; primary and secondary antibody responses, B- and T-lymphocyte function and NK-cell cytotoxicity ('NK activity') (26).

Selye defined a general adaptation syndrome whereby stress was counteracted after the alarm reaction had ceased (27). However, this general adaptation syndrome was subsequently found to have different efferent pathways, depending on the type of stress. One single general adaptation mechanism was no longer a completely tenable concept, and as a result the term 'stress' expanded to cover practically anything (and by definition, it could not be otherwise).

Too comprehensive a definition of stress implies that any disease is a stressor. Other, less aversive experiences and even some pleasant ones, however, are also to be included in the 'stress list'. It is, therefore, logical that if psychoimmunological mechanisms are important for stress, they will also be important for disease. Disease is, after all, a particular state of the organism adapting to environmental demands and is, therefore, a function of both the organism and the environment. The body responds to a disease as a whole and the end result of the *noxa*-organism interaction depends on the level of function of the organism, as well as on the type of *noxa*. The level of function of the organism results from many variables, amongst which are parameters such as attention and arousal on the psychological side, and immune surveillance on the physiological side. Therefore, the same quantity of a noxious agent can have very different effects on the body, depending on its state of alertness (in a broad sense). An 'alert' person, for example, may be affected less by a given disease, simply by being more able to detect its onset, and therefore, promptly refer themselves to a physician. However, it should not be forgotten that the noxious agent is important as well, and sometimes the nature of this is such that psychological or immunological reaction(s) to the disease may be rendered unimportant.

Experimental approaches to the psychoimmunology of stress often deal with subtle concepts that can rarely be standardized, even in those using animal models. Tables 1 and 2 summarize research (28–97) into the effects of various stressors on the immune system of animals and humans respectively. From a glance, it is apparent that there is little overlap in the stress models and experimental designs used. This is natural, given the fact that human beings should not be treated harshly to induce stress (like a salmon kept out of water for 3 minutes (29)). Furthermore, the human psyche, besides being more complex than in most other animals, is more easily communicated in terms of spoken language; a fact that imposes quite different rules and limitations on the design of experiments. What then is the relevance, if any, of studies of animal stress to the effects of human stress? There are things animals cannot tell us. For example, how certain types of stress are actually perceived by the animal (52). What does social isolation or overcrowding in a cage mean to them? Apparently, in humans loneliness can lead to immunosuppression (98–100). Do individually caged rats perceive something similar to the feeling of loneliness perceived by humans? If yes, can immunological changes in rats be expected to be similar in nature to those encountered in humans? Individually housed rodents (71, 72) and birds (31) showed increased immunocompetence, whereas animals caged in groups of two or eight animals are less immunocompetent than animals housed in groups of four per cage. Taken together, these data could suggest that grouping affects immunity, therefore, psychosocial factors could be important in determining protection from disease. But again, why should one animal be better than two in a cage, and four be just right, but eight be too many? And how can we translate this finding into useful information about human disease? We cannot even extend it to other rat strains, as strain-related differences are found regarding hormone responses and immune changes in responses to stress (47, 101).

Besides criticism about extrapolating from animal data to the human condition, another factor which hampers the validation of psychoimmunological studies concerns the fleeting nature of some immunological responses and the lack of sufficiently frequent follow-up. Transversal experimental designs to explore the most dangerous aspects of the stress response, that is its long-term effects are usually inadequate. Acute stress is not the same as chronic stress, since the former might serve as some form of training for an intact organism, and the more it deals with the stress factor successfully, overcoming it promptly, the more it may be prepared to face a subsequent stress. Chronic stress, on the other hand, may lead to fatigue of the stress-responding system, thereby leading to permanent impairment and to the acquisition of stress-dealing patterns which are maladaptive. The structuring of these patterns may establish new equilibria within the organism that render it more susceptible to disease in general, since all diseases impinge on the stress–response system of the body at the beginning.

**Table 1** A summary of recent studies of the immunological effects of stress: animal studies

| Type of stress | Animal | Result | Reference |
|---|---|---|---|
| Electric shock and water change | Mollusc (*Mytilus edulis*) | Haemocytic opioid-induced mobilization | Stefano *et al.* 1990 (28) |
| Transport, manipulation, unsuitable environment | Salmon | Decreased antibody-forming ability and increased susceptibility to infection in acutely stressed animals that parallels a rise in cortisol (4 hours); enhanced immunity after 24 hours | Maule *et al.* 1989 (29) |
| Social (confrontation) | Fish (subordinate) | μ-opioid-induced immune suppression | Faisal *et al.* 1989 (30) |
| Social isolation | Japanese quail chicks | High social reinstatement: quails show increased heterophil/ lymphocyte ratios | Mills *et al.* 1993 (31) |
| Food deprivation | Mouse | Thymic and spleen atrophic changes; early transient increase in NK cells and macrophage respiratory burst; increased T-cell count, but decreased B-cell count | Nakamura *et al.* 1990 (32) |
| Physical restraint | Mouse | Decreased NK-cell activity and specific response to Herpes simplex-1 virus | Bonneau *et al.* 1991 (33) |
| Physical restraint | Mouse | Inhibition of specific T-lymphocyte memory against Herpes simplex virus | Bonneau *et al.* 1991 (34) |
| Physical restraint | Mouse | Elicited significant corticosterone secretion, transiently suppressed expression of MHC class II glycoproteins (Ia) by peritoneal macrophages of Mycobacterial infection-susceptible animals | Zwilling *et al.* 1990 (35) |
| Physical restraint | Mouse | Corticosterone suppresses MHC class-II (Ia) glycoproteins after 2 hours | Zwilling *et al.* 1990 (36) |
| Physical restraint, inescapable shock | Mouse | Decrease of mature/immature T-cell ratio attenuated by pretreatment with diazepam or naloxone | Teshima *et al.* 1991 (37) |
| Intense acute restraint | Mouse | Long-term decrease in IgE production | Loureiro and Wada 1993 (38) |

**Table 1**  (*continued*)

| Type of stress | Animal | Result | Reference |
|---|---|---|---|
| Physical restraint | Mouse | Decreased cellular anti-viral immunity; reduced IL-2 secretion; humoral immune response unaffected | Sheridan *et al.* 1991 (39) |
| Physical restraint | Swine | Cortisol secretion more sensitive to ACTH in animals that could turn around, but not move freely; no immunological alterations detected (of the few investigated) | Becker *et al.* 1989 (40) |
| Physical restraint | Rat | Corticosteroid receptors (type-I and -II) decreased in the hippocampus, but not in lymphoid tissues | Miller *et al.* 1990 (41) |
| Physical restraint | Rat | Decrease in primary and secondary antibody response was further enhanced by naltrexone | Ray *et al.* 1992 (42) |
| Physical exercise | Mouse | Reduced mitogenesis after treadmill in untrained mice, probably due to increase in T-suppressor cells | Randall Simpson *et al.* 1989 (43) |
| Rotational | Mouse | Normal, but not adrenalectomized, mice showed reduced lymphocyte plaque forming cell response to sheep red blood cells | Esterling and Rabin 1987 (44) |
| Cold swim | Rat | Single session reduced T-cell proliferation, an effect that was blocked by pretreatment with an opioid antagonist; this effect undergoes tolerance with repeated sessions | Ferry *et al.* 1991 (45) |
| Cold swim | Mouse | Reduced thymocyte and splenocyte counts, decreased T-cell blastogenesis, and reduced NK-cell activity. Increased PGE2 secretion by peritoneal macrophages from stressed mice; and decreased IFN-$\alpha$-induced Ia expression. Increased IL-1 in stressed mice | Cheng *et al.* 1990 (46) |

**Table 1** (*continued*)

| Type of stress | Animal | Result | Reference |
|---|---|---|---|
| Electric foot-shock | Mouse | Strain-related effects. Generally, enhanced mitogenic response to ConA, but the mouse strain that did not show such response presented leucopenia | Lysle *et al.* 1990 (47) |
| Electric foot-shock, light or odour | Mouse | Plaque-forming cell response and antibody titre decreased after 3 days | Zalcman *et al.* 1991 (48) |
| Electric foot-shock | Rat | Shock induced suppression of both mitogenic response of peripheral blood T-cells and of splenic T-cells; adrenalectomy prevented the former, whereas $\beta$-blockers attenuated the latter | Cunnick *et al.* 1990 (49) |
| Electric foot-shock | Mouse | Depression of secondary, but not primary (at least, not consistently) immune response | Moynihan *et al.* 1990 (50) |
| Electric foot-shock | Rat | Intermittent inescapable shock decreased response to ConA and PHA, but not IgM-plaque forming cell response to sheep red blood cells, while eliciting a 20-fold increase in cortisol plasma levels | Jessop *et al.* 1989 (51) |
| Prenatal maternal (foot-shock or psychological) and postnatal (electric foot-shock) | Rats (pups) | Electric foot-shock induced a prolonged decrease of antibody response in the offspring, whereas psychological stress was transient; postnatal foot-shock was found to be immunosuppressive in control offspring but not in offspring of psychologically stressed rats | Sobrian *et al.* 1992 (52) |
| Inescapable shock | Rat | Antibody formation to sheep red blood cells enhanced in high locomotor activity animals (i.e. responding to novelty stress) | Sandi *et al.* 1992 (53) |
| Electric foot-shock | Rat (male) | Paraventricular nucleus (PVN) lesions attenuated the increases in plasma ACTH and corticosterone in both acutely and chronically stressed animals; central injection of | Rivest and Rivier 1991 (54) |

**Table 1**   (*continued*)

| Type of stress | Animal | Result | Reference |
|---|---|---|---|
| | | IL-1$\beta$ decreased LH and increased ACTH and corticosterone secretion; PVN lesions did not influence LH decrease but abolished the HPA response | |
| Electric foot-shock; odour; light | Mouse | Reduced splenic plaque-forming cell (PFC) response and plasma antibody titres | Zalcman *et al.* 1991 (55) |
| Electric foot-shock-infection | Mouse | Foot-shock decreases specific immunity to herpes simplex-1 virus and cytotoxic T-lymphocyte response in herpes-infected animals | Kusnecov *et al.* 1992 (56) |
| Brain lesion | Rat | Lesion of the amygdala did not result in NK-cell activity changes | Grijalva *et al.* 1990 (57) |
| Surgery and general anaesthesia | Rat | Opioid-mediated NK-cell activity reduced | Beilin *et al.* 1992 (58) |
| Surgery | Mouse | Chronic midazolam decreased the detrimental effects of laparatomy on lymphocyte counts and mitogenic responses | Freire-Garabal *et al.* 1992 (59) |
| Surgery | Mouse | Surgical stress-induced susceptibility to infection is attenuated by chronic diazepam | Freire-Garabal *et al.* 1991 (60) |
| Audiogenic | Mouse | Chronic buspirone reduces stress-induced spleen and thymic atrophic changes and the drop in peripheral T-lymphocyte counts | Freire-Garabal *et al.* 1991 (61) |
| Audiogenic | Mouse | Chronic clonazepam reduced stress-induced thymic and spleen atrophy and fall in peripheral T-lymphocyte counts | Freire-Garabal *et al.* 1991 (62) |
| Audiogenic | Rat | Suppression of splenic lymphocyte responsiveness on the first day and habituation after 4 days, despite persistent ACTH and corticosterone elevations | Sandi *et al.* 1992 (63) |

**Table 1**  (*continued*)

| Type of stress | Animal | Result | Reference |
|---|---|---|---|
| Audiogenic | Mouse | Depressed primary, but enhanced secondary immune response | Kim 1989 (64) |
| Neurogenic | Rat | Increased corticosterone response to ACTH and cytokines (effects were additive) | Torres Aleman *et al*. 1988 (65) |
| Novelty (cage switch) | Rat | Rise in TNF levels and in body temperature; the latter was further increased by anti-TNF antiserum | Long *et al*. 1990 (66) |
| Novelty (transport and new housing) | Swine | Increased susceptibility to infection, as shown by increased TNF-α after 4–10 days | Artursson *et al*. 1989 (67) |
| Social (conflict) | Mouse | Enhanced phagocytosis, attenuated by opioids and enhanced by μ-opioid antagonists and abolished by HPA axis disruption; no effect on proliferative T- and B-cell responses | Lyte *et al*. 1990 (68) |
| Social (crowding) | Mouse | Mice housed in groups of 8 or 2 per cage had decreased lymphocyte counts with respect to mice housed in groups of 4 in a cage | Peng *et al*. 1989 (69) |
| Social (competition) | Rat | Decreased antibody production in territory-defending rats; lowest antibody levels in submissive animals | Fleshner *et al*. 1989 (70) |
| Social (isolation) | Rat | Enhanced peripheral blood and splenic lymphocyte responses | Jessop *et al*. 1987 (71) |
| Social isolation and crowding | Mouse | Individually housed mice display greater phagocytotic and chemotactic capacity, produce more macrophage colony stimulating factor (CSF), and release more IL-1 from peritoneal macrophages | Salvin *et al*. 1990 (72) |
| Unfamiliar social grouping | Rhesus monkey | Increased cortisol, and decreased T-helper and T-suppressor lymphocytes 24 hours after group formation; | Gust *et al*. 1991 (73) |

**Table 1** (*continued*)

| Type of stress | Animal | Result | Reference |
|---|---|---|---|
| | | decrease in lymphocytes apparent after several weeks only in non-dominant animals | |
| Social (peer separation) | Squirrel monkey | 3-hour separation from peers induced decreased response to ConA after 3–24 hours and to PHA after 2 days; cortisol was found to be increased throughout. After one week, all alterations subsided | Friedman *et al.* 1991 (74) |

Longitudinal study designs are needed to study chronic stress (102). Such studies are more difficult to perform, since they suffer from high subject attrition (often due to the delicate nature of the stressor; for example, bereavement or life-threat) and they require complex designs that are likely to increase variability. Despite these inconveniences, chronic stressor studies have yielded surprisingly uniform data on the immunodepressant potential of various stressors such as bereavement (actual or anticipated) (103), threat of loss (104), divorce (105, 106), loneliness (107), life threatening disease (108, 109), and unemployment (110).

## 3   Interactions between neural, endocrine, and immune molecules

Animal studies have proved useful in elaborating something of the cellular and humoral mechanisms by which the organism responds to disease, especially when the type of study needed cannot be performed on man. Examples of this include neuroendocrine studies involving receptor identification in the central nervous system (CNS) or brain peptide interactions. Communication between cells is important in processing information from outside the body, and for setting the values of controlled variables in the internal environment. Cell-to-cell communication is mediated by various means. This usually involves peptides being released for local or systemic use. Peptide action distant from the site of production is largely responsible for the co-ordination of cell functions, maintenance of homoeostasis, or promotion of morphogenesis. Most distantly acting peptides are produced by APUD (amine precursor uptake and decarboxylation) cells. These cells constitute a diffuse system which secretes peptides for paracrine, synaptic, and endocrine purposes. These peptides may be co-localized in these cells or they may also

**Table 2**   A summary of recent studies of the immunological effects of stress: human studies

| Stress | Sample | Result | Reference |
|---|---|---|---|
| Surgery and anaesthesia | Patients having coronary artery bypass grafting | NK-cell activity increased before surgery, decreased after anaesthesia, and increased during cardiopulmonary bypass. After surgery, NK-cell activity, PHA response, and lymphocyte counts decreased for 3 days. Immune changes were related to cortisol levels | Tonnesen *et al.* 1987 (75) |
| Surgery | Patients | Transient glucocorticoid receptor increased | Krasznai *et al.* 1989 (76) |
| Surgery, and general or epidural anaesthesia | Patients undergoing herniorrhaphy | Immune response changes (leucocyte migration) only in patients subjected to general anaesthesia | Edwards *et al.* 1990 (77) |
| Surgery | Patients with aortic aneurysm | Persistent increase in IFN production | Baigrie *et al.* 1992 (78) |
| Surgery | Patients undergoing upper abdominal operations | Increased ACTH, cortisol, and cytokine (TNF and IL-6) plasma levels. Epidural block up to upper thoracic spine did not affect stress response; extension to the lower thoracic segment abolished stress response | Naito *et al.* 1992 (79) |
| Electric and audiogenic | Healthy men subjected to escapable or inescapable shock | Decreased, post-stress mitogenic response to ConA and monocyte percentages with escapable shock | Weisse *et al.* 1990 (80) |
| Glucose challenge | Healthy ageing men | Life events and depressive symptoms positively correlate with thymosin-1 (only post-challenge) | Aldwin *et al.* 1991 (81) |
| Chronic pain | Patients with temporomandibular pain/dysfunction | Mitogenic responses to PWM and ConA decreased with increased demoralization; response to ConA decreased with high pain levels | Marbach *et al.* 1990 (82) |

**Table 2**  (*continued*)

| Stress | Sample | Result | Reference |
|---|---|---|---|
| Parturition | Pregnant women | Decreased salivary IgA; state anxiety accounted for part of IgA variance | Annie and Groer 1991 (83) |
| Birth (maternal stress) | Neonates delivered after labour vs. neonates delivered after caesarean section vs. adults | Mothers' labour decreased total and helper T-lymphocytes in neonates | Pittard *et al.* 1989 (84) |
| Unhealthy lifestyle | Healthy adult men | Decreased NK-cell number and activity with men with unhealthy lifestyles | Kusaka *et al.* 1992 (85) |
| Chronic life threat | Healthy individuals living near damaged nuclear plant | Decreased lymphocyte counts, B-lymphocytes, T suppressors, NK cells, and antibody production. Increased neutrophil numbers | McKinnon *et al.* 1989 (86) |
| Depression or threat | Depressed patients and healthy controls | Decreased NK-cell activity | Irwin *et al.* 1990 (87) |
| Mental stress, with adrenaline vs. placebo infusion | Healthy men | Biphasic lymphocyte response to adrenaline; mental stress decreased 2-adrenoceptors, but lymphocyte function was unaffected | Larsson *et al.* 1989 (88) |
| Mental stress | Healthy young men | Increase in NK-cell number; decreased T-helper/ T-suppressor ratio; reduced mitogenesis | Bachen *et al.* 1992 (89) |
| Life stress | Healthy adults | Social support decreased stress-induced immunodepression | Thomas *et al.* 1985 (90) |
| Life events | Type-1 diabetic patients vs. controls | Fewer total life events in diabetics, but at least one effect precedes onset of illness; decreased response to PHA in patients who experienced a recent life event vs. those who did not | Vialettes *et al.* 1989 (91) |
| Daily uplifts and hassles | Healthy volunteers | Fewer uplifts and more hassles, anger, and tension increases susceptibility to the common cold | Evans and Edgerton 1991 (92) |

**Table 2** (*continued*) ·

| Stress | Sample | Result | Reference |
|--------|--------|--------|-----------|
| Ranger training course | Healthy men | Increased VIP secretion, increased VIP-induced cAMP levels in monocytes and suppression of their respiratory bursts | Wiik *et al.* 1989 (93) |
| Social (family) stress | Families (parents and at least one child, aged 1–18 years) | High scores on the FACES II scale for cohesion and adaptability correlated with frequency of influenza B infection | Clover *et al.* 1989 (94) |
| Social stress (5-day seminar on self-awareness) | Medical students | Increased T-suppressor cell response to PHA and IL-2 stimulation; decreased total T-lymphocytes. Changes correlated with achievement orientation | Kropiunigg *et al.* 1989 (95) |
| Academic | Medical students | No modification of cortisol across the three timé-points investigated (one month prior to examination, immediately, and 10 days after). Mitogenic responses to ConA and PWM, and IFN production decreased, and IL-1 increased, only just after examinations | Dobbin *et al.* 1991 (96) |
| Academic | Healthy medical students | Incomplete reactivation of latent Epstein–Barr virus | Glaser *et al.* 1991 (97) |

co-localize with classical neurotransmitters. Apparently, glial elements and some neurones belong to this system. Similar cells may also be found in lymphoid tissues, so it is not surprising that the latter may produce signalling peptides. Moreover, since they produce these peptides or receive them from peripheral nerves, immune cells also bear receptors for these peptides, together with those for classical neurotransmitters. However, lymphoid cell-expressed receptors for neurotransmitters are not necessarily identical to those in the CNS (111).

APUD peptides were first isolated in the gastrointestinal tissues and termed gastrointestinal peptides. They retained some of the nomenclature associated with this early classification, even after they were also found to be produced by some neurones. Similarly, neuropeptides that were first found to exist in lymphoid tissues were grouped under the fashionable name of 'immuno-peptides', and when found to act in the brain, were not immediately attributed a neuromodulatory role. Despite mRNA for interleukins (ILs) being found in neurones (112), their neuromodulatory function has yet to be accepted. This is another example of scientific rigidity induced by adherence to early nomenclature and classification.

At present, the major link between the CNS and the immune system is the hypothalamus. This is the site of production of 'stress' hormone-releasing factors, and is where most of the neuromodulatory effects of ILs and interferons (IFNs) occur. IL-1 stimulates the median eminence and the para-ventricular nucleus to induce the release of corticotrophin-releasing factor (CRF) (113–115), which in turn releases adrenocorticotrophin (ACTH) and β-endorphin; the most important peripheral effectors of the hypothalamic–pituitary–adrenal (HPA) axis. It is not clear whether IL-1 actually releases ACTH indirectly via its influence on vasopressin, an ACTH secretagogue (115, 116). Another 'immunopeptide' which influences the activity of the HPA axis is IL-6 which enhances ACTH release directly from the pituitary. Further-more, IL-6 was shown to be released by pituitary folliculo-stellate cells upon stimulation with IL-1 (117). This peptide also stimulates the release of thyrotrophin at the pituitary level (118). Other 'immune molecules' able to promote ACTH release include tumour necrosis factor (TNF)-α, thymosin fraction 5 (TF-5) (114), and IFN-α (119).

The effects of molecules associated with the immune system on the growth hormone axis are mediated largely via their influence on growth hormone (GH) releasing factors. IL-β1 stimulates growth hormone releasing hormone (GHRH) release from the hypothalamus and GH from the anterior pituitary. However, doses of IL-1β inhibit GH release, presumably through activation of CRF release (120). IFN-γ transiently inhibits GH release from the rat pituitary (at low concentrations), although by releasing somatostatin in the hypothalamus, the suppressive action of IFN-γ on GH release is protracted (121). Both the above hypothalamic peptides have immunological effects. GHRH and CRF are both capable of increasing target cell $3'–5'$ cyclic adenosine monophosphate (cAMP) and can affect NK activity. CRF decreases such activity, whereas GHRH shows a biphasic effect (122).

Various studies have suggested that IL-1α and IL-1β may be present in neurons and function as neuromodulators, IL-1β being the most widely expressed. It is distributed mostly in the hypothalamus (the paraventricu-lar nucleus—*pars magnocellularis*; suprachiasmatic nucleus and median eminence), but is evident in other CNS sites as well (cortex, hippocampus, and possibly the thalamus). IL-1α is also found, albeit at lower concentrations compared with IL-1β, in the anterior hypothalamus and hippocampus (123). The two peptides do not easily cross the blood–brain barrier, therefore their central actions are due either to indirect actions mediated via neural or glial compartments of the CNS, or to actions on brain sites not protected by such a barrier.

Peptides which are known to act on cells of the immune system via receptor-mediated mechanisms include cholecystokinin, somatostatin, GRP/bombesin-like, vasoactive intestinal polypeptide (VIP), prolactin (protein), tachykinins, neurotensin, pro-opiomelanocortin-derived peptides, dynorphin, α-neoendorphin, and calcitonin gene-related peptide (see ref. 124, for review). Receptors for 'neuropeptides' and neurotransmitters found on immune cells include those for noradrenaline, dopamine, serotonin, GAGA/benzodiazepine, acetylcholine, and the recently discovered cannabinoid receptor (125).

With this panoply of communication molecules, the immune and nervous systems are able to communicate their changing states to each other, so that they both adapt to (or cope with) environmental needs with minimal loss of information. Their communication is relevant to the way the organism interacts to external stimuli and, therefore, to disease (which can be viewed as a stressor). Environmental stressors tend to be translated into molecular terms which could potentially be harmful to the body. However, the transcripts of such molecular insults impinging on an organism usually bear testimony to the effect of the stressor and are likely to reproduce the same bodily state on repetition of the stimulus. It is due to evolution that innate healing mechanisms operate in organisms which are fit for survival. Therefore, such an organism is likely to counteract a noxious stimulus and is also likely to enhance a functional state which can be associated with well-being, since the stressor has been dealt with successfully. This forms the basis of the process called 'conditioning'.

# 4 Conditioning and brain–immune interactions

Conditioning is the process whereby the organism pairs a response to a stimulus (called an unconditioned stimulus) to another one which is not specifically related to the original response, but which somehow repeatedly occurred during the unconditioned stimulus–response triggering. The computer-like, predictive nature of the brain is responsible for this phenomenon. The phenomenon can best be explained by accepting Hebb's model of synaptic functioning, which involves state-dependent responses. By extending this model of functioning to the immune system, we are in a position to understand why a second antigenic presentation may elicit an enhanced and accelerated antibody response; the immune system, as with any other bodily system is capable of a learned or 'conditioned' response.

If we admit that the body reacts to environmental stimuli as a whole, it is easy to understand that the state of a given subsystem may markedly influence the overall state of the system, and that each of the subsystem states provides a host of possible conditionable responses to an unconditioned stimulus. Thus, anything may elicit a conditioned response, therefore, conditioning *must* be one of the ways the immune and the nervous system interact. Furthermore, stressors bear a higher conditioning (or extinguishing) potential than most stimuli, so they are more likely to produce learned states which make up the overall response of the system to them. If maladaptive responses are learned, as is supposed to occur in such diseases as cancer, they have to be unlearned, so that they allow adaptive (good coping) mechanisms to take over and deal with the environment. However, it is difficult to say which parts of an individual's response to environmental stimuli are defective. Moreover, if these maladaptive behaviour patterns are long established, they can reach a balance with the disease state, that is, they constitute a new, stable equilibrium state. So, it is to be expected that most chronic patients are 'unwilling' to break the vicious circle of their disease process, not because they are non-compliant (hence 'guilty') but simply because they cannot afford to do otherwise. It should be borne in mind that the longer a disease process takes to establish itself, the longer and harder the healing process. At present, after analysing the findings of numerous studies, it is possible to highlight just a few common behavioural correlates of favourable or unfavourable predictors of disease outcome (for some patients at least).

Drugs are good candidates for conditioning signals, especially psycho-active drugs, in that they easily constitute internal cues or discriminative stimuli. Alcohol, benzodiazepines, $5\text{-}HT1_A$ agonists, and other drugs are internal stimuli. This means they can associate themselves with a particular immunological state which could contrast with their direct immunomodu-latory action on leukocytes themselves. This consideration may help us to understand the occurrence of some apparently paradoxical phenomena, besides explaining the fact that both immunological enhancement and suppres-sion may be conditioned (for review, see refs 126, 127, and 128). Camphor odour-conditioned, poly I:C-induced NK-cell activation could be reversed by naltrexone, a weak $\mu$-opioid antagonist (129) indicating an opioid mediation of the effect.

Conditioning paradigms may also be used to understand the physiological mechanisms of action of immunological molecules. Conditioned taste aversion has been used to clarify whether the anorectic effect of IFN-$\alpha$ could be related to taste aversion; it emerged that the mechanisms of the two phenomena are different (130). The fact that the expression of the protein for the proto-oncogene, c-fos, in the rat forebrain was conditioned by stressful stimuli might open new pathways to understanding central pathways of the stress response (131).

The features of stress conditioning which are pertinent to clinical medicine are manifold, but essentially consist of understanding that relativity is an intrinsic property of living organisms, and that the commonplace belief that immunosuppression is due to exposure to corticosteroids is an oversimplification and incorrect (126). Potential clinical areas for the thoughtful application of psychoimmunological techniques include those requiring the enhancement (cancer, AIDS) and suppression (graft vs. host reaction) of the immune system (132).

# 5   Psychoimmunology and psychiatric disorders

Psychiatric disorders are often accompanied by immunological abnormalities. Moreover, supraphysiological concentrations of immunoregulatory peptides can induce clinically diagnosed, psychopathological manifestations. This is another point in favour of the brain–immune system cross-talk concept. However, for psychoimmunological mechanisms to be described as being involved in the pathogenesis of psychiatric disorders, a causal relationship needs to be established. As mentioned previously, stress may permanently impair immunity, provided that the stressor is not overcome. Most serious psychiatric disorders have a chronic course, with exacerbations and partial remissions, and are, therefore, particularly likely to involve immunological abnormalities. The similarity of immune abnormalities induced by various psychiatric disorders lends credence to the view that this may be a non-specific stress-linked phenomenon.

## 5.1 SCHIZOPHRENIA

Schizophrenia is the most multifaceted of the psychiatric disorders. The concept of an abnormal type or 'P' lymphocyte (see Table 3) emerged during the early sixties (133). Another approach was epidemiological and involved coincidences between influenza or other viral epidemics and peak incidence of schizophrenia (see ref. 134, for a review). However, the immunological abnormalities of schizophrenia (Table 3) remain diverse and highly variable.

Based on the results of the most recent investigations of immunological abnormalities in schizophrenia (135–154), no consistent immunological abnormality is apparent. Therefore, one is tempted to speculate that non-specific, stress-related alterations may occur in this condition.

## 5.2 DEPRESSION

Immunological abnormalities accompanying depressive disorders have been thoroughly investigated in recent years. Table 4 shows the most recent studies performed in this area (138, 155–184). The most consistent findings cite this as a stress–response. Depressives, as opposed to schizophrenics, have high

**Table 3**  A summary of recent studies of immunological changes associated with schizophrenia

| Sample | Findings | Reference |
|---|---|---|
| Florid schizophrenics vs. drug-responsive schizophrenics vs. healthy controls | Stronger lymphocyte response to PHA and PWM, higher total and helper-lymphocyte counts, non-significant decrease in antibody response (except for tuberculin) and T-suppressor function in schizophrenics vs. controls prior to drug treatment; mitogenic responses further increased during drug treatment | Müller *et al.* 1991 (135) |
| Patients with schizophrenia vs. patients with schizoaffective psychosis vs. healthy controls | Schizophrenics and schizoaffective psychotics have higher total T-lymphocytes and T-helper cells than controls; these measures positively correlate with total psychotic symptomatology, as assessed through the BPRS, and with negative symptom scores, as assessed by means of the SANS, only after positive therapeutic response to neuroleptics | Müller *et al.* 1993 (136) |
| Neuroleptic drug-naïve vs. neuroleptic-free vs. matched healthy controls | No significant difference between groups for IL-2 and IFN-$\gamma$ serum concentrations; IFN-$\alpha$ not detected in any subject | Gattaz *et al.* 1992 (137) |
| Schizophrenic vs. depressive patients vs. two matched healthy control groups | NK-cell cytotoxicity decreased in depressive patients but not in schizophrenics, as compared to their respective control groups; hospitalization did not influence NK-cell cytotoxicity | Caldwell *et al.* 1991 (138) |
| Chronic schizophrenic patients vs. healthy controls | Reduced lymphocyte response to PHA and OKT3 in both drug-free and neuroleptic-treated chronic schizophrenics | Monteleone *et al.* 1991 (139) |
| Acute, recently diagnosed schizophrenic males | Low peripheral T-lymphocyte number; increased T helpers; unaltered T-helper/T-suppressor ratio; increased immature T-cell number | Rogoznikova 1991 (140) |
| Acute schizophrenics | Normalization of T-lymphocyte counts, reduction of undifferentiated cells, increased theophylline sensitivity of lymphocytes after insulin shock; enhanced lymphocyte pattern normalization with added neuroleptics; persistence or rise of the proportion of immature T cells with treatment was predictive of poor prognosis and a correlate of psychopathology | Rogoznikova 1991 (141) |

**Table 3** (*continued*)

| Sample | Findings | Reference |
|---|---|---|
| Treatment-resistant schizophrenics vs. healthy controls | Response to PHA, circulating immune complexes, T- and B-lymphocytes, null-cells and double-cells differ between schizophrenics and controls. Immunomodulator (xin shen ling) normalized all immunological parameters, but B-cell counts; furthermore, its continuous use after 3 years was associated with 5 relapses in 20 patients discharged from hospital | Ma *et al*. 1991 (142) |
| Florid schizophrenics vs. healthy controls | Lower neopterin (macrophage/T-cell activator) levels at baseline in schizophrenic patients, as compared with controls; neopterin levels increased with drug treatment and this correlated positively with decrease in psychopathology | Sperner-Unterweger *et al*. 1992 (143) |
| Schizophrenic patients vs. their relatives vs. healthy controls | High affinity $^3$H-spiroperidol (selective dopamine D2/5-HT$_{2/1C}$ receptor blocker) uptake by lymphocytes abnormally high only in 14% of patients and 5% of their parents; high affinity $^3$H-spiroperidol by lymphocytes does not appear to be useful as a vulnerability marker | Griffiths *et al*. 1992 (144) |
| Schizophrenic patients vs. healthy controls | 'P' lymphocytes (cells with basophilic cytoplasm, often vacuolated, a frequently irregular nucleus and high nucleus-to-cytoplasm ratio) represent a significant proportion of the lymphocyte population of schizophrenic patients (20%) and a negligible portion of control lymphocytes | Hirata-Hibi and Hayashi 1992 (145) |
| Schizophrenics vs. healthy controls | No evidence of retroviral infection in any of the subjects, as assessed by peripheral lymphocyte exposure to ionizing radiation and subsequent co-culture with indicator cells | Coggiano *et al*. 1991 (146) |
| Schizophrenic vs. depressive patients vs. healthy controls | Anti-brain antibodies to rabbit brains react with neuronal tissue in one third of schizophrenics compared with less than 4% in depressives and with 0% in controls | Shima *et al*. 1991 (147) |
| Schizophrenic patients vs. patients with inflammatory disease vs. healthy controls | About 50% of schizophrenic patients, compared with 8% of patients with inflammatory disorders and 0% of healthy controls, have neural antibodies to a neuroblastoma protein, identified as the 60 kDa P1 mitochondrial human heat-shock protein | Kilidireas *et al*. 1992 (148) |

**Table 3**  (*continued*)

| Sample | Findings | Reference |
|---|---|---|
| Schizophrenic patients vs. healthy controls | Significantly higher frequencies of HLA Class III allotypes BF*F, BF*SO7 and C4A*4 in schizophrenic patients, as compared with controls; no significant differences between patients and controls regarding C2 allotypes | Wang *et al.* 1992 (149) |
| Systematically assessed pedigrees | No linkage of schizophrenia to 5q11-q13 chromosome | Hallmayer *et al* 1992 (150) |
| Schizophrenic patients vs. healthy controls | No significant difference in mutant frequency resulting from mutation at the hprt locus in human T-lymphocytes, as well as in DNA repairing ability between schizophrenics and controls | Magin *et al.* 1991 (151) |

rates of impairment of dexamethasone suppression and resultant hyper-secretion of cortisol. High cortisol levels, especially with disrupted circadian patterns, are widely considered as sufficient *per se* to explain immunodepression. However, not all aspects of immunity are depressed by cortisol. Natural killer (NK) activity, which is the most consistently affected immune cell function in depressives, depends on the status of CNS opioid mechanisms (185) rather than cortisol levels. On the other hand, it should be remembered that ACTH, the pituitary effector of the corticosteroid response, is co-secreted with $\beta$-endorphin in near-equimolar amounts the same pituitary cells. It is possible, therefore, that increased $\beta$-endorphin could account for the effects of depression on NK-cells, but again, consistent $\beta$-endorphin elevations have yet to be shown in depression. One curious finding regarding $\beta$-endorphin is the higher frequency of an IgG directed against $\beta$-endorphin in the plasma of depressive patients than in healthy controls (186).

Smith also proposed an immunological model involving such cytokines as IL-1 in the pathogenesis of depression (187). The evidence, however, is not convincing. For Weisse (188), such immunological abnormalities characterize dysphoric mood rather than depressive disorders. An interesting finding that should prompt new research on the therapeutic potential of immuno-peptides is the finding that a thymic peptide preparation, thymopentin, as an adjunct to imipramine, improved depressive symptomatology whilst improving immune responsiveness (increased total and helper T-lymphocyte numbers and IL-2 levels (189)).

**Table 4** Summary of recent studies of immunological changes associated with depression

| Sample | Findings | Reference |
|---|---|---|
| Patients with severe depression vs. healthy controls | Healthy controls showed decreased PWM-induced B-cell proliferation and increased dexamethasone-induced inhibition of spontaneous leukocyte proliferation after metyrapone; depressed patients failed to respond | Rupprecht *et al.* 1991 (155) |
| Patients with severe depression before and after recovery (patients as their own controls) vs. healthy controls | No difference in glucocorticoid receptor number or affinity between patients (when depressed and after recovery) and controls; no significant ACTH or cortisol changes; no influence of antidepressant drugs on glucocorticoid receptor binding characteristics | Miller *et al.* 1991 (156) |
| Depressed patients vs. matched controls | Depressed patients had lower proliferative responses than controls who had less depression, anergia, and total BPRS scores, as well as fewer obsessions and compulsions and less psychomotor agitation than did patients | Darko *et al.* 1991 (157) |
| Depressed in-patients vs. healthy hospital staff controls | Patients with major depression had lower mitogenic responses to ConA and PHA with respect to controls and to other diagnoses of depressive disorder (atypical, dysthymic, or atypical bipolar disorder) | Levy *et al.* 1991 (158) |
| Patients with major depression vs. subjects anticipating bereavement vs. healthy controls | In depressive patients, scores on the Hamilton Depression Rating Scale and the Beck Depression Inventory correlated inversely with mitogenic response to PHA, whereas in the loss-anticipating subjects, such a correlation was positive | Spurrell and Creed 1993 (159) |
| Patients with major depression, with and without co-morbid panic disorder, vs. matched healthy controls | Higher T-cell counts and mitogenic response to PHA in co-morbid major depression/panic disorder patients with respect to depressives without panic disorder; higher mitogenic response to PHA and ConA in co-morbid major depression/panic disorder patients with respect to healthy controls; co-morbidity for panic disorder loads on the immunological alteration factor of affective disorder patients | Andreoli *et al.* 1992 (160) |
| Depressed patients | Dexamethasone suppression test (DST)-non-suppressors had more hypertension and a lower per cent blood lymphocyte count | Pfohl *et al.* 1991 (161) |
| Patients with major depression | Positive correlation between anxiety scores and T-helper/T-suppressor-cytotoxic cell ratio only in DST non-suppressors | Charles *et al.* 1992 (162) |
| Patients with severe major depression vs. healthy controls | No difference between patients and controls as for lectin-induced blastogenesis; patients showed less dexamethasone-induced reduction of | Rupprecht *et al.* 1991 (163) |

**Table 4**  (*continued*)

| Sample | Findings | Reference |
|---|---|---|
| | mitogenic response to PHA, but not to PWM or to ConA, and this effect was inversely correlated with *in vivo* ACTH afternoon levels; these results are compatible with reduced glucocorticoid receptor sensitivity in major depression | |
| Depressed outpatients vs. healthy controls | No difference in NK-cell activity between groups as a whole, but significantly higher NK-cell activity in female depressed patients, compared with female controls; no correlation between cortisol secretion and NK activity in any of the groups | Wodarz *et al.* 1991 (164) |
| Clinically recovered depressive patients (follow-up) | Mitogenic responses unchanged; *in vitro* glucocorticoid-sensitivity (dexamethasone) of lectin-induced lymphocyte blastogenesis not impaired; mitogenic response-inhibiting potency of dexamethasone correlated with *in vivo* ACTH afternoon levels; abnormalities in glucocorticoid receptor sensitivity are thus limited to the clinically active phase of depressive disorder | Wodarz *et al.* 1992 (165) |
| Depressed in-patients vs. healthy controls | Predexamethasone and postdexamethasone serum dipeptidyl-peptidase IV (enzyme related to IL-2) activity is lower in major depressives as compared with healthy controls, in melancholic patients as compared with minor depressives, and men as compared with women | Maes *et al.* 1992 (166) |
| Patients with major depression, with or without melancholia/ psychosis and patients with minor depression | Patients with major depression and melancholia/psychosis had weaker mitogenic responses than other patients; mitogenic responses inversely correlated with base-line cortisol and post-dexamethasone $\beta$-endorphin levels; urinary free cortisol correlates positively with responses to PHA and PWM | Maes *et al.* 1991 (167) |
| Patients with major depression, with or without melancholia, and patients with minor depression | The depressive state is characterized by higher total leucocyte, monocyte, class II MHC HLA-DR, and memory T-cell (CD4$^+$CD45RA) numbers; major depressives showed an increase in CD25$^+$ (IL-2 receptor) cells; major depressives with accompanying melancholic features had increased total T-, B- and T-suppressor/cytotoxic cell counts, and a lower T-helper to T-suppressor/cytotoxic ratio, compared with the other groups of patients | Maes *et al.* 1992 (168) |
| Depressed in-patients vs. healthy controls | The depressive state is characterized by a higher percentage of T-helper cells and a lower percentage of T-suppressor (CD8$^+$CD57$^-$ cells; | Maes *et al.* 1992 (169) |

**Table 4** (*continued*)

| Sample | Findings | Reference |
|---|---|---|
| | melancholics had more T-memory cells ($CD4^+CD45^-$) and T-helper cells | |
| Depressed in-patients vs. healthy controls | Pre-dexamethasone, enhanced mitogenic responses in minor depressives, as compared with controls and with major depressives; mitogenic responses inversely correlate with severity of depression; melancholics accumulate more IL-1$\beta$ in PHA culture supernatant than healthy controls. Post-dexamethasone, the latter showed less blast transformation, IL-1$\beta$ and soluble IL-2 receptor release by PBMCs in culture supernatants than for depressive patients | Maes *et al.* 1991 (170) |
| Patients with major depression, with or without melancholia, and patients with minor depression vs. healthy controls | The depressive state was characterized by increased serum circulating levels of soluble IL-2 receptor compared with the healthy state; anticardiolipin antibody was higher in melancholics than in healthy controls and minor depressives; antinuclear antibodies were more frequent in depressed patients than in healthy controls; anticardiolipin and antinuclear antibodies positively correlated with one another; the former also correlated positively with soluble IL-2 receptors | Maes *et al.* 1991 (171) |
| Depressed patients vs. healthy controls | Depressives had increased numbers of HLADR+ and CD19+ B-cells and a higher percentage of HLADR+ and CD21+ B-cells with respect to controls; melancholics had higher numbers of CD21+ cells and CD19+ cell percentage | Maes *et al.* 1992 (172) |
| Drug-free major depressives vs. healthy controls | Depressives had a higher number and percentage of CD25+ (IL-2) receptor-bearing) cells, higher concentrations of serum circulating soluble IL-2 receptors, higher supernatant soluble IL-2 receptors after PHA challenge, and a higher number of CD4+ cells (T helpers) | Maes *et al.* 1990–91 (173) |
| Depressed in-patients vs. healthy controls | NK-cell activity was much inhibited in melancholic depressives and intermediately blunted in minor depressives; it also correlated inversely with severity of illness and is not affected by steroids | Maes *et al.* 1992 (174) |
| Depressed in-patients vs. healthy controls | Major depressives exhibit a degree of leucocytosis which was greater than that found in minor depressives; healthy controls had no leucocytosis. Leukocytosis, which is due to both neutrophilia and monocytosis, was more pronounced in men | Maes *et al.* 1992 (175) |

**Table 4** (*continued*)

| Sample | Findings | Reference |
|---|---|---|
| Depressed patients vs. healthy controls | Reduced number of Leu-11 (CD16$^+$) (natural killer effector) cells and NK-cell activity and dissociation between Leu-11 cell percentage and NK-cell activity in depressive subjects; these differences may be attributed to sex, since only depressed men differed from healthy men in this respect. CD16$^+$ lymphocyte counts were inversely correlated with depressive scores on the Hamilton Depression Rating Scale in depressive men | Evans *et al.* 1992 (176) |
| Patients with major depression vs. healthy controls | Blunted circadian variation of NK-cell number and activity in patients with major depression with respect to controls | Petitto *et al.* 1992 (177) |
| Depressed patients vs. healthy controls | Sleep electroencephalogram parameters (total sleep time, sleep efficiency, and duration of non-REM sleep) positively correlated with NK-cell activity in both patients and controls | Irwin *et al.* 1992 (178) |
| Depressive vs. schizophrenic patients vs. two matched healthy control groups | NK-cell cytotoxicity decreased in depressive patients but not in schizophrenics, as compared with their respective control groups; hospitalization did not influence NK-cell cytotoxicity | Caldwell *et al.* 1991 (138) |
| Patients with major depression vs. patients with the chronic fatigue syndrome vs. healthy controls | Major depressives and healthy subjects had normal lymphocyte response to PHA and no reduction of delayed-type hypersensitivity skin responses as compared with subjects with the chronic fatigue syndrome | Lloyd *et al.* 1992 (179) |
| Healthy aged subjects with immunological or endocrine abnormalities linked to depression | Mitotic response to PHA was reduced in elderly as compared with adult subjects, and was significantly lower and inversely correlated with depression scores in the depressed aged subjects; the sample had low IL-2, IL-4, and IFN-$\gamma$ levels, with the depressed subpopulation displaying the lowest values; non-depressed aged subjects had normal IL-2-stimulated NK-cell activity; scores on a depression scale correlated inversely with IL-2- and IFN-$\alpha$-stimulated NK-cell activity | Guidi *et al.* 1991 (180) |
| Healthy aged subjects with immunological or endocrine abnormalities linked to depression | Reduced cutaneous delayed hypersensitivity in the aged, but no correlation with psychological status; reduced CD4$^+$/CD8$^+$ cell ratio, CD4$^+$/CD45R$^+$ cell subset, B-lymphocyte percentage, and CD16$^+$ in non-depressed aged, as compared to adult controls; Leu7$^+$ cells were significantly higher in the non-depressed compared with depressed aged subjects; Leu7$^+$ | Bartoloni *et al.* 1991 (181) |

**Table 4** (*continued*)

| Sample | Findings | Reference |
|---|---|---|
| | cell levels correlate inversely with depression scores; percentages of $CD16^+/Leu7^+$ cells were increased in the subgroup of depressed aged and positively correlated with age; urinary free cortisol level was higher in the depressed aged | |
| Adolescent patients with major depression vs. healthy controls | No differences in NK-cell activity between patients and controls, but significant correlations of depressive scores on the Reynolds Adolescent Depression Scale with NK-cell activity | Shain *et al.* 1991 (182) |
| Subjects diagnosed as depressives vs. college students screened for type I allergic disorders | Type I (IgE-mediated hay fever, asthma, eczema, hives) subjects reported significantly worse mood after the flu than did non-allergic subjects, clinical depression-prone individuals have more allergies than non-depressives | Bell *et al.* 1991 (183) |
| Case report on an elderly depressed woman | Psychotic behaviour after withdrawal of protracted corticosteroid treatment; reinstated therapy reversed this trend | Hassanyeh *et al.* 1991 (184) |

## 5.3 OTHER PSYCHIATRIC DISORDERS

Only recently has interest focused on the possible immunological abnormalities in psychiatric disorders other than schizophrenia and depression, and this is entirely due to the recent expansion of psychoimmune research. Data obtained to date (190–200) are not sufficiently detailed or consistent to allow any clear conclusions to be drawn (Table 5). However, the finding of differential behaviour of glucocorticoid receptors in post-traumatic stress disorder with respect to depression is very interesting (190). This could be taken to mean that neuroendocrine impairment in post-traumatic stress disorder is less than is the case with depression. Or it might be inferred that post-traumatic disorder is still an acute stress disorder that the organism tries to overcome. Further studies are needed to extend this finding to other possible impaired immunological functions in patients with this disorder.

Other findings worthy of mention are those that relate to schizoaffective disorder, which is accompanied by hyperglobulinaemia and phobic disorders, where there is a clear tendency to develop allergies. These results are difficult to explain and might have been biased by poor patient selection. Generally, the immune parameters measured in these studies are not those investigated for depression or schizophrenia.

**Table 5** Recent studies of immunological changes associated with psychiatric disorders other than schizophrenia or depression

| Disorder and sample | Findings | Reference |
|---|---|---|
| Post-traumatic stress disorder (PTSD) patients vs. healthy controls | Glucocorticoid receptors higher in PTSD patients than in normals; receptor circadian variations wider than in normals; changes opposite to those found in depression | Yehuda *et al.* 1991 (190) |
| Schizoaffective disorder vs. healthy controls vs. schizophrenics | Increased IgA, IgM, and IgG levels in schizoaffective patients | Balaita *et al.* 1992 (191) |
| Anxiety disorder patients (generalized anxiety disorder; panic disorder; obsessive compulsive disorder) vs. other psychiatric disorders | Lymphocyte $^3$H-PK11195 (peripheral benzodiazepine ligand) binding density lower in generalized anxiety disorder and obsessive-compulsive disorder | Rocca *et al.* 1991 (192) |
| Patients with panic disorder vs. controls | Higher IgA levels in patients | Ramesh *et al.* 1991 (193) |
| Patients with panic disorder before and after treatment vs. healthy controls | No difference in mitogenic response to PHA or in lymphocyte $\beta$-endorphin concentration | Brambilla *et al* 1992 (194) |
| Patients with phobic anxiety treated with behaviour therapy | Phobic patients more allergic | Schmidt-Traub 1991 (195) |
| Women with anorexia nervosa, restricted or bulimic anorectics vs. age-matched controls | No difference between the two groups in mitogenic response to PHA, or pre- and post-CRF levels | Brambilla *et al.* 1993 (196) |
| Patients with anorexia nervosa vs. healthy controls | Increased spontaneous production of TNF *in vitro* by peripheral monocytes from patients, but plasma levels undetectable; decreased cell-mediated cytotoxicity in patients; no difference in IFN levels | Schattner *et al.* 1990 (197) |
| Patients who attempted suicide vs. healthy controls | Increased soluble IL-2 receptor plasma concentrations, not related to treatment, nor correlating with endocrine measures; the only correlation was with urinary catecholamines and cerebrospinal fluid 3,4-MHPG (noradrenaline metabolite) | Nässberger and Träskman-Bendz 1993 (198) |
| Autistic children vs. controls (normal children, children with Down syndrome, and other mental deficiency) | Higher frequency of anti-myelin basic protein in patients with respect to controls | Singh *et al.* 1993 (199) |

# 6 Psychopharmacology, the CNS, and the immune system

Given the close interplay between these systems, and the bidirectional influences of their products, it might be expected that drugs acting on structures of one will also act on structures of the other.

## 6.1 IMMUNOLOGICAL EFFECTS OF PSYCHOPHARMACOLOGICAL AGENTS

Since drugs acting within the CNS are delivered to the brain through the blood, they usually come into contact with, and bind to, cells of the immune system, since the latter often possess similar receptors to those the psychopharmacological agents occupy in the CNS. Despite this extended potential of psychopharmacological agents, little work has been done in this area. This is because drugs used in psychiatry do not usually cause immunological problems (with the exception of clozapine, lithium, and carbamazepine for which thorough haematological control is warranted). On the contrary, in depression and schizophrenia, their use is often accompanied by reversal of existing immune alterations which can herald, at times, clinical improvement. For these reasons, psychopharmacological agents were not subjected to close scrutiny to assess their long-term or subclinical immunological effects. Such an approach is not fully legitimate, since immunological modifications are often subtle, yet they are thought to account for the induction of most undesirable disorders. Pre-marketing toxicological studies are unlikely to detect very subtle modifications, so it is surprising that no systematic study of the effects of psychopharmacological agents on immunity has been undertaken to date.

The most commonly prescribed drugs, benzodiazepines, are not uniform in their effects on immunity. They may indirectly enhance chemotaxis of mononuclear cells (201). Diazepam inhibits phagocytosis and antibody production, whereas alprazolam enhances T-lymphocyte-dependent responses (202). The effects of diazepam are probably mediated through peripheral benzodiazepine receptors, whereas those of alprazolam could be due to its central action to increase the ratio of $\alpha/\beta$ adrenoceptors. $\beta$-Adrenoceptors are expressed by $CD56^+/CD57^+$ leucocytes (NK cells mainly) and probably mediate immunological effects of some drugs (203). It is not yet known, however, whether these receptors are influenced by alprazolam. Inverse benzodiazepine agonists (anxiogenic $\beta$-carbolines) depress the immune response (204). In particular, N-methyl-$\beta$-carboline-3-carboxamide was found to suppress cytotoxic T-lymphocyte activity (205) and NK activity (206); these effects were antagonized by flumazenil, a benzodiazepine receptor antagonist. Some of the immunological effects of anxiogenic $\beta$-carbolines may be mediated through the inhibition of benzodiazepine receptors located in the

CNS. Ethyl-$\beta$-carboline-3-carboxylate, when microinfused into the locus ceruleus, produces decreases in IL-2 synthesis and NK activity, whereas infusion into the hippocampus resulted in decreased NK activity (207). The benzodiazepine receptor antagonist, flumazenil, blocked the effect of the inverse agonist on NK activity and the benzodiazepine receptor agonist, diazepam, more so, thus pointing to the existence of a GABA-A/benzodiazepine-mediated immune potentiation that emerges only when immunity is depressed (since the administration of flumazenil or diazepam alone had no effect on immune parameters).

Neuroleptic drugs increase both total T-cell and helper T-cell counts at low doses and lowers these at high doses (208). Clozapine, compared with other neuroleptics, has no effect and does not differ from other neuroleptics in its effects on PHA or ConA-induced proliferative responses (209). However, neuroleptic-induced symptom resolution in schizophrenic patients is often paralleled by an improvement in immune parameters. This might be due to the prolactin-releasing effect of classical neuroleptics as this pituitary hormone is known to enhance some aspects of immunity (210).

Response to viruses can be either enhanced, lowered, or unaffected by neuroleptics, depending on the virus (211). This effect is thought to be due to phenothiazine effects on nucleic acids (212, 213). Thioridazine, at therapeutic dosages on the other hand, inhibits T-cell proliferation and IL-2 production *in vitro* (214).

The evidence for neuroleptic effects on immune function is thus far from conclusive. Given the immune-enhancing properties of dopaminergic agents (for example, amphetamine increases NK activity) (215), they too deserve to be studied more closely.

Aside from the clinically correlated improvements in mood and immune status, anti-depressant drugs are not known to have immunostimulating properties on their own. Chronic maprotiline, but not desipramine treatment, depressed mouse NK activity, both *in vitro* and *in vivo* (216). One of the best elucidated mechanisms of anti-depressant action involves synaptic inhibition of serotonin re-uptake, a mechanism that acutely increases intrasynaptic serotonin availability. Both serotonergic and antiserotenergic agents decrease the plaque-forming cell response to sheep red blood cells. Serotonin antagonist-induced immunosuppression could be attributed to a direct 5-HT$_{2/1C}$ mechanism (217), whereas a serotonin-agonist induced one could be related to stress (218) since serotonin is a central CRF releaser. We may similarly interpret as a stress effect the case report of a fluoxetine-induced reactivation of herpes simplex infection (219).

To summarize, besides drugs that are well known to affect immunity, such as lithium, clozapine, valproate, and carbamazepine, other psychotropic drugs are little investigated with respect to their potential immunological effects.

**Table 6** Human disorders for which psychoimmunological hypotheses have been advanced

| Disease | Reference |
| --- | --- |
| Diabetes (type 1) | Robinson *et al.* 1989 (234)* |
| Multiple sclerosis | Grant *et al.* 1989 (235)*, Foley *et al.* 1988 (236)*, Garland and Zis 1991 (237), Grant *et al.* 1989 (238)*, Sternberg *et al.* 1992 (232)*, Chandarana *et al.* 1987 (239)*, Nakarama *et al.* 1992 (240), Katon *et al.* 1991 (241), Zautra *et al.* 1989 (242), McFarlane and Brooks 1990 (243)*, Soroka 1991 (244)* |
| Systemic lupus erythematosus | Lim *et al.* 1991 (245)*, Hinrichsen *et al.* 1989 (246), Wekking *et al.* 1991 (247) |
| Sjögren's syndrome | Drosos *et al.* 1989 (248) |
| Primary fibrositis | Wolfe *et al.* 1984 (249) |
| Hypersomnia | Bell *et al.* 1978 (250), Katon *et al.* 1991 (241)* |
| Chronic fatigue syndrome | Hickie *et al.* 1992 (251)* |
| Myasthenia gravis | Rohr 1992 (252), Lützenkirchen 1977 (253) |
| Grave's disease | Harsh *et al.* 1992 (254)* |
| Infantile asthma | Bender *et al.* 1991 (255) |
| Psoriasis | Blomquist and Sakki 1991 (256)#, Farber *et al.* 1990 (257)* |
| Atopic eczema | Blomquist and Sakki 1991 (256)# |
| Alopecia universalis | Teshima *et al.* 1991 (258) |
| Myofacial-pain dysfunction | Marbach *et al.* 1990 (259), Schleifer *et al.* 1990 (260) |
| AIDS (acquired immune deficiency syndrome) | Hassan and Douglas 1990 (261)*, Levy *et al.* 1989 (262), Antoni *et al.* 1991 (263) |
| Cancer progression (general) | Zanker and Kroczek 1991 (264), Bovbjerg 1991 (265) |
| Breast cancer | Levy *et al.* 1990, (266)*, Fredrikson *et al.* 1993 (267)* |
| Gynaecologic cancer | Teshima *et al.* 1991 (268)*, Antoni and Goodkin 1989 (269)* |
| Cancer (unspecified) | Lechin *et al.* 1990 (270)*, Toge *et al.* 1989 (271) |

* Stress-related mechanism.
# Mechanism related to alexithymia.


## 6.2 NEURAL EFFECTS OF IMMUNOMODULATORY AGENTS

Immunomodulators used in anti-tumour therapy have long been known to cause adverse psychological effects (220, 221). IFN-$\alpha$ was found to possess behavioural effects in as much as it decreased locomotor activity (222) and induced memory impairment (223). The behavioural effects of IFNs are mediated through stimulation of central IFN receptors, where IFNs act to induce neuroexcitatory, but not neurotoxic, effects (224). IL-1 acts on a central receptor to induce sedation and fever, whereas TNF is endowed with an antipyretic effect (225). IL-2 may induce psychotic-like reactions, but its main effect is induction of sleep, possibly mediated through $\mu$-opioid receptor enhancement and concomitant presynaptic $\alpha_2$-adrenoceptor stimulation (which inhibits adrenergic activity in the locus ceruleus) (226). These peptides also reduce feeding behaviour, as does muramyl dipeptide (227). Thymic peptides and levamisol showed behavioural effects that parallel their immunostimulating influence, (189–228) and may prove useful in increasing responsiveness of depressive patients to anti-depressants.

The full range of behavioural effects induced by immunomodulating molecules is far from fully established although it is expected that this line of research will prove to be extremely fruitful in years to come. Of the twelve ILs isolated to date, five (IL-1, -2, -4, -6, and -8) show behavioural effects compatible with an action at a CNS level; a list which is clearly set to increase.

## 7  Psychoimmunology in clinical medicine

Psychoimmunological mechanisms are increasingly thought to contribute to the pathogenesis of many disorders. Table 6 comprises some such disorders. In most of these, an important role for stress is acknowledged and the link with psychic parameters supported by the effects of psychotropic agents on such 'physical' measures as tumour growth (229), in which immune status is also crucial, at least in animal models (230). As a result, the concept of a disease subcategory, termed 'stress system disorders' (231) has evolved. This includes all disorders stemming from an impaired ability of the organism to adapt to environmental stimulation, maintain its homoeostasis, and ensure survival. According to this formulation, the 'stress system' consists of various axes 'responsible for reproduction, growth, and immunity' (231). Inflammatory disorders with an autoimmune component as well as important psychological correlates, as, for example, rheumatoid arthritis, enter this frame (232), for which there have been suggestions that drugs acting on CRF (233), a neuropeptide whose secretion is defective in depression, might be useful.

An intact HPA axis is an essential requirement for an appropriate response to any stressor, including disease. Intervention at the CRF level could set free the organism's innate healing abilities. It is improbable, however, that it could constitute a cure for all the disorders listed in Table 6, even though these have been related to stress (or to alexithymia, at least in one case) (234–271). Alexithymia is a psychological construct which measures the extent to which a subject has no words to express emotions. It is regrettable that the immunological correlates of psychological constructs like alexithymia, internal–external locus of control, self-efficacy, and the like, have not been investigated to date.

Not all suggestions of psychoneuroimmune links and alterations in stress-related disorders are new. Given the enormous social potential that a psychoneuroimmunological approach could have for disease susceptibility and cure, it is rather disappointing that more research on this has not been carried out in recent years. For most of the disorders listed in Table 6, psychological assessment was included in only 1 per cent (or fewer) of clinical studies performed; the inclusion of both psychological *and* immunological measures markedly reduces this meagre number yet further. Studies that investigate possible correlations between immunological and psychological variables in a given disease are those that contribute to the development of psychoneuroimmunology as a fully scientific discipline. The proportion of these studies is relatively small. Thus, whatever their potential relevance, their impact on the treatment of most diseases is negligible at present.

The impact of psychoneuroimmunology on the prevention and/or treatment of human disease can be measured only in terms of changing medical thinking and other social attitudes (for example, towards recognizing the role of psychosocial factors towards personal habits such as smoking, diet, or work, and towards changing environmental policy). At present, very few people think in terms of psyche–lymphocyte interactions. At present, those that do are mainly research workers, psychotherapists, experimental study volunteers, and in the worst of cases, poorly supervised or supported cancer patients. The direction in which they alter immune cell activity may not always be predictable, or may not produce the desired effect (272, 273).

## 8   Summary and conclusion

Although the observation of psyche–brain–immune interactions is as old as the recognition of the existence of the immune system itself, this has only been expressed in a written form and considered a science in the last few decades. The brain interacts with the immune system in a plethora of ways, and the possibility that the activity of some central nuclei or neural networks might influence immunity has yet to be identified. A complex interaction takes place at the hypothalamic–pituitary level, where neuroimmunoendocrine signals are integrated; molecules released by immune cells influence hypothalamic neuronal activity, and the release of hypothalamic releasing factors and pituitary hormones. The latter is largely responsible for immunological modulation, achieved through target hormones (for example, adrenal or sexual steroids) or through direct influence on immune cells (for example, the effects of $\beta$-endorphin, CRF, ACTH, and GH on lymphocytes and NK-cells).

Another mechanism operates via the innervation of lymphoid tissues, such as the thymus, tonsils, spleen, and enteric lymphoid system. The CNS controls the activity of the peripheral nervous system which, in turn, releases neurotransmitters or neuromodulators to modify the activity of immune cells, either directly or indirectly. Furthermore, immunopeptides act on brain centres which express receptors for them, such as in the limbic system, thereby modulating emotional behaviour; thereby completing the loop.

Given the importance of neuroendocrine axes in psychoimmune interactions, particular emphasis has been placed in past studies on stress and its mechanisms in causing susceptibility to disease (for example cancer, infection, autoimmunity). However, animal and human physiological systems do not necessarily overlap; therefore, extrapolation from conditions in one to the other is difficult.

Some psychiatric illnesses cause an abnormal secretion of such immune molecules as TNF, IFNs, and ILs which can act on the CNS, or immune complexes directed against brain tissue. Moreover, some psychiatric symptoms can be elicited by the neurotropism of infectious agents; in this respect, psychological mechanisms may not be centrally involved, although there is evidence that various personality traits may be important in determining the outcome of such infections (for example infection with the human immunodeficiency virus). Some psychiatric disorders may also induce immunological abnormalities, but not to the point of true or detectable immunological correlates of these disorders (although for depression such correlates might exist). As with other diseases, psychoimmunological considerations are seldom incorporated into the design of experimental clinical studies, and the cross-influence of psychotropic and immunomodulating medications has yet to be fully defined.

Psychoimmunological considerations are appropriate whenever diseases are thought to be related to stress (this would in fact encompass practically any disease, since all insults to body integrity are stressors). However, despite the considerable relevance of psychoimmunology to human disease, its actual impact on clinical practice remains negligible. A change of attitudes is urgently needed to allow this relatively new, but exciting discipline to blossom fully.

# 9 References

1. Solomon, G. F. and Moos, R. H. (1964). Emotions, immunity, and disease. A speculative theoretical integration. *Arch. Gen. Psychiatry,* **11**, 657–674.
2. Ader, R. (ed.) (1981). *Psychoneuroimmunology.* Academic Press, New York.
3. Ader, R., Felten, S. L., and Cohen, N. (eds) (1991). *Psychoneuroimmunology* (2nd edn). Academic Press, New York.

4. Angell, M. (1985). Disease as a reflection of the psyche (editorial). *N. Engl. J. Med.*, **312**, 1570–1572.

5. Casileth, B. R., Lusk, E. J., Miller, D. S., Brown, L. L., and Miller, C. (1985). Psychosocial correlates of survival in advanced malignant disease. *N. Engl. J. Med.*, **312**, 1551–1555.

6. Funch, D. P. (1985). Psychosocial variables and the course of cancer (letter). *N. Engl. J. Med.*, **313**, 1354.

7. Fiore, N. A. (1985). Psychosocial variables and the course of cancer (letter). *N. Engl. J. Med.*, **313**, 1354–1355.

8. Vitaliano, P. P., Lipscomb, P. A., and Carr, J. E. (1985). Psychosocial variables and the course of cancer (letter). *N. Engl. J. Med.*, **313**, 1355.

9. Levy, S. M., Winkelstein, A., Rabin, B. S., Lippman, M., and Cohen, S. (1985). Psychosocial variables and the course of cancer (letter). *N. Engl. J. Med.*, **313**, 1355–1356.

10. Williams, R. B., Jr., Benson, H., and Follick, M. J. (1985). Disease as a reflection of the psyche (letter). *N. Engl. J. Med.*, **313**, 1356–1357.

11. Livnat, S. and Felten, D. L. (1985). Disease as a reflection of the psyche (letter). *N. Engl. J. Med.*, **313**, 1357.

12. Brooks, J. O. III (1985). Disease as a reflection of the psyche (letter). *N. Engl. J. Med.*, **313**, 1357–1358.

13. Adler, R. H. (1985). Disease as a reflection of the psyche (letter). *N. Engl. J. Med.*, **313**, 1358.

14. Pepper, G. M. (1985). Disease as a reflection of the psyche (letter). *N. Engl. J. Med.*, **313**, 1358.

15. Bagenal, F. S., Easton, D. F., Harris, E., Chilvers, C. E. D., and McElwain, T. J. (1990). Survival of patients with breast cancer attending Bristol Cancer Help Centre. *Lancet*, **336**, 606–610.

16. Chilvers, C. E. D., Easton, D. F., Bagenal, F. S., Harris, E., and McElwain, T. J. (1990). Bristol Cancer Help Centre (reply to letter). *Lancet*, **336**, 1185–1188.

17. Hayes, R. J., Smith, P. G., and Carpenter, L. (1990). Bristol Cancer Help Centre (letter). *Lancet*, **336**, 1185.

18. Sheard, T. A. B. (1990). Bristol Cancer Help Centre (letter). *Lancet*, **336**, 1185–1186.

19. Sheard, T. A. B. (1990). Bristol Cancer Help Centre (letter). *Lancet*, **336**, 683.

20. Bourke, I. and Goodare, H. (1991). Bristol Cancer Help Centre. Bristol Survey Support Group (letter). *Lancet*, **338**, 1401–1402.

21. Goodare, K. J. (1992). Bristol Cancer Help Centre (letter). *Lancet*, **340**, 248.

22. Hall, N. R. S. and O'Grady, M. P. (1991). In *Psychoneuroimmunology* (2nd edn) (eds R. Ader, S. L. Felten, and N. Cohen), pp. 1067–1080. Academic Press, New York.

23. McGoldrick, K. E. (1989). Psychoneuroimmunology: blaming the victim? *J. Am. Med. Wom. Assoc.*, **44** (5), 134.

24. Selye, H. (1950). *Stress*. Acta, Montreal.

25. Selye, H. (1936). A syndrome produced by diverse nocuous agents. *Nature*, **138**, 32.

26. Monjan, A. A. (1981). Stress and immunologic competence: studies in animals. In *Psychoneuroimmunology* (ed. R. Ader), pp. 185–228. Academic Press, New York.

27. Selye, H. (1946). The general adaptation syndrome and the diseases of adaptation. *J. Clin. Endocrinol.*, **6**, 117–230.

28. Stefano, G. B., Cadet, P., Dokun, A., and Scharrer, B. (1990). A neuro-immunoregulatory-like mechanism responding to stress in the marine bivalve *Mytilus edulis. Brain Behav. Immun.*, **4**, 323–329.

29. Maule, A. G., Tripp, R. A., Kaattari, S. L., and Schreck, C. B. (1989). Stress alters immune function and disease resistance in chinook salmon (*Oncorhynchus tshawytscha*). *J. Endocrinol.*, **120**, 135–142.

30. Faisal, M., Chiappelli, F., Ahmed, I. I., Cooper, E. L., and Weiner, H. (1989). Social confrontation 'stress' in aggressive fish is associated with an endogenous opioid-mediated suppression of proliferative response to mitogens and non-specific cytotoxicity. *Brain Behav. Immun.*, **3**, 223–233.

31. Mills, A. D., Jones, R. B., Faure, J. M., and Williams, J. B. (1993). Responses to isolation in Japanese quail genetically selected for high or low sociality. *Physiol. Behav.*, **53**, 183–189.

32. Nakamura, K., Aoike, A., Hosokawa, T., Rokutan, K., Koyama, K., Nishi, Y., Yoshida, A., and Kawai, K. (1990). Effect of food-restriction stress on immune response in mice. *J. Neuroimmunol.*, **30**, 23–29.

33. Bonneau, R. H., Sheridan, J. F., Feng, N. G., and Glaser, R. (1991). Stress-induced suppression of herpes simplex virus (HSV)-specific cytotoxic T-lymphocyte and natural killer cell activity and enhancement of acute pathogenesis following local HSV infection. *Brain Behav. Immun.*, **5**, 170–192.

34. Bonneau, R. H., Sheridan, J. F., Feng, N. G., and Glaser, R. (1991). Stress-induced effects on cell-mediated innate and adaptive memory components of the murine immune response to herpes simplex virus infection. *Brain Behav. Immun.*, **5**, 274–295.

35. Zwilling, B. S., Brown, D., Christner, R., Faris, M., Hilburger, M., McPeek, M. *et al.* (1990). Differential effect of restraint stress on MHC class II expression by murine peritoneal macrophages. *Brain Behav. Immun.*, **4**, 330–338.

36. Zwilling, B. S., Dinkins, M., Christner, R., Faris, M., Griffin, A., Hilburger, M. *et al.* (1990). Restraint stress-induced suppression of major histocompatibility complex class II expression by murine peritoneal macrophages. *J. Neuroimmunol.*, **29**, 125–130.

37. Teshima, H., Sogawa, H., Kihara, H., and Nakagawa, T. (1991). Influence of stress on the maturity of T-cells. *Life Sci.*, **49**, 1571–1581.

38. Loureiro, I. and Wada, C. Y. (1993). Influence of stress on IgE production. *Physiol. Behav.*, **53**, 417–420.

39. Sheridan, J. F., Feng, N., Bonneau, R. H., Allen, C. M., Huneycutt, B. S., and Glaser, R. (1991). Restraint stress differentially affects anti-viral cellular and humoral immune responses in mice. *J. Neuroimmunol.*, **31**, 245–255.

40. Becker, B. A., Christenson, R. K., Ford, J. J., Nienaber, J. A., DeShazer, J. A., and Hahn, G. L. (1989). Adrenal and behavioral responses of swine restricted to varying degrees of mobility. *Physiol. Behav.*, **45**, 1171–1176.

41. Miller, A. H., Spencer, R. L., Stein, M., and McEwen, B. S. (1990). Adrenal

steroid receptor binding in spleen and thymus after stress or dexamethasone. *Am. J. Physiol.*, **259**, E405–E412.

42. Ray, A., Mediratta, P. K., and Sen, P. (1992). Modulation by naltrexone of stress-induced changes in humoral immune responsiveness and gastric mucosal integrity in rats. *Physiol. Behav.*, **51**, 293–296.

43. Randall Simpson, J. A., Hoffman-Goetz, L., Thorne, R., and Arumugam, Y. (1989). Exercise stress alters the percentage of splenic lymphocyte subsets in response to mitogen but not in response to interleukin-1. *Brain Behav. Immun.*, **3**, 119–128.

44. Esterling, B. and Rabin, B. S. (1987). Stress-induced alteration of T-lymphocyte subsets and humoral immunity in mice. *Behav. Neurosci.*, **101**, 115–119.

45. Ferry, A., Weill, B., Amiridis, I., Laziry, F., and Rieu, M. (1991). Splenic immunomodulation with swimming-induced stress in rats. *Immunol. Lett.*, **29**, 261–264.

46. Cheng, G. J., Morrow-Tesch, J. L., Beller, D. I., Levy, E. M., and Black, P. H. (1990). Immunosuppression in mice induced by cold water stress. *Brain Behav. Immun.*, **4**, 278–291.

47. Lysle, D. T., Cunnick, J. E., and Rabin, B. S. (1990). Stressor-induced alteration of lymphocyte proliferation in mice: evidence for enhancement of mitogenic responsiveness. *Brain Behav. Immun.*, **4**, 269–277.

48. Zalcman, S., Kerr, L., and Anisman, H. (1991). Immunosuppression elicited by stressors and stressor-related odors. *Brain Behav. Immun.*, **5**, 262–273.

49. Cunnick, J. E., Lysle, D. T., Kucinski, B. J., and Rabin, B. S. (1990). Evidence that shock-induced immune suppression is mediated by adrenal hormones and peripheral beta-adrenergic receptors. *Pharmacol. Biochem. Behav.*, **36**, 645–651.

50. Moynihan, J. A., Ader, R., Grota, L. J., Schachtman, T. R., and Cohen, N. (1990). The effects of stress on the development of immunological memory following lose-dose antigen priming in mice. *Brain Behav. Immun.*, **4**, 1–12.

51. Jessop, J. J., West, G. L., and Sobotka, T. J. (1989). Immunomodulatory effects of footshock in the rat. *J. Neuroimmunol.*, **25**, 241–249.

52. Sobrian, S. K., Vaughn, V. T., Block, E. F., and Burton, L. E. (1992). Influence of prenatal maternal stress on the immunocompetence of the offspring. *Pharmacol. Biochem. Behav.*, **43**, 537–547.

53. Sandi, C., Borrell, J., and Guaza, C. (1992). Behavioral factors in stress-induced immunomodulation. *Behav. Brain Res.*, **48**, 95–98.

54. Rivest, S. and Rivier, C. (1991). Influence of the paraventricular nucleus of the hypothalamus in the alteration of neuroendocrine functions induced by intermittent footshock or interleukin. *Endocrinology*, **129**, 2049–2057.

55. Zalcman, S., Kerr, L., and Anisman, H. (1991). Immunosuppression elicited by stressors and stressor-related odors. *Brain Behav., Immun.*, **5**, 262–273.

56. Kusnecov, A. V., Grota, L. J., Schmidt, S. G., Bonneau, R. H., Sheridan, J. F., Glaser, R. *et al.* (1992). Decreased herpes simplex viral immunity and enhanced pathogenesis following stressor administration in mice. *J. Neuroimmunol.*, **38**, 129–138.

57. Grijalva, C. V., Levin, E. D., Morgan, M., Roland, B., and Martin, F. C. (1990). Contrasting effects of centromedial and basolateral amygdaloid lesions

on stress-related responses in the rat. *Physiol. Behav.*, **48**, 495–500.

58. Beilin, B., Shavit, Y., Cohn, S., and Kedar, E. (1992). Narcotic-induced suppression of natural killer cell activity in ventilated and nonventilated rats. *Clin. Immunol. Immunopathol.*, **64**, 173–176.
59. Freire-Garabal, M., Belmonte, A., Balboa, J. L., and Nuñez, M. J. (1992). Effects of midazolam on T-cell immunosuppressive response to surgical stress in mice. *Pharmacol. Biochem. Behav.*, **43**, 85–89.
60. Freire-Garabal, M., Couceiro, J., Balboa, J. L., Nuñez, M. J., Fernandez-Rial, J. C., Cimadevila, B. *et al.* (1991). Effects of diazepam on the resistance, on the development of immunity and on the passive transfer of immunity to Listeria monocytogenes in mice submitted to surgical stress. *Acta Ther.*, **17**, 355–362.
61. Freire-Garabal, M., Belmonte, A., and Suarez-Quintanilla, J. (1991). Effects of buspirone on the immunosuppressive response to stress in mice. *Arch. Int. Pharmacodyn. Ther.*, **314**, 160–168.
62. Freire-Garabal, M., Jose-Meizoso, M., Rodriguez-Bujan, L., and Belmonte, A. (1991). Effects of clonazepam on T-cell immunosuppressive response to stress in mice. *Res. Commun. Psychol. Psychiatry Behav.*, **16**, 65–78.
63. Sandi, C., Cambronero, J. C., Borrell, J., and Guaza, C. (1992). Effects of HPA hormones on adapted lymphocyte responsiveness to repeated stress. *Brain Res. Bull.*, **28**, 581–585.
64. Kim, K. J. (1989). Effect of sound stress on immune response (Engl. abstr.). *Kanho Hakhoe Chi.*, **19** (2), 135–146.
65. Torres Aleman, I., Barasoain, I., Borrell, J., and Guaza, C. (1988). Immmune activation and psychoneurogenic stress modulate corticosterone-releasing effects of lymphokines and ACTH. *Am. J. Physiol.*, **255**, R839–R845.
66. Long, N. C., Vander, A. J., Kunkel, S. L., and Kluger, M. J. (1990). Antiserum against tumor necrosis factor increases stress hyperthermia in rats. *Am. J. Physiol.*, **258** (3 Pt. 2), R591–R595.
67. Artursson, K., Wallgren, P., and Alm, G. V. (1989). Appearance of interferon-alpha in serum and signs of reduced immune function in pigs after transport and installation in a fattening farm. *Vet. Immunol. Immunopathol.*, **23**, 345–353.
68. Lyte, M., Nelson, S. G., and Baissa, B. (1990). Examination of the neuroendocrine basis for the social conflict-induced enhancement of immunity in mice. *Physiol. Behav.*, **48**, 685–691.
69. Peng, X., Lang, C. M., Drozdowicz, C. K., and Ohlsson-Wilhelm, B. M. (1989). Effect of cage population density on plasma corticosterone and peripheral lymphocyte populations of laboratory mice. *Lab. Anim.*, **23**, 302–306.
70. Fleshner, M., Laudenslager, M. L., Simons, L., and Maier, S. F. (1989). Reduced serum antibodies associated with social defeat in rats. *Physiol Behav.*, **45**, 1183–1187.
71. Jessop, J. J., Gale, K., and Bayer, B. M. (1987). Enhancement of rat lymphocyte proliferation after prolonged exposure to stress. *J. Neuroimmunol.*, **16**, 261–271.
72. Salvin, S. B., Rabin, B. S., and Neta, R. (1990). Evaluation of immunologic assays to determine the effects of differential housing on immune reactivity. *Brain Behav. Immun.*, **4**, 180–188.

73. Gust, D. A., Gordon, T. P., Wilson, M. E., Ahmed-Ansari, A., Brodie, A. R., and McClure, H. M. (1991). Formation of a new social group of unfamiliar female rhesus monkeys affects the immune and pituitary adrenocortical systems. *Brain Behav. Immun.*, **5**, 296–307.

74. Friedman, E. M., Coe, C. L., and Ershler, W. B. (1991). Time-dependent effects of peer separation on lymphocyte proliferation responses in juvenile squirrel monkeys. *Dev. Psychobiol.*, **24**, 159–173.

75. Tonnesen, E., Brinklov, M. M., Christensen, N. J., Olesen, A. S., and Madsen, T. (1987). Natural killer cell activity and lymphocyte function during and after coronary artery bypass grafting in relation to the endocrine stress response. *Anesthesiology*, **67**, 526–533.

76. Krasznai, A., Krajcsi, P., Aranyi, P., and Horvath, I. (1989). Effects of operations on lymphocyte glucocorticoid receptors. *Acta Chir. Hung.*, **30**, 39–43.

77. Edwards, A. E., Smith, C. J., Gower, D. E., Williams, C. P., Ferguson, B. J. M., Gough, J. *et al.* (1990). Anaesthesia, trauma, stress and leucocyte migration: Influence of general anaesthesia and surgery. *Eur. J. Anaesthesiol.*, **7**, 185–196.

78. Baigrie, R. J., Lewis, C. E., Lamont, P. M., Morris, P. J., and McGee, J. O. (1992). Effect of major surgery on the release of interferon gamma by peripheral blood mononuclear cells: an investigation at the single cell level using the reverse haemolytic plaque assay. *Cytokine*, **4**, 63–65.

79. Naito, Y., Tamai, S., Shingu, K., Shindo, K., Matsui, T., Segawa, H. *et al.* (1992). Responses of plasma adrenocorticotropic hormone, cortisol, and cytokines during and after upper abdominal surgery. *Anesthesiology*, **77**, 426–431.

80. Weisse, C. S., Pato, C. N., McAllister, C. G., Littman, R., Breier, A., Paul, S. M. *et al.* (1990). Differential effects of controllable and uncontrollable acute stress on lymphocyte proliferation and leukocyte percentages in humans. *Brain Behav. Immun.*, **4**, 339–351.

81. Aldwin, C. M., Spiro, A., III, Clark, G., and Hall, N. (1991). Thymic peptides, stress, and depressive symptoms in older men: a comparison of different statistical techniques for small samples. *Brain Behav. Immun.*, **5**, 206–218.

82. Marbach, J. J., Schleifer, S. J., and Keller, S. E. (1990). Facial pain, distress, and immune function. *Brain Behav. Immun.*, **4**, 243–254.

83. Annie, C. L. and Groer, M. (1991). Childbirth stress. An immunologic study. *J. Obstet. Gynecol. Neonatal. Nurs.*, **20**, 391–397.

84. Pittard, W. B., III, Schleich, D. M., Geddes, K. M., and Sorensen, R. U. (1989). Newborn lymphocyte subpopulations: the influence of labor. *Am. J. Obstet. Gynecol.*, **160**, 151–154.

85. Kusaka, Y., Kondou, H., and Morimoto, K. (1992). Healthy lifestyles are associated with higher natural killer cell activity. *Prev. Med.*, **21**, 602–615.

86. McKinnon, W., Weisse, C. S., Reynolds, C. P., Bowles, C. A., and Baum, A. (1989). Chronic stress, leukocyte subpopulations, and humoral response to latent viruses. *Health Psychol.*, **8**, 389–402.

87. Irwin, M., Patterson, T., Smith, T. L., Caldwell, C., Brown, S. A., Gillin, J. C., and Grant, I. (1990). Reduction of immune function in life stress and depression. *Biol. Psychiatry*, **27**, 22–30.

88. Larsson, P. T., Martinsson, A., Olsson, G., and Hjemdahl, P. (1989). Altered

adrenoceptor responsiveness during adrenaline infusion but not during mental stress: differences between receptor subtypes and tissues. *Br. J. Clin. Pharmacol.*, **28**, 663–674.

89. Bachen, E. A., Manuck, S. B., Marsland, A. L., Cohen, S., Malkoff, S. B., Muldoon, M. F. *et al.* (1992). Lymphocyte subset and cellular immune responses to a brief experimental stressor. *Psychosom-Med.*, **54**, 673–679.

90. Thomas, P. D., Goodwin, J. M., and Goodwin, J. S. (1985). Effect of social support on stress-related changes in cholesterol level, uric acid level, and immune function in an elderly sample. *Am. J. Psychiatry*, **142**, 735–737.

91. Vialettes, B., Ozanon, J. P., Kaplansky, S., Farnarier, C., Sauvaget, E., Lassmann-Vague, V., Bernard, D., and Vague, P. (1989). Stress antecedents and immune status in recently diagnosed type I (insulin dependent) diabetes mellitus. *Diabete. Metab.*, **15**, 45–50.

92. Evans, P. D. and Edgerton, N. (1991). Life-events and mood as predictors of the common cold. *Br. J. Med. Psychol.*, **64** (Pt. 1), 35–44.

93. Wiik, P., Haugen, A. H., Lvhaug, D., Byum, A., and Opstad, P. K. (1989). Effect of VIP on the respiratory burst in human monocytes *ex vivo* during prolonged strain and energy deficiency. *Peptides*, **10**, 819–823.

94. Clover, R. D., Abell, T., Becker, L. A., Crawford, S., and Ramsey, C. N., Jr. (1989). Family functioning and stress as predictors of influenza B infection. *J. Fam. Pract.*, **28**, 535–539.

95. Kropiunigg, U., Hamilton, G., Roth, E., and Simmel, A. (1989). Selektive Wirkung von Persönlichkeitsmerkmalen und psychosozialem Stress auf die T-Lymphozyten-Subpopulationen. *Psychother. Psychosom. Med. Psychol.*, **39** (1), 18–25.

96. Dobbin, J. P., Harth, M., McCain, G. A., Martin, R. A., and Cousin, K. (1991). Cytokine production and lymphocyte transformation during stress. *Brain Behav. Immun.*, **5**, 339–348.

97. Glaser, R., Pearson, G. R., Jones, J. F., Hillhouse, J., Kennedy, S., Mao, H. Y. *et al.* (1991). Stress-related activation of Epstein–Barr virus. *Brain Behav. Immun.*, **5**, 219–232.

98. Kiecolt-Glaser, J. K., Garner, W., Speicher, C., Penn, G. M., Holliday, J., and Glaser, R. (1984). Psychosocial modifiers of immunocompetence in medical students. *Psychosom. Med.*, **46**, 7–14.

99. Kiecolt-Glaser, J. K., Ricker, D., George, J., Messick, G., Speicher, C. E., Garner, W. *et al.* (1984). Urinary cortisol levels, cellular immunocompetency, and loneliness in psychiatric inpatients. *Psychosom. Med.*, **46**, 15–23.

100. Glaser, R., Kiecolt-Glaser, J. K., Speicher, C. E., and Holliday, J. E. (1983). Stress, loneliness, and changes in herpesvirus latency. *J. Behav. Med.*, **8**, 249–260.

101. Glowa, J. R., Sternberg, E. M., and Gold, P. W. (1992). Differential behavioral response in LEW/N and F344/N rats: effects of corticotropin releasing hormone. *Prog. Neuro-Psychopharmacol. Biol. Psychiatry*, **16**, 549–560.

102. Biondi, M. and Pancheri, P. (1993). Clinical research strategies in psychoneuroimmunology: a review of 46 human research studies (1972–1992). In *Stress, the Immune System, and Psychiatry*, (eds B. Leonard and K. Miller). John Wiley, Chichester. In press.

103. Irwin, M., Daniels, M., Bloom, E. T., and Weiner, H. (1986). Life events, depression, and natural killer cell activity. *Psychopharmacol. Bull.*, **22**, 1093–1096.

104. Udelman, D. L. (1982). Stress and immunity. *Psychother. Psychosom.*, **37**, 176–184.

105. Kiecolt-Glaser, J. K., Kennedy, S., Malkoff, S., Fisher, L., Speicher, C. E., and Glaser, R. (1988). Marital discord and immunity in males. *Psychosom. Med.*, **50**, 213–229.

106. Schleifer, S. J., Keller, S. E., Camerino, M., Thornton, J. C., and Stein, M. (1983). Suppression of lymphocyte stimulation following bereavement. *J. Am. Med. Assoc.*, **250**, 374–377.

107. Kiecolt-Glaser, J. K., Ricker, D., George, J. E., Messik, G., Speicher, C. E., Garner, W. *et al.* (1984). Urinary cortisol levels, cellular immunocompetency, and loneliness in psychiatric inpatients. *Psychosom. Med.*, **46**, 15–23.

108. Levy, S. M., Herberman, R. B., Whiteside, T., Sanzo, K., Lee, J., and Kirkwood, J. (1990). Perceived social support and tumor estrogen/progesterone receptor status as predictors of natural killer cell activity in breast cancer patients. *Psychosom. Med.*, **52**, 73–85.

109. Fawzy, F. I., Kemeny, M. E., Fawzy, N. W., Elashoff, R., Morton, D., Cousins, N. *et al.* (1990). A structured psychiatric intervention for cancer patients. II. Changes over time in immunological measures. *Arch. Gen. Psychiatry*, **47**, 729–735.

110. Arnetz, B. B., Wasserman, J., Petrini, B., Brenner, S. O., Levi, L., Eneroth, P. *et al.* (1987). Immune function in unemployed women. *Psychosom. Med.*, **49**, 3–11.

111. Stefano, G. B., Zhao, X., Bailey, D., Metlay, M., and Leung, M. K. (1989). High affinity dopamine binding to mouse thymocytes and *Mytilus edulis* (Bivalvia) hemocytes. *J. Neuroimmunol.*, **21**, 67–74.

112. Cunningham, E. T., Jr. and De Souza, E. B. (1993). Interleukin 1 receptors in the brain and endocrine tissues. *Immunol. Today*, **14**, 171–176.

113. Tsagarakis, S., Gillies, G., Rees, L. H., Besser, M., and Grossman, A. (1989). Interleukin-1 directly stimulates the release of corticotrophin releasing factor from rat hypothalamus. *Neuroendocrinology*, **49**, 98–101.

114. Spinedi, E., Hadid, R., Daneva, T., and Gaillard, R. C. (1992). Cytokines stimulate the CRH but not the vasopressin neuronal system: evidence for a median eminence site of interleukin-6 action. *Neuroendocrinology*, **56**, 46–53.

115. Watanobe, H. and Takebe, K. (1993). Intrahypothalamic perfusion with interleukin-1-beta stimulates the local release of corticotropin-releasing hormone and arginine-vasopressin and the plasma adrenocorticotropin in freely moving rats: A comparative perfusion of the paraventricular nucleus and the median eminence. *Neuroendocrinology*, **57**, 593–599.

116. Chulyan, H. E., Saphier, D., Rohn, W. M., and Dunn, A. J. (1992). Noradrenergic innervation of the hypothalamus participates in adrenocortical responses to interleukin-1. *Neuroendocrinology*, **56**, 106–111.

117. Vankelecom, H., Carmeliet, P., Van Damme, J., Billiau, A., and Denef, C. (1989). Production of interleukin-6 by folliculo-stellate cells of the anterior

pituitary gland in a histiotypic cell aggregate culture system. *Neuroendocrinology*, **49**, 102–106.

118. Lyson, K., Mihlenkovic, L., and McCann, S. M. (1991). The stimulatory effect of interleukin 6 on corticotropin-releasing hormone and thyrotropin-releasing hormone release *in vitro*. *Prog. NeuroEndocrinImmunol.*, **4**, 161–165.

119. Gisslinger, H., Svoboda, T., Clodi, M., Gilly, B., Ludwig, H., Havelec, L. *et al.* (1993). Interferon-α stimulates the hypothalamic-pituitary-adrenal axis *in vivo* and *in vitro*. *Neuroendocrinology*, **57**, 489–495.

120. Payne, L. C., Obal, F., Jr., Opp, M. R., and Krueger, J. M. (1992). Stimulation and inhibition of growth hormone secretion by interleukin-1β: the involvement of growth hormone-releasing hormone. *Neuroendocrinology*, **56**, 118–123.

121. Gonzales, M. C., Aguila, M. C., and McCann, S. M. (1991). *In vitro* effects of recombinant human γ-interferon on growth hormone release. *Prog. NeuroEndocrinImmunol.*, **4**, 222–227.

122. Pawlikowski, M., Zelazowski, P., Döhler, K., and Stepien, H. (1988). Effects of two neuropeptides, somatoliberin (GRF) and corticoliberin (CRF), on human lymphocyte natural killer activity. *Brain Behav. Immun.*, **2**, 50–56.

123. Koenig, J. I. (1991). Presence of cytokines in the hypothalamic–pituitary axis. *Prog. NeuroEndocrinImmunol.*, **4**, 143–153.

124. Stead, R. H., Tomioka, M., Pezzati, P., Marshall, J., Croitoru, K., Perdue, M. *et al.* (1991). Interaction of the mucosal immune and peripheral nervous systems. In *Psychoneuroimmunology* (2nd edn) (eds R. Ader, D. L. Felten, and N. Cohen), pp. 177–207. Academic Press, San Diego.

125. Bouaboula, M., Rinaldi, M., Carayon, P., Carillon, C., Delpech, B., Shire, D. *et al.* (1993). Cannabinoid-receptor expression in human leukocytes. *Eur. J. Biochem.*, **214**, 173–180.

126. Ader, R. and Cohen, N. (1991). The influence of conditioning on immune responses. In *Psychoneuroimmunology* (2nd edn) (eds R. Ader, D. L. Felten, and N. Cohen), pp. 611–646. Academic Press, San Diego.

127. Gorczynski, R. M. (1991). Conditioned immunosuppression: analysis of lymphocytes and host-environment of young and aged mice. In *Psychoneuroimmunology* (2nd edn) (eds R. Ader, D. L. Felten, and N. Cohen), pp. 647–662. Academic Press, San Diego.

128. Dyck, D. G. and Greenberg, A. H. (1991). Immunopharmacological tolerance as a conditioned response: dissecting the brain-immune pathways. In *Psychoneuroimmunology* (2nd edn) (eds R. Ader, D. L. Felten, and N. Cohen), pp. 663–684. Academic Press, San Diego.

129. Solvason, H. B., Hiramoto, R. N., and Ghanta, V. K. (1989). Naltrexone blocks the expression of the conditioned elevation of natural killer cell activity in BALB/c mice. *Brain Behav. Immun.*, **3**, 247–262.

130. Segall, M. A. and Crnic, L. S. (1990). A test of conditioned taste aversion with mouse interferon-alpha. *Brain Behav. Immun.*, **4**, 223–231.

131. Pezzone, M. A., Lee, W.-S., Hoffman, G. E., and Rabin, B. S. (1992). Induction of c-Fos immunoreactivity in the rat forebrain by conditioned and unconditioned aversive stimuli. *Brain Res.*, **597**, 41–50.

132. Kusnecov, A., King, M. G., and Husband, A. J. (1989). Immunomodulation by behavioural conditioning. *Biol. Psychol.*, **28**, 25–39.

133. Fessel, W. J. and Hirata-Hibi, M. (1963). Abnormal leukocytes in schizophrenia. *Arch. Gen. Psychiatry*, 9, 601–613.
134. DeLisi, L. E. (1987). Immunologic studies of schizophrenic patients. In *Viruses, Immunity, and Mental Disorders* (eds E. Kurstak, Z. J. Lipowski, and P. V. Morozov), pp. 271–283. Plenum Medical, New York.
135. Müller, N., Ackenheil, M., Hofschuster, E., Mempel, W., and Eckstein, R. (1991). Cellular immunity in schizophrenic patients before and during neuroleptic treatment. *Psychiatry. Res.*, 37, 147–160.
136. Müller, N., Hofschuster, E., Ackenheil, M., and Eckstein, R. (1993). T-cells and psychopathology in schizophrenia: relationship to the outcome of neuroleptic therapy. *Acta Psychiatr. Scand.*, 87, 66–71.
137. Gattaz, W. F., Dalgalarrondo, P., and Schröder H. C. (1992). Abnormalities in serum concentrations of interleukin-2, interferon-alpha and interferon-gamma in schizophrenia not detected. *Schizophr. Res.*, 6, 237–241.
138. Caldwell, C. L., Irwin, M., and Lohr, J. (1991). Reduced natural killer cell cytotoxicity in depression but not in schizophrenia. *Biol. Psychiatry*, 30, 1131–1138.
139. Monteleone, P., Valente, B., Maj, M., and Kemali, D. (1991). Reduced lymphocyte response to PHA and OKT3 in drug-free and neuroleptic-treated chronic schizophrenics. *Biol. Psychiatry*, 30, 201–204.
140. Rogoznikova, O. A. (1991). Sostoianie T-sistemy immuniteta u bol'nykh s vpervye diagnosti-rovannoi pristupoobraznoi shizofreniei (Status of the T-lymphocyte system of immunity in patients with newly diagnosed paroxysmal schizophrenia) (Engl. abstr.). *Zh. Nevropatol. Psikhiatrii*, 91 (8), 47–49.
141. Rogoznikova, O. A. (1991). Dinamika izmenenii pokazatelei T-sistemy immuniteta u bol'nykh s vpervye diagnostirovannoi pristupoobrazno-progredientnoi shizofreniei v protsesse lecheniia (Dynamics of the changes in the indicators of the T-system of immunity in patients with newly diagnosed paroxysmal progressive schizophrenia during its treatment) (Engl. abstr.). *Zh. Nevropatol. Psikhiatrii*, 91 (10), 42–45.
142. Ma, Q. H., Ju, Y. L., and Zhang, Z. L. (1991). Immunological study of inefficiency schizophrenics with deficiency syndrome treated with xin shen ling (Engl. abstr.). *Chung Hsi I. Chieh Ho Tsa Chih*, 11 (4), 215–217, 219.
143. Sperner-Unterweger, B., Barnas, C., Fuchs, D., Kemmler, G., Wachter, H., Hinterhuber, H. *et al.* (1992). Neopterin production in acute schizophrenic patients: an indicator of alterations of cell-mediated immunity. *Psychiatry Res.*, 42, 121–128.
144. Griffiths, R. S., Chung-a-on, K. O., Griffiths, K. D., Payne, J. W., and Davies, J. I. (1992). The sequestration of [3H]spiperone by lymphocytes in schizophrenics and their first-degree relatives: a limited vulnerability marker? *J. Psychiatr. Res.*, 26, 77–84.
145. Hirata-Hibi, M. and Hayashi, K. (1992). The anatomy of the P lymphocyte. *Schizophr. Res.*, 8, 257–262.
146. Coggiano, M. A., Alexander, R. C., Kirch, D. G., Wyatt, R. J., and Kulaga, H. (1991). The continued search for evidence of retroviral infection in schizophrenic patients. *Schizophr. Res.*, 5, 243–247.
147. Shima, S., Yano, K., Sugiura, M., and Tokunaga, Y. (1991). Anticerebral

antibodies in functional psychoses. *Biol. Psychiatry*, **29**, 322–328.

148. Kilidireas, K., Latov, N., Strauss, D. H., Gorig, A. D., Hashim, G. A., Gorman, J. M. *et al.* (1992). Antibodies to the human 60 kDa heat-shock protein in patients with schizophrenia. *Lancet*, **340**, 569–572.

149. Wang, C., Jian, B.-X., Jiang, X.-D., and Zhao, X.-Z. (1992). Investigation of allotypes of HLA class III (C2, BF and C4) in patients with schizophrenia. *Chin. Med. J. (Engl.)*, **105** (4), 316–318.

150. Hallmayer, J., Maier, W., Ackenheil, M., Ertl, M. A., Schmidt, S., Minges, J. *et al.* (1992). Evidence against linkage of schizophrenia to chromosome 5q11-q13 markers in systematically ascertained families. *Biol. Psychiatry*, **31**, 83–94.

151. Magin, G. K., Robison, S. H., Breslin, N., Wyatt, R. J., and Alexander, R. C. (1991). DNA repair and mutant frequency in schizophrenia. *Mutat. Res.*, **255**, 241–246.

152. Smith, R. S. (1991) Is schizophrenia caused by excessive production of interleukin-2 and interleukin-2 receptors by gastrointestinal lymphocytes? *Med. Hypotheses*, **34**, 225–229.

153. Smith, R. S. (1992). The GI T-lymphocyte theory of schizophrenia: some new observations. *Med. Hypotheses*, **37**, 27–30.

154. Wodarz, N., Fritze, J., Kornhuber, J., and Riederer, P. (1992). 3H-spiroperidol binding to human peripheral mononuclear cells: methodological aspects. *Biol. Psychiatry*, **31**, 291–303.

155. Rupprecht, R., Wodarz, N., Kornhuber, J., Wild, K., Schmitz, B., Braner, H. U. *et al.* (1991). In vivo and in vitro effects of glucocorticoids on lymphocyte proliferation in depression. *Eur. Arch. Psychiatry Clin. Neurosci.*, **241**, 35–40.

156. Miller, A. H., Asnis, G. M., Lackner, C., Halbreich, U., and Norin, A. J. (1991). Depression, natural killer cell activity, and cortisol secretion. *Biol. Psychiatry*, **29**, 878–886.

157. Darko, D. F., Wilson, N. W., Gillin, J. C., and Golshan, S. (1991). A critical appraisal of mitogen-induced lymphocyte proliferation in depressed patients. *Am. J. Psychiatry*, **148**, 337–344.

158. Levy, E. M., Borrelli, D. J., Mirin, S. M., Salt, P., Knapp, P. H., Peirce, C. *et al.* (1991). Biological measures and cellular immunological function in depressed psychiatric inpatients. *Psychiatry Res.*, **36**, 157–167.

159. Spurrell, M. T. and Creed, F. H. (1993). Lymphocyte response in depressed patients and subjects anticipating bereavement. *Br. J. Psychiatry*, **162**, 60–64.

160. Andreoli, A., Keller, S. E., Rabaeus, M., Zaugg, L., Garrone, G., and Taban, C. (1992). Immunity, major depression, and panic disorder comorbidity. *Biol. Psychiatry*, **31**, 896–908.

161. Pfohl, B., Rederer, M., Coryell, W., and Stangl, D. (1991). Association between post-dexamethasone cortisol level and blood pressure in depressed inpatients. *J. Nerv. Ment. Dis.*, **179**, 44–47.

162. Charles, G., Machowski, R., Brohee, D., Wilmotte, J., and Kennes, B. (1992). Lymphocyte subsets in major depressive patients. Influence of anxiety and corticoadrenal overdrive. *Neuropsychobiology*, **25**, 94–98.

163. Rupprecht, R., Kornhuber, J., Wodarz, N., Lugauer, J., Gobel, C., Riederer, P. *et al.* (1991). Lymphocyte glucocorticoid receptor binding during depression and after clinical recovery. *J. Affect. Disord.*, **22**, 31–35.

164. Wodarz, N., Rupprecht, R., Kornhuber, J., Schmitz, B., Wild, K., Braner, H. U. *et al.* (1991). Normal lymphocyte responsiveness to lectins but impaired sensitivity to in vitro glucocorticoids in major depression. *J. Affective Disord.*, **22**, 241–248.

165. Wodarz, N., Rupprecht, R., Kornhuber, J., Schmitz, B., Wild, K., and Riederer, P. (1992). Cell-mediated immunity and its glucocorticoid-sensitivity after clinical recovery from severe major depressive disorder. *J. Affective Disord.*, **25**, 31–38.

166. Maes, M., De Meester, I., Vanhoof, G., Scharpe, S., Bosmans, E., Vandervorst, C. *et al.* (1991). Decreased serum dipeptidyl peptidase IV activity in major depression. *Biol. Psychiatry*, **30**, 577–586.

167. Maes, M., Bosmans, E., Suy, E., Minner, B., and Raus, J. (1991). A further exploration of the relationships between immune parameters and the HPA-axis activity in depressed patients. *Psychol. Med.*, **21**, 313–320.

168. Maes, M., Lambrechts, J., Bosmans, E., Jacobs, J., Suy, E., Vandervorst, C. *et al.* (1992). Evidence for a systemic immune activation during depression: results of leukocyte enumeration by flow cytometry in conjunction with monoclonal antibody staining. *Psychol. Med.*, **22**, 45–53.

169. Maes, M., Stevens, W., DeClerck, L., Bridts, C., Peeters, D., Schotte, C. *et al.* (1992). Immune disorders in depression: higher T helper/T suppressor-cytotoxic cell ratio. *Acta Psychiatr. Scand.*, **86**, 423–431.

170. Maes, M., Bosmans, E., Suy, E., Vandervorst, C., DeJonckheere, C., and Raus, J. (1991). Depression-related disturbances in mitogen-induced lymphocyte responses and interleukin-1 beta and soluble interleukin-2 receptor production. *Acta Psychiatr. Scand.*, **84**, 379–386.

171. Maes, M., Bosmans, E., Suy, E., Vandervorst, C., Dejonckheere, C., and Raus, J. (1991). Antiphospholipid, antinuclear, Epstein–Barr and cytomegalovirus antibodies, and soluble interleukin-2 receptors in depressive patients. *J. Affective Disord.*, **21**, 133–140.

172. Maes, M., Stevens, W. J., DeClerck, L. S., Bridts, C. H., Peeters, D., Schotte, C. *et al.* (1992). A significantly increased number and percentage of B-cells in depressed subjects: results of flow cytometric measurements. *J. Affective Disord.*, **24**, 127–134.

173. Maes, M., Bosmans, E., Suy, E., Vandervorst, C., De Jonckheere, C., and Raus, J. (1990–91). Immune disturbances during major depression: upregulated expression of interleukin-2 receptors. *Neuropsychobiology*, **24**, 115–120.

174. Maes, M., Stevens, W., Peeters, D., DeClerck, L., Scharpe, S., Bridts, C. *et al.* (1992). A study on the blunted natural killer cell activity in severely depressed patients. *Life Sci.*, **50**, 505–513.

175. Maes, M., Van der Planken, M., Stevens, W. J., Peeters, D., DeClerck, L. S., Bridts, C. H. *et al.* (1992). Leukocytosis, monocytosis and neutrophilia: hallmarks of severe depression. *J. Psychiatr. Res.*, **26**, 125–134.

176. Evans, D. L., Folds, J. D., Petitto, J. M., Golden, R. N., Pedersen, C. A., Corrigan, M. *et al.* (1992). Circulating natural killer cell phenotypes in men and women with major depression. Relation to cytotoxic activity and severity of depression. *Arch. Gen. Psychiatry*, **49**, 388–395.

177. Petitto, J. M., Folds, J. D., Ozer, H., Quade, D., and Evans, D. L. (1992). Abnormal diurnal variation in circulating natural killer cell phenotypes and

cytotoxic activity in major depression. *Am. J. Psychiatry*, **149**, 694–696.

178. Irwin, M., Smith, T. L., and Gillin, J. C. (1992). Electroencephalographic sleep and natural killer activity in depressed patients and control subjects. *Psychosom. Med.*, **54**, 10–21.

179. Lloyd, A., Hickie, I., Hickie, C., Dwyer, J., and Wakefield, D. (1992). Cell-mediated immunity in patients with chronic fatigue syndrome, healthy control subjects and patients with major depression. *Clin. Exp. Immunol.*, **87**, 76–79.

180. Guidi, L., Bartoloni, C., Frasca, D., Antico, L., Pili, R., Cursi, F. *et al.* (1991). Impairment of lymphocyte activities in depressed aged subjects. *Mech. Ageing Dev.*, **60**, 13–24.

181. Bartoloni, C., Guidi, L., Frasca, D., Antico, L., Pili, R., Cursi, F. *et al.* (1991). Immune parameters in a population of institutionalized elderly subjects: influence of depressive disorders and endocrinological correlations. *Mech. Ageing Dev.*, **60**, 1–12.

182. Shain, B. N., Kronfol, Z., Naylor, M., Goel, K., Evans, T., and Schaefer, S. (1991). Natural killer cell activity in adolescents with major depression. *Biol. Psychiatry*, **29**, 481–484.

183. Bell, I. R., Jasnoski, M. L., Kagan, J., and King, D. S. (1991). Depression and allergies: survey of a nonclinical population. *Psychother. Psychosom.*, **55**, 24–31.

184. Hassanyeh, F., Murray, R. B. and Rodgers, H. (1991). Adrenocortical suppression presenting with agitated depression, morbid jealousy, and a dementia-like state. *Br. J. Psychiatry*, **159**, 870–872.

185. Rabin, B. S., Cunnick, J. E., and Lysle, D. T. (1990). Stress-induced alteration of immune function. *Prog. NeuroEndocrinImmunol.*, **3**, 116–124.

186. Roy, B. F., Rose, J. W., McFarland, H. F., McFarlin, D. E., and Murphy, D. L. (1986). Anti-beta-endorphin immunoglobulin G in humans. *Proc. Natl. Acad. Sci. USA*, **83**, 8739–8743.

187. Smith, R. S. (1991). The macrophage theory of depression. *Med. Hypotheses*, **35**, 298–306, **36**, 178.

188. Weisse, C. S. (1992). Depression and immunocompetence: a review of the literature. *Psychol. Bull.*, **111**, 475–489.

189. Aguglia, E., Biondi, M. R., and Azzarelli, O. (1991). Valutazione dell'efficacia della timopentina (sintomodulina) in associazione all'imipramina nel trattamento della depressione maggiore. *Neuropsicofarmacologia del Comportamento*, **4** (3), 1–9.

190. Yehuda, R., Lowy, M. T., Southwick, S. M., Shaffer, D., and Giller, E. L., Jr. (1991). Lymphocyte glucocorticoid receptor number in posttraumatic stress disorder. *Am. J. Psychiatry*, **148**, 499–504.

191. Balaita, C., Iscrulescu, C., and Sarbulescu, A. (1992). Serum immunoglobulin levels in schizoaffective disorders (manic and depressive). *Rom. J. Neurol. Psychiatry*, **30** (1), 63–71.

192. Rocca, P., Ferrero, P., Gualerzi, A., Zanalda, E., Maina, G., Bergamasco, B. *et al.* (1991). Peripheral-type benzodiazepine receptors in anxiety disorders. *Acta Psychiatr. Scand.*, **84**, 537–544.

193. Ramesh, C., Yeragani, V. K., Balon, R., and Pohl, R. (1991). A comparative

study of immune status in panic disorder patients and controls. *Acta Psychiatr. Scand.*, **84**, 396–397.

194. Brambilla, F., Bellodi, L., Perna, G., Battaglia, M., Sciuto, G., Diaferia, G. *et al.* (1992). Psychoimmunoendocrine aspects of panic disorder. *Psychoneurobiology*, **26**, 12–22.

195. Schmidt-Traub, S. (1991). Angst und immunologische Störung: Phobien, generalisiertes Angstsyndrom und Panikattacken psycho-immunologisch betrachtet in hypothesengenerierender. *Absicht. Z. Psychol.*, **199**, 19–34.

196. Brambilla, F., Ferrari, E., Panerai, A., Manfredi, B., Petraglia, F., Catalano, M. (1993). Psychoneuroimmunoendocrine investigation in anorexia nervosa. *Neuropsychobiology*, **27**, 9–16.

197. Schattner, A., Steinbock, M., Tepper, R., Schonfeld, A., Vaisman, N., and Hahn, T. (1990). Tumour necrosis factor production and cell-mediated immunity in anorexia nervosa. *Clin. Exp. Immunol.*, **79**, 62–66.

198. Nässberger, L. and Träskman-Bendz, L. (1993). Increased soluble interleukin-2 receptor concentrations in suicide attempters. *Acta Psychiatr. Scand.*, **88**, 48–52.

199. Singh, V. K., Warren, R. P., Odell, J. D., Warren, W. L., and Cole, P. (1993). Antibodies to myelin basic protein in children with autistic behavior. *Brain Behav. Immun.*, **7**, 97–103.

200. Egger, J., Carter, C. M., Graham, P. J., Gumley, D., and Soothill, J. F. (1985). Controlled trial of oligoantigenic treatment in the hyperkinetic syndrome. *Lancet*, i, 540–545.

201. Ruff, M. R. and Pert, C. B. (1987). Human monocyte chemotaxis to neuropeptides. In *Hypothalamic Dysfunction in Neuropsychiatric Disorders* (eds D. Nerozzi, F. K. Goodwin, and E. Costa), pp. 247–260. Raven Press, New York.

202. Covelli, V., Munno, I., Decandia, P., Altamura, M., Cannuscio, B., Maffione, A. B. *et al.* (1991). Effects of benzodiazepines on the immune system. *Acta Neurol. (Naples)*, **13**, 418–423.

203. Landmann, R. (1992). Beta-adrenergic receptors in human leukocyte subpopulations. *Eur. J. Clin. Invest.*, **22** (1 Suppl.), 30–36.

204. Arora, P. K., Hanna, E. E., Paul, S. M., and Skolnick. P. (1987). Suppression of the immune response by benzodiazepine receptor inverse agonists. *J. Neuroimmunol.*, **15**, 1–9.

205. Arora, P. K., Hanna, E. E., and Skolnick, P. (1991). Suppression of cytotoxic T-lymphocyte (CTL) activity by FG 7142, a benzodiazepine receptor 'inverse agonist'. *Immunopharmacology*, **21**, 91–98.

206. Petitto, J. M., Skolnick, P., and Arora, P. K. (1989). Suppression of natural killer cell activity by FG 7142, a benzodiazepine receptor 'inverse agonist'. *Brain Behav. Immun.*, **3**, 39–46.

207. Libri, V., Del Gobbo, V., Villani, N., Agosto, R., Caliò, R., and Nisticò, G. (1991). Microinfusion of ethyl-$\beta$-carboline-3-carboxylate in the locus ceruleus reduces both interleukin 2 production and natural killer cell activity. *Prog. NeuroEndocrinImmunol.*, **4**, 79–85.

208. Ganguli, R., Rabin, B., Raghu, U., and Ulrich, R. S. (1987). T-lymphocytes

in schizophrenics and normals and the effects of varying antipsychotic dosage. In *Viruses, Immunity, and Mental Disorders* (eds E. Kurstak, Z. J. Lipowski, and P. V. Morozov), pp. 321–326. Plenum Medical, New York.

209. Rapaport, M. H., McAllister, C. G., Kirch, D. G., and Pickar, D. (1990). The effects of typical and atypical neuroleptics on mitogen-induced T-lymphocyte responsiveness. *Biol. Psychiatry*, **29**, 715–717.

210. Bernton, E. W., Bryant, H. U., and Holaday, J. W. (1991). Prolactin and immune function. In *Psychoneuroimmunology* (2nd edn) (eds R. Ader, D. L. Felten, and N. Cohen), pp. 403–428. Academic Press, San Diego.

211. Pogady, J. and Libiková, H. (1982). Influence upon the immune response and cytotoxicity of psychotropic drugs. *Activ. Nerv. Super.*, **24**, 269–270.

212. Baker, G. A., Santalo, R., and Blumenstein, J. (1977). Effect of psychotropic agents upon the blastogenic response of human T-lymphocytes. *Biol. Psychiatry*, **12**, 159–169.

213. Barbu, V., Mazière, J. C., Maindrault, F., Mazière, C., Rampini, C., Roux, C. *et al.* (1987). Effect of AY 9944 and chlorpromazine on concanavalin A-induced stimulation of human lymphocytes. *Biochem. Pharmacol.*, **36**, 353–356.

214. Androsova, L. V. and Sekirina, T. P. (1991). Izmenenie funktsional'noi aktivnosti T-limfotsitov pod vliianiem stelazina. (Changes in the functional activity of T-lymphocytes after administration of stelazine) (Engl. abstr.). *Zh. Nevropatol. Psikhiatrii*, **91** (8), 87–89.

215. Swerdlow, N. R., Hauger, R., Irwin, M., Koob, G. F., Britton, K. T., and Pulvirenti, L. (1991). Endocrine, immune, and neurochemical changes in rats during withdrawal from chronic amphetamine intoxication. *Neuropsychopharmacology*, **5**, 23–31.

216. Eisen, J. N., Irwin, J., Quay, J., and Livnat, S. (1989). The effect of antidepressants on immune function in mice. *Biol. Psychiatry*, **26**, 805–817.

217. Surman, O. S. (1993). Possible immunological effects of psychotropic medication. *Psychosomatics*, **34**, 139–143.

218. Boranic, M., Pericic, D., Poljak-Blazi, M., and Sverko, V. (1984). Suppression of the immune response by drugs interfering with the metabolism of serotonin. *Experientia*, **40**, 1153–1155.

219. Reed, S. M. and Glick, J. W. (1991). Fluoxetine and reactivation of the herpes simplex virus (letter). *Am. J. Psychiatry*, **148**, 949–950.

220. Rohatiner, S. Z. A., Priom, P. F., Burton, A. C., Smith, A. T., Balkwill, F. R., and Lister, T. A. (1983). Central nervous toxicity of interferon. *Br. J. Cancer*, **47**, 419–422.

221. McDonald, E. M., Mann, A. H., and Thomas, H. C. (1987). Interferons as mediators of psychiatric morbidity. An investigation in a trial of recombinant alpha-interferon in hepatitis-B carriers. *Lancet*, **ii**, 1175–1178.

222. Weinberger, S. B., Schulteis, G., Fernando, A. G., Bakhit, C., and Martinez, J. L., Jr. (1988). Decreased locomotor activity produced by repeated, but not single, administration of murine-recombinant interferon-gamma in mice. *Life Sci.*, **42**, 1085–1090.

223. Iivainen, M., Laaksonen, R., Niemi, M.-L., Farkkila, M., Bergstrom, L., Mattson, K. *et al.* (1985). Memory and psychomotor impairment following

high-dose interferon treatment in amyotrophic lateral sclerosis. *Acta Neurol. Scand.*, **72**, 475–480.

224. Born, J., Spath-Schwalbe, E., Pietrowsky, R., Porzsolt, F., and Fehm, H. L. (1989). Neurophysiological effects of recombinant interferon-gamma and -alpha in man. *Clin. Physiol. Biochem.*, **7**, 119–127.

225. Long, N. C., Vander, A. J., Kunkel, S. L., and Kluger, M. J. (1990). Antiserum against tumor necrosis factor increases stress hyperthermia in rats. *Am. J. Physiol.*, **258** (3 Pt. 2), R591–R595.

226. Nisticò, G. and de Sarro, G. (1990). Locus ceruleus: site of soporific effects of interleukin-2 in rats. *Prog. NeuroEndocrinImmunol.*, **3**, 43–48.

227. Langhans, W., Balkowski, G., and Savoldelli, D. (1991). Differential feeding responses to bacterial lipopolysaccharide and muramyl dipeptide. *Am. J. Physiol.*, **261** (3 Pt. 2), R659–R664.

228. Vinar, O., Poch, T., and Vinarová, E. (1987). Levamisol counteracts the resistance to antidepressants. *Activ. Nerv. Super.*, **29**, 239–241.

229. Basso, A. M., Depiante-Depaoli, M., and Molina, V. A. (1992). Chronic variable stress facilitates tumoral growth: Reversal by imipramine administration. *Life Sci.*, **50**, 1789–1796.

230. Ben-Eliyahu, S., Yirmiya, R., Liebeskind, J. C., Taylor, A. N., and Gale, R. P. (1991). Stress increases metastatic spread of a mammary tumor in rats: evidence for mediation by the immune system. *Brain Behav. Immun.*, **5**, 193–205.

231. Chrousos, G. P. and Gold, P. W. (1992). The concepts of stress and stress system disorders: Overview of physical and behavioral homeostasis. *J. Am. Med. Assoc.*, **267**, 1244–1252.

232. Sternberg, E. M., Chrousos, G. P., Wilder, R. L., and Gold, P. W. (1992). The stress response and the regulation of inflammatory disease. *Ann. Intern. Med.*, **117**, 854–866.

233. Sternberg, E. M., Young, W. S., III, Bernardini, R., Calogero, A. E., Chrousos, G. P., Gold, P. W. *et al.* (1989). A central nervous system defect in biosynthesis of corticotropin-releasing hormone is associated with susceptibility to streptococcal cell wall-induced arthritis in Lewis rats. *Proc. Natl. Acad. Sci. USA*, **86**, 4771–4775.

234. Robinson, N., Lloyd, C. E., Fuller, J. H., and Yateman, N. A. (1989). Psychosocial factors and the onset of type 1 diabetes. *Diabetic Med.*, **6**, 53–58.

235. Grant, I., Brown, G. W., Harris, T., McDonald, W. I., Patterson, T., and Trimble, M. R. (1989). Severely threatening events and marked life difficulties preceding onset or exacerbation of multiple sclerosis. *J. Neurol. Neurosurg. Psychiatry*, **52**, 8–13.

236. Foley, F. W., Miller, A. H., Traugott, U., LaRocca, N. G., Scheinberg, L. C., Bedell, J. R. *et al.* (1988). Psychoimmunological dysregulation in multiple sclerosis. *Psychosomatics*, **29**, 398–403.

237. Garland, E. J. and Zis, A. P. (1991). Multiple sclerosis and affective disorders. *Can. J. Psychiatry*, **36**, 112–117.

238. Grant, I., Brown, G. W., Harris, T., McDonald, W. I., Patterson, T., and Trimble, M. R. (1989). Severely threatening events and marked life difficulties preceding onset or exacerbation of multiple sclerosis. *J. Neurol. Neurosurg. Psychiatry*, **52**, 8–13.

239. Chandarana, P. C., Eals, M., Steingart, A. B., Bellamy, N., and Allen, S. (1987). The detection of psychiatric morbidity and associated factors in patients with rheumatoid arthritis. *Can. J. Psychiatry*, **32**, 356–361.
240. Nakamura, H., Yoshino, S., Fujimori, J., Koiwa, M., and Shiga, H. (1992). (Psychosomatic medicine in rheumatoid arthritis) (Engl. abstr.). *Nippon Rinsho*, **50**, 558–562.
241. Katon, W. J., Buchwald, D. S., Simon, G. E., Russo, J. E., and Mease, P. J. (1991). Psychiatric illness in patients with chronic fatigue and those with rheumatoid arthritis. *J. Gen. Intern. Med.*, **6**, 277–285.
242. Zautra, A. J., Okun, M. A., Robinson, S. E., Lee, D., Roth, S. H., and Emmanual, J. (1989). Life stress and lymphocyte alterations among patients with rheumatoid arthritis. *Health Psychol.*, **8**, 1–14.
243. McFarlane, A. C. and Brooks, P. M. (1990). Psychoimmunology and rheumatoid arthritis: concepts and methodologies. *Int. J. Psychiatry Med.*, **20**, 307–322.
244. Soroka, N. F. (1991). Psikhologicheskie osobennosti lichnosti bol'nykh revmatoidnym artritom (The psychological personality characteristics of patients with rheumatoid arthritis) (Engl. abstr.). *Revmatologiia (Moscow)*, (N 3), 15–17.
245. Lim, L. C., Lee, T. E., Boey, M. L. (1991). Psychiatric manifestation of systemic lupus erythematosus in Singapore. A cross-cultural comparison. *Br. J. Psychiatry*, **159**, 520–523.
246. Hinrichsen, H., Barth, J., Ferstl, R., and Kirch, W. (1989). Einfluß von akustischem Stress auf immunregulatorische Zellen bei Patientinnen mit systemischem Lupus erythematodes (SLE), Patienten mit Sarkoidose und gesunden Vergleichspersonen. *Schweiz. Med. Wochenschr.*, **119**, 1771–1773.
247. Wekking, E. M., Nossent, J. C., van Dam, A. P., and Swaak, A. J. (1991). Cognitive and emotional disturbances in systemic lupus erythematosus. *Psychother. Psychosom.*, **55**, 126–131.
248. Drosos, A. A., Angelopoulos, N. V., Liakos, A., and Moutsopoulos, H. M. (1989). Personality structure disturbances and psychiatric manifestations in primary Sjögren's syndrome. *J. Autoimmun.*, **2**, 489–493.
249. Wolfe, F., Cathey, M. A., Kleinheksel, S. M., Amos, S. P., Hoffman, R. G., Young, D. Y. *et al.* (1984). Psychological status in primary fibrositis and fibrositis associated with rheumatoid arthritis. *J. Rheumatol.*, **11**, 500–506.
250. Bell, I. R., Guilleminault, C., and Dement, W. C. (1978). Hypersomnia, multiple-system symptomatology, and selective IgA deficiency. *Biol. Psychiatry*, **13**, 751–757.
251. Hickie, I., Lloyd, A., and Wakefield, D. (1992). Immunological and psychological dysfunction in patients receiving immunotherapy for chronic fatigue syndrome. *Aust. N.-Z. J. Psychiatry*, **26**, 249–256.
252. Rohr, W. (1992). Handlungs- und Gedankenzwänge bei Patienten mit Myasthenia gravis. *Schweiz. Arch. Neurol. Psychiatr.*, **143**, 105–115.
253. Lützenkirchen, J. (1977). Psychosomatik der Myasthenie. *Z. Psychosom. Med. Psychoanal.*, **23**, 363–370.
254. Harsch, I., Paschke, R., and Usadel, K. H. (1992). The possible etiological role of psychological disturbances in Graves' disease. *Acta Med. Austriaca*, **19** (suppl. 1), 62–65.

255. Bender, B. G., Lerner, J. A., and Poland, J. E. (1991). Association between corticosteroids and psychologic change in hospitalized asthmatic children. *Ann. Allergy*, **66**, 414–419.

256. Blomquist, K. and Sakki, M. L. (1991). Children with dermatological disease and their mothers. *Acta Derm. Venereol. (Stockholm)*, **Suppl. 156**, 28–36.

257. Farber, E. M., Lanigan, S. W., and Rein, G. (1990). The role of psychoneuroimmunology in the pathogenesis of psoriasis. *Cutis*, **46**, 314–316.

258. Teshima, H., Sogawa, H., Mizobe, K., Kuroki, N., and Nakagawa, T. (1991). Application of psychoimmunotherapy in patients with alopecia universalis. *Psychother. Psychosom.*, **56**, 235–241.

259. Marbach, J. J., Schleifer, S. J., and Keller, S. E. (1990). Facial pain, distress, and immune function. *Brain Behav. Immun.*, **4**, 243–254.

260. Schleifer, S. J., Marbach, J., and Keller, S. E. (1990). Psychoneuroimmunology: potential relevance to chronic orofacial pain. *Anesth. Prog.*, **37**, 93–98.

261. Hassan, N. F. and Douglas, S. D. (1990). Stress-related neuroimmunomodulation of monocyte-macrophage functions in HIV-1 infection. *Clin. Immunol. Immunopathol.*, **54**, 220–227.

262. Levy, E. M., Cottrell, M. C., and Black, P. H. (1989). Psychological and immunological associations in men with AIDS pursuing a macrobiotic regimen as an alternative therapy: a pilot study. *Brain Behav. Immun.*, **3**, 175–182.

263. Antoni, M. H., Schneiderman, N., Klimas, N., LaPerriere, A., Ironson, G., and Fletcher, M. A. (1991). Disparities in psychological, neuroendocrine, and immunologic patterns in asymptomatic HIV-1 seropositive and seronegative gay men. *Biol. Psychiatry*, **29**, 1023–1041.

264. Zanker, K. S. and Kroczek, R. (1991). Looking along the track of the psychoneuroimmunologic axis for missing links in cancer progression. *Int. J. Sports Med.*, **12** (suppl. 1), S58–S62.

265. Bovbjerg, D. H. (1991). Psychoneuroimmunology. Implications for oncology? *Cancer*, **67** (3, suppl.), 828–832.

266. Levy, S. M., Herberman, R. B., Whiteside, T., Sanzo, K., Lee, J., and Kirkwood, J. (1990). Perceived social support and tumor estrogen/progesterone receptor status as predictors of natural killer cell activity in breast cancer patients. *Psychosom. Med.*, **52**, 73–85.

267. Fredrickson, M., Fürst, C. J., Lekander, M., Rotstein, S., and Blomgren, H. (1993). Trait anxiety and anticipatory immune reactions in women receiving adjuvant chemotherapy for breast cancer. *Brain Behav. Immun.*, **7**, 79–90.

268. Teshima, H., Noda, F., Nakagawa, T., Kamura, T., Matsuyama,T., and Nakano, H. (1991) Psychosomatic approach to patients with gynecologic cancer. *Fukuoka Igaku Zasshi*, **82**, 499–507.

269. Antoni, M. H. and Goodkin, K. (1989). Host moderator variables in the promotion of cervical neoplasia—II. Dimensions of life stress. *J. Psychosom. Res.*, **33**, 457–467.

270. Lechin, F., Van Der Dijs, B., Vitelli-Florez, G., Lechin-Baez, S., Azocar, J., Cabrera, A. *et al.* (1990). Psychoneuroendocrinological and immunological parameters in cancer patients: Involvement of stress and depression. *Psychoneuroendocrinology*, **15**, 435–451.

271. Toge, T., Kegoya, Y., Yamaguchi, Y., Baba, N., Kuninobu, H., Takayama,

T. *et al.* (1989). (Surgical stress and immunosuppression in cancer patients) (Engl. abstr). *Gan. To. Kagaku Ryoho*, **16** (4 Pt. 2–1), 1115–1121.

272. Zachariae, R., Kristensen, J. S., Hokland, P., Ellegaard, J., Metze, E., and Hokland, M. (1990). Effect of psychological intervention in the form of relaxation and guided imagery on cellular immune function in normal healthy subjects. An overview. *Psychother. Psychosom.*, **54**, 32–39.

273. Rider, M. S. and Achterberg, J. (1989). Effect of music-assisted imagery on neutrophils and lymphocytes. *Biofeedback Self Regul.*, **14**, 247–257.

# 2

# Neural and endocrine links between the brain and the immune system

D. L. BELLINGER, K. S. MADDEN, S. Y. FELTEN, AND
D. L. FELTEN

# 1   Introduction

Evidence from many fields of research including psychology, epidemiology, neurobiology, pharmacology, and immunology has demonstrated that the immune system is not autonomously regulated, but rather is influenced by signalling from the central nervous system (CNS). Changes in immune function can be induced by classical behavioural conditioning, stressful stimuli, and other psychosocial factors. Furthermore, lesions in distinct regions of the brain can alter immunity in the periphery, and changes in neurotransmitter turnover and firing rates occur in parallel with the development, progression, and decline of an immune response. Removal of the pituitary gland or other neuroendocrine organs produces striking changes in lymphoid tissue morphology and in immune reactivity. Both neuropeptidergic and noradrenergic nerves innervate lymphoid tissue in both primary and secondary lymphoid organs. Conversely, there is abundant evidence demonstrating that cytokines (intercellular signals) and other immune mediators can influence functions carried out by the CNS, including sleep induction, fever production, and altered feeding behavior. Cytokines administered in high doses can lead to the development of neuropsychiatric disorders. Collectively, these findings provide overwhelming evidence for bidirectional communication between the nervous and immune systems of the body. Immunomodulation by the CNS occurs via two pathways, (1) neuroendocrine outflow and (2) direct innervation of lymphoid organs by autonomic nerves. In this chapter, we describe the pathways, summarize the literature regarding their role in immune modulation, and discuss some of the implications of neural–immune modulation in health and illness.

# 2   Central neural circuits involved in signalling the immune system

Studies examining the effects of psychosocial factors and stressors on a variety of immune measures have revealed CNS-mediated changes in immune functions that can alter health status. Likewise, behavioural conditioning of immune responses has indicated that the CNS is capable of detecting alterations in immune responses and, subsequent to detection, is able to initiate a change in immune response upon re-exposure to the conditioned stimulus. These studies point toward the participation of neural circuitry in the modulation of immune reactivity, but do not reveal the specific circuitry that may be involved. The nature of all the channels of communication between the brain and the immune system, and the functional significance of these interrelationships have yet to be established. However, the central control of neuroendocrine and autonomic outflow is well documented. Neuroendocrine outflow from the brain occurs via the release of hormones from the anterior and posterior pituitary under the control of the hypothalamus, limbic forebrain, and brain stem circuitry, the so-called hypothalamo–pituitary–endocrine target organ axis. Nerve terminals from cell bodies in the magnocellular paraventricular and supraoptic nuclei secrete neurohormones such as vasopressin and oxytocin directly into the systemic circulation in the posterior pituitary. Nerve terminals from a number of hypothalamic and other 'visceral' nuclei secrete releasing or inhibiting factors, and other hormones into the hypophyseal portal blood at the median eminence. From this portal system, these hormones bathe target cells in the anterior pituitary to influence the release of anterior pituitary hormones such as adrenal corticotropic hormone (ACTH), thyroid-stimulating hormone (TSH), follicle-stimulating hormone (FSH), luteinizing hormone (LH), growth hormone (GH), and prolactin. Apart from their many classic endocrine effects, these hormones also act as signal molecules through which the CNS communicates with the immune system.

Autonomic neural connections consisting of a two-neuron chain for both the sympathetic and parasympathetic subdivisions link the spinal cord and brain stem with target organs that include cardiac muscle, smooth muscle, and exocrine (secretory) glands. More recently, additional target sites in the body for noradrenergic sympathetic nerves, such as hepatocytes, brown fat cells, and cells of the immune system have been recognized. The autonomic preganglionic neurons in the spinal cord and brain stem terminate on autonomic postganglionic neurons in autonomic ganglia distributed throughout the body, which in turn project their axons to end on target cells. Autonomic preganglionic neurons are under direct regulation by the cerebral cortex, limbic forebrain structures, specific regions of the hypothalamus, and brain stem autonomic and reticular nuclei. These areas include nucleus solitarius, raphe nuclei, tegmental noradrenergic nuclei, paraventricular nucleus of the hypothalamus, lateral hypothalamus, posterior hypothalamus, dorsal hypothalamus, central amygdaloid nucleus, and frontal, cingulate, and insular cortical areas that are mainly zones of the limbic cortex. In addition, indirect regulation of autonomic outflow arises from regions such as the parabrachial nuclei, central gray, and reticular formation of the brain stem, numerous hypothalamic nuclei and cell groups, limbic forebrain areas such as the hippocampal formation and septum, and cortical association areas. The central autonomic system has an integrated circuitry with extensive ascending and descending connections among the regions mentioned above, and is intimately involved in visceral, autonomic, and neuroendocrine regulation. This is also the major circuitry suspected to play a key role in responding to signal molecules from the immune system, and regulating CNS outflow to the immune system. Cortical and limbic regions may be involved in altered immune responses to stressors, behavioural conditioning, and psychosocial factors. These are sites that respond to administration of cytokines, immunization by altered neuronal activity, and altered monoamine metabolism. Furthermore, it is these brain regions that possess the highest density of glucocorticoid (GC) receptors and regulate the balance of neuroendocrine and autonomic outflow.

Signalling between the nervous and immune systems occurs bidirectionally through short, intermediate, and long communication loops using chemical mediators such as hormones, neurotransmitters, and cytokines that interact with receptors present on target cells of both systems. Binding of these mediators with specific receptors activates common second messenger systems, changes receptor expression for specific signal molecules on the cell surface, and/or alters membrane permeability. Signal molecules can interact with one another or with the target cell providing integrated responses when acting on neurons or lymphocytes. The following section summarizes some of the evidence for direct CNS interactions with the immune system (for review, see ref. 1).

## 2.1 CNS MODULATION OF IMMUNE FUNCTION

One of the strategies used to study CNS sites involved in modulation of the immune system has been to produce stereotactically placed electrolytic lesions. With this approach investigators have been able to demonstrate the role of the CNS in the absence of specifically lesioned circuitry, and provide insights into the potential circuitry involved in brain–immune interactions (albeit largely in rodents rather than humans). Regions of the hypothalamus have been the most extensively examined. The anterior hypothalamus appears to be either directly or indirectly involved in the stimulation of both humoral and cell-mediated immune functions. Discrete lesions in anterior hypothalamus resulted in decreased nucleated splenocytes (2–4), reduced proliferation of T-cells in response to the mitogen concanavalin A (Con A) (2, 4–6), thymic involution (2), decreased natural killer (NK) cell activity (7, 8), reduced antibody production (9), altered tumour cell growth (10), and inhibited development of lethal anaphylactic response (11). Most of these responses were transient in nature, and some of the responses were reversible with hypophysectomy (HypoX) indicating that the effects are mediated through neuroendocrine mechanisms (5, 9).

Ablation studies in other sites in the hypothalamus have produced more variable results. Lesions in the medial hypothalamus were reported to decrease T-and B-cell number (3) and to enhance graft rejection (12). Roszman and colleagues (6), however, detected no alterations in immune functions with lesions placed in this hypothalamic site. Lesions in the posterior hypothalamus decreased T-helper/T-suppressor cell ratio (3) and enhanced tumour growth (10). Lesions in medial or posterior hypothalamus did not alter the development of lethal anaphylaxis (11).

These studies indicate that the anterior hypothalamus and possibly other hypothalamic regions can influence immune reactivity. However, interpretation of the data is limited due to the difficulty in accurate placement of the lesion in small discrete hypothalamic nuclei which often contain many subsets of chemically specific neurons that can be compact or scattered in the nucleus. In addition, this approach is limited because of the abundance of fibres passing through the hypothalamus which may or may not be damaged when nuclei are lesioned. The involvement of discrete projections and chemically identified neurons in the hypothalamus awaits further studies with techniques that have a higher degree of resolution and specificity.

Further evidence for the involvement of the hypothalamus in immune modulation comes from electrical recordings of neuronal firing rates in discrete nuclear regions. An extensive body of early Soviet literature has documented electrophysiological responses in the hypothalamus, limbic forebrain structures, and midbrain reticular formation in response to antigenic challenge (reviewed in English by Korneva *et al*. ref. 13). Besedovsky and co-workers (14) demonstrated enhanced neuronal firing rates in the ventromedial nucleus of the hypothalamus at the peak of an antibody response following immunization. Antigenic challenge also increased neuronal firing rates in the preoptic/anterior hypothalamic area at peak antibody production (day 5) and suppressed neuronal activity in the paraventricular nucleus of the hypothalamus during the first 3 days after immunization followed by enhancement in neuronal activity by day 6. Secondary immunization resulted in a similar pattern of neuronal firing in the preoptic/anterior hypothalamus, but the response was not as abrupt or as robust as that observed with primary immunization. It is believed that changes in neuronal firing patterns in specific regions of the brain result from the release of cytokines from cells of the immune system that can interact either directly or indirectly with neurons in these brain regions. Differences in responsiveness to primary and secondary immunization may reflect the differences in cytokine secretion that occurs under these two conditions.

Discrete lesions in the limbic forebrain structures also produce changes in immune reactivity. The direction of change in immune responses is generally in favour of enhancement. Ablations of the dorsal hippocampus and amygdaloid complex transiently increased splenocyte and thymocyte number, and mitogen-induced T-cell proliferation (2, 5). These effects were reversible by HypoX (5), suggesting mediation via neuroendocrine routes. Lesions in these sites, however, did not affect the development and progression of experimental allergic encephalomyelitis (EAE) and graft rejection. Following lesions of the lateral septal area and its connections to the hippocampus, Nance and co-workers (15) reported chronic alteration in T-cell mediated responses. Because of the extensive connections between these limbic structures and the hypothalamus, alterations in immune functions could result from either altered neuroendocrine or autonomic outflow.

Based on ablation studies, brain stem autonomic nuclei also modulate immune responses. Delayed-type hypersensitivity (DTH) responses were inhibited by lesions in the caudal reticular formation of the medulla and pons (16), and enhanced by lesions in the rostral medial reticular formation and raphe nuclei (17). Thymic involution also resulted from lesions in the reticular formation. Because the reticular formation is a diffuse network of neurons and connections that link together many neuronal systems, identification of the chemically specific neurons involved in modulating immune function is not possible. Felten and colleagues (1) have suggested the possible involvement of monoaminergic systems with these reticular formation lesions, since noradrenergic and serotonergic cell bodies in the caudal reticular formation and rostral raphe nuclei, respectively, project extensively to the hypothalamus and some limbic structures. These two monoaminergic systems regulate numerous visceral and neuroendocrine events, and clearly are involved in both affective and cognitive processes. In addition to the influence of these monoaminergic systems on the hypothalamus and limbic structures through ascending connections, these systems also exert descending control of autonomic preganglionic neurons in the brain stem and spinal cord. Thus, removal of these connections would alter autonomic outflow as well.

Following central administration of 6-hydroxydopamine (6-OHDA) into the cisterna magna, a neurotoxin specific for noradrenergic nerve fibres, Cross and co-workers (18) reported enhancement of suppressor T-cell activity in immunized rodents. Further support for the involvement of the monoaminergic system in the modulation of immune functions comes from neurochemical measurement of monoamines from specific brain sites following immunization. Besedovsky *et al.* (19) demonstrated a decrease in noradrenaline (NA) levels in the hypothalamus at the time of peak antibody response (day 4) to a primary antigen challenge. Furthermore, 2 hours after administration of supernatants from cultures of Con A-stimulated lymphocytes, hypothalamic NA content decreased suggesting that cytokine secretion from lymphocytes may be responsible for altered monoamine content. Turnover studies have indicated that decreased hypothalamic NA content following immunization is accompanied by increased NA turnover (20, 21). Neurochemical measurement of monoamines from specifically microdissected regions of hypothalamus and other CNS sites revealed that an altered monoamine content was specific both to certain brain regions and the time course of the antibody response. NA content in the paraventricular nucleus of the hypothalamus (but not in the supraoptic nucleus, the anterior or medial hypothalamus) decreased at the peak of the antibody response (day 4), and at the peak time of secretion of GC (22). Changes in monoamine metabolism and electrophysiological activity in the paraventricular nucleus in response to immunologic stimuli provides a potential mechanism for mediating the activity of the corticotrophin-releasing hormone (CRH)–ACTH–GC axis, which is known to modulate lymphocyte responses. Decreased NA and serotonin (5-HT) content in the dorsal hippocampus, and increased 5-HT content in the nucleus solitarius, were also found during the rising phase of the immune response. No alterations in monoamine content were observed in other discrete brain regions, or during the declining phase of the immune response. These studies lend additional support to the idea that the immune system, presumably through secretion of one or more cytokines, is able to communicate with specific hypothalamic, limbic forebrain, and brain stem autonomic nuclei, either directly or indirectly, and induce specific changes in the metabolism of central monoamines. These are key regulatory neurotransmitters involved in visceral, autonomic, and neuroendocrine process, as well as inter-neuronal activity.

Decreased proliferation of thymocytes was reported following discrete lesions in ventral and medial aspects of the parabrachial nuclei (23). These nuclei contribute to the circuitry linking brain stem autonomic nuclei such as the nucleus solitarius with hypothalamus and such limbic forebrain structures as the amygdala. This suggests that these nuclei may process both afferent and efferent information related to autonomic regulation, and influence hypothalamic and limbic influences on the neuroendocrine system.

Reported changes in immune parameters to psychosocial factors, stressors, and behavioural conditioning suggest the involvement of the cerebral cortex, particularly the frontal, cingulate, and temporal regions. These cortical regions have direct projections to the limbic forebrain, hypothalamus, brain stem, visceral nuclei, and autonomic preganglionic neurons. Various studies by Renoux and colleagues (24–26) indicate a role for the cerebral cortex in the modulation of immune responses and that this system may be lateralized (for review, see ref. 27). Large lesions in the left cerebral hemisphere in mice exhibited decreased T-cell numbers, T-cell response and NK cell activity, whilst B-cell and macrophage functions remained unaffected. Lesions in the right cerebral cortex appeared to have the opposite effect, which could be due to modulation of efferent signals arising from the left cerebral cortex. These findings were subsequently confirmed by Newlands and co-workers (28).

# 3  Direct innervation of lymphoid organs

## 3.1  NORADRENERGIC SYMPATHETIC INNERVATION

The autonomic nervous system, through its innervation of lymphoid organs, provides a direct route for communication between the nervous and immune systems. Noradrenergic sympathetic innervation of both primary and secondary lymphoid organs has been well described using fluorescence histochemistry for localization of catecholamines (CA), and using immunocytochemical (ICC) staining for tyrosine hydroxylase (TH), the rate-limiting enzyme in the synthesis of NA (29–52). This innervation is regional and specific, distributing along the vasculature and in the parenchyma adjacent to cells of the immune system. Other studies collectively provide evidence that NA fulfils the criteria for neurotransmission in lymphoid organs with cells of the immune system as targets. In summary, these studies demonstrate: (i) the presence of noradrenergic innervation in lymphoid compartments (29–52); (ii) the release and availability of NA from nerve terminals upon sympathetic nerve stimulation (35, 52–54); (iii) the presence of adrenoceptors on a variety of cells of the immune system, including T- and B-lymphocytes, thymocytes, macrophages, mast cells, and granulocytes (49, 55–65) (reviewed by 66); and (iv) predictable immune responses to manipulation of noradrenergic innervation, and NA and its receptors (40, 41, 43, 48, 67–72) (reviewed in refs 40 and 48).

Anatomical studies have demonstrated noradrenergic sympathetic innervation of both the smooth muscle of blood vessels, and the parenchyma of specific lymphoid compartments within primary and secondary lymphoid organs (34, 36–44, 46–52). Within the parenchyma, noradrenergic nerves distributed to zones of T- and B-lymphocytes, and accessory cells including the lymphoid compartment where macrophages reside. In spleen, noradrenergic nerves coursed along the central arteriole and its branches, and extended from these vascular plexuses into the surrounding periarteriolar lymphatic sheath (PALS), a zone where T-lymphocytes predominate. Noradrenergic fibres also coursed adjacent to arterioles, or in nerve bundles, into the marginal zone and parafollicular zone where macrophages and B-lymphocytes reside. In spleens from adult rodents, few noradrenergic nerves were present in the follicle, a B-lymphocyte compartment. In the red pulp, noradrenergic nerves resided along the venous sinuses and in the capsuler/trabecular system; few fibres coursed from these compartments into the parenchyma of the red pulp.

Evidence of the release and availability of NA for interaction with target cells has been provided from studies showing: (i) increased NA content in splenic venous blood following sympathetic nerve stimulation (54); (ii) depletion of NA following intraperitoneal (i.p.) administration of 6-OHDA or removal of sympathetic ganglion that supplies noradrenergic nerves to lymphoid organs (35, 52); and (iii) measurement of nanomolar concentrations of NA following *in vivo* dialysis of the spleen (53). These findings suggest that noradrenergic nerves are capable of providing high splenic NA concentrations, and support a paracrine role for NA in the splenic microenvironment.

The possibility that noradrenergic nerves also may interact with cells of the immune system through a mode other than via the paracrine secretion of NA is indicated from ICC studies performed at the ultrastructural level. In spleen sections stained for TH and examined with electron microscopy (46), we showed the presence of TH+ nerve terminals adjacent to lymphocytes in the PALS and adjacent to lymphocytes and macrophages in the marginal zone. Appositions between TH+ nerve terminals and lymphocytes and macrophages were characterized by a gap junction of about 6 nm with relatively large regions of membrane apposition and no specialization of either pre- or post-junctional membranes. In contrast, noradrenergic sympathetic terminals whose targets were presumably smooth muscle cells of the central arteriole were interposed by a basement membrane within a gap of about 250 nm. The presence of TH+ nerve terminals closely apposed to lymphocytes and macrophages suggests direct interaction between TH+ nerve terminals and cells of the immune system: however, the directionality of this interaction remains unclear. $\beta$-Adrenoceptor ($\beta$AR) expression on these cell types supports nerve-to-immune cell signalling; conversely it is likely that presumed target cells secrete signal molecules that can interact with closely apposed nerve terminals.

With direct ligand binding assays, $\beta$AR expression has been demonstrated on leukocytes (T- and B-lymphocytes, neutrophils, basophils and macrophages) and on accessory cells of the immune system (mast cells) (49, 55–65) (reviewed in ref. 66). $\beta$AR on lymphocytes and accessory cells of the immune system are linked with adenylate cyclase and the generation of cAMP. $\beta$AR on lymphocytes from young adult rodents appear to be regulated in a similar manner to other tissues innervated by noradrenergic sympathetic nerves, with the presence of $\beta$AR agonists and antagonists resulting in down-regulation and up-regulation of $\beta$AR, respectively. Furthermore, the presence of $\alpha$-adrenoceptors ($\alpha$AR) on human lymphocytes (73) and activated murine macrophages (74) has been documented by ligand binding studies. Pharmacological studies in rodents demonstrating changes in immune parameters mediated via $\alpha$AR suggest the presence of $\alpha$AR on cells of the immune system (48, 75).

A complex role for noradrenergic innervation in immunomodulation has been highlighted by various functional studies. Several approaches have been taken to evaluate the effect of CA on immunological reactivity, including the use of relatively selective adrenergic agents *in vitro*, infusion of adrenergic agents *in vivo*, and the surgical or chemical destruction of sympathetic nerves that distribute to lymphoid organs. Based on these studies several roles have been proposed for NA modulation of immune reactivity, including regulation of proliferation and differentiation of lymphocytes (70, 71), lymphocyte trafficking (68, 69, 72), and immunocompetence (29, 40, 48, 52, 75–77) (reviewed in refs. 40, 48). T- and B-lymphocyte reactivity *in vitro*, including mitogen- and cytokine-induced proliferation (78–81), cytotoxic T-lymphocyte (CTL) activity (82), cytokine production (83), and antibody production (80, 84, 85) were inhibited by $\beta$AR stimulation. Sanders and Munson (86–88) showed that application of NA (or other $\beta_2$-agonists) to unfractionated mouse splenocytes at the start of their culture enhanced the plaque-forming cell (PFC) response approximately two- to fourfold on day 5, the peak of the immune response, in a dose-dependent manner. This effect was blockable in the presence of propranolol within 6 hours of culturing splenocytes. Furthermore, $\beta$-blockade revealed an $\alpha$AR-mediated enhancement of the primary immune response on day 4, and suppression on day 5. Adrenergic agonists potentiated CTL activity; an effect mediated by both $\alpha$AR and $\beta$AR. Findings from our laboratory (40, 48) have recently demonstrated that the addition of nanomolar to micromolar concentrations of adrenergic agonists to mixed-lymphocyte cultures enhanced their CTL activity by 25–350 per cent.

Macrophage and NK cell functions can also be modified by CA and other adrenergic agents. CA suppressed the killing of virus-infected cells and tumour cells by interferon-gamma (INF$\gamma$)-stimulated macrophages (89, 90), and increased synthesis of complement components in human monocytes (91). Reported effects of CA on NK activity *in vitro* were variable (enhancement (92), suppression (93)). We have not detected significant changes in murine NK cell function using a variety of adrenergic agonists *in vitro* (S. Livnat of this laboratory, unpublished observation). However, chemical sympathectomy (SympX) in adult mice enhanced NK cell activity *in vitro* (standard[51] Cr-release assay) and *in vivo* (as measured by clearance of intravenously injected radiolabelled-tumour cells from the lung), suggesting that noradrenergic innervation suppresses NK cell activity *in vivo* (94).

Adrenaline (A) hastened the peak and the decline of the PFC response of splenocytes by day 1 when given 6 hours prior to immunization, but inhibited the primary antibody response at all time points examined when administered 2–4 days before immunization (95). Adoptive transfer of splenocytes either exposed to $10^{-5}$ M A for 1 hour *in vitro* or six hours of A administration *in vivo* into syngeneic, irradiated recipients resulted in the enhancement of a primary antibody response to a sheep red blood cell (SRBC) challenge compared with recipients of untreated splenocytes.

Infusion of A in humans produced a transient increase in the number of circulating lymphocytes and monocytes, and decreased mitogen-induced

T-lymphocyte proliferation (96–98). In rodents, intracardiac injection of either NA or isoproterenol increased lymphocyte and granulocyte release from the spleen following blockade by pretreatment with phentolamine and propranolol, respectively. Treatment of SympX rodents with NA enhanced leukocyte release from the spleen. In guinea pigs previously immunized with SRBC, release of PFC from the spleen at the peak day of the secondary immune response was enhanced dramatically after intracardiac injection of A and was sustained beyond the peak day of the response leading to a decrease in spleen PFC number. Findings described above could not be attributed to changes in vascular smooth muscle contractility and altered blood flow, suggesting that CA can modulate lymphocyte migration.

We and others have investigated sympathetic modulation of immune reactivity *in vivo* using sympathetic denervation strategies. Destruction of noradrenergic nerves can be achieved by systemic injection of 6-OHDA, or by surgical removal of sympathetic ganglion that distribute to lymphoid organs. The consequences of noradrenergic depletion in the spleen are as follows. Denervation with 6-OHDA at birth and surgical SympX in adults augmented primary and secondary antibody response (52, 75). Chemical Sympx in adults suppressed primary and secondary antibody responses (40, 48, 76, 77). Chemical SympX with 6-OHDA in adult rodents abrogated primary immune responses in spleens challenged systemically by 80 per cent of intact animals, and in popliteal lymph nodes challenged by foot pad injection by 97 per cent of untreated levels (41, 43, 48). Further studies from our laboratories (40, 48, 94, 99–101) based on chemical SympX in adult rodents, showed that chemical SympX results in suppression of DTH responses to contact sensitizing agents, reduced CTL responses that were accompanied by lowered interleukin-2 (IL-2) production, enhanced NK cell activity *in vivo* and *in vitro*, augmented B-lymphocyte proliferative responses in lymph nodes, and a complex pattern of mitogen responses in spleen and specific lymph nodes. Suppression of DTH was blocked by preventing uptake of the neurotoxin into the nerve terminals with desmethylimipramine, a tricyclic uptake inhibitor of NA. This response was not blocked by propranolol, administered concomitantly with the 6-OHDA, indicating that the effect is not mediated through the release of NA from damaged noradrenergic terminals and interaction with postsynaptic receptors on lymphocytes. Sympathetic denervation also significantly influenced cellular trafficking (100). Lymphocytes from nondenervated donors migrated in larger numbers to inguinal and axillary lymph nodes of chemically SympX recipients, while lymph node cells taken from SympX donors exhibited decreased migration to lymph nodes in nondenervated recipients. These findings suggest that noradrenergic innervation of secondary lymphoid organs in young adult rodents is necessary for competent immune reactivity.

## 3.2 NEUROPEPTIDERGIC INNERVATION OF LYMPHOID ORGANS

Using ICC for a number of neuropeptides, we have demonstrated the presence of nerves in the spleen, thymus, and lymph nodes which are immunoreactive for substance P (SP), calcitonin gene-related peptide (CGRP), vasoactive inteslinal polypeptide (VIP), and neuropeptide Y (NPY) at the light microscopic level (30, 102–105). Radioimmunoassay studies confirmed relatively high levels of SP, VIP, and NPY in these lymphoid organs. NPY+ nerves were present in a distribution that overlapped noradrenergic nerves in the spleen, thymus, and lymph nodes (106–108). Studies from our laboratory which examined NPY concentration and ICC staining following chemical SympX have indicated that NPY colocalizes with NA in the spleen and thymus (108). Further evidence to support colocalization of NPY and NA in these lymphoid organs came from pilot studies from our laboratories showing a parallel decline in NPY+ nerves and noradrenergic nerves in spleens from ageing Fischer 344 (F344) rats (106). VIP-immunoreactive fibres in the spleen, thymus, and mesenteric lymph nodes were present in a much lower density than NPY+ nerves, and localized to different compartments (102). Other investigators have provided evidence for VIP innervation of gut-associated lymphoid tissue (109–111).

We have recently demonstrated both SP+ and CGRP+ nerves in the rat thymus, spleen, and lymph nodes (104, 105, 112). The distribution of SP+ and CGRP+ nerves in the spleen and thymus were overlapping, and differed from that of NA/NPY. In the spleen, SP+/CGRP+ nerves coursed along the large venous sinuses and trabeculae, in the parenchyma of the red pulp and marginal zone, and to a lesser extent along large central arterioles and in the adjacent periarteriolar lymphatic sheaths. ICC for SP/CGRP in the rat thymus, revealed SP+/CGRP+ nerves abundant in the capsule and in interlobular septa often adjacent to mast cells, and among CD8+ cortical thymocytes. SP+/CGRP+ nerves also were found along the vasculature at the corticomedullary junction. In lymph nodes, SP+/CGRP+ nerves resided at the hilus, beneath the capsule, in the corticomedullary junction, the medullary region, and the internodular region. CGRP+ fibres were more numerous than SP+/CGRP+ fibres in the spleen.

Neuropeptides present in lymphoid organs also may derive from sources other than peripheral nerves. Neuropeptide availability may result from synthesis and release of neuropeptides from the hypothalamic–pituitary axis (as a hormone or prehormone), either via the circulation or directly from synthesis by cells of the immune system (113, 114). The target cells of peptidergic nerve fibres in lymphoid organs may be cells of the immune system, accessory or supportive cells, and/or vascular beds.

Receptors specific for a variety of neuropeptides, including VIP, SP, and opiate peptides have been demonstrated on cells of the immune system (reviewed in ref. 112). Functional responses following interaction of VIP with VIP receptors on lymphocytes are mediated via cAMP-dependent protein kinase (111, 115). SP receptors are coupled with the phosphotidylinositol pathway, activation of protein kinase C (PKC), and calcium mobilization (116, 117). SP receptors on lymphocytes appear to be different from those on mast cells; the carboxy-terminal end of the SP molecule is important in ligand binding on lymphocytes (118), while the amino acid-terminal end is necessary for release of mediators of inflammation (119).

Opioid receptors appear to be divided into two general classes: classical receptors ($\mu$ and $\delta$ where naloxone and morphine can displace binding of opiate peptides (120–122)), and non-typical opioid receptors that bind opiate peptides not displaceable by naloxone or morphine (123–126). The second messenger system coupled with opioid receptors is dependent upon the specific opioid peptide, type of receptor on the target cell, and type of immunocyte.

There is abundant evidence supporting modulation of immune responses by neuropeptides. VIP inhibits mitogen-induced proliferation of lymphocytes from murine Peyer's patches and spleen (127, 128), suppresses NK cell activity (129), and alters antibody production (128). VIP also influences the migration of T-lymphocytes into gut-associated lymphoid tissue (130, 131) and mesenteric lymph nodes (132, 133). Pre-incubation of rat T-lymphocytes from Peyer's patches with VIP in concentrations that down regulate VIP receptors on T-lymphocytes prevents homing of desensitized T-lymphocytes to Peyer's patches following adoptive transfer of these cells into a syngeneic host (130). VIP also appears to be involved in vasodilatation of vascular beds during local inflammatory responses (134, 135).

SP stimulates mitogen-induced proliferation of lymphocytes (118, 128), plays a major role in local inflammation via dilatation of vascular beds (136, 137), and stimulates mast cells and basophils to release histamine and other mediators, such as leukotrienes (119, 134, 138). Neurotensin prevents SP-induced release of histamine by competing for SP receptors on target cells, and SOM blocks release of SP from peripheral nerve endings (135, 139). Somatostatin (SOM) also modulates several immune functions *in vitro*, including concentration-dependent modulation of the spontaneous proliferation of murine splenocytes (140), inhibition of mitogen-stimulated proliferation of murine splenocytes (141), human T-lymphocytes and the human lymphoblast cell line, Molt-4b (142), and reduction in colony-stimulating activity of murine splenocytes (143). SOM is a major mediator of immediate hypersensitivity through its stimulation of leucocyte and monocyte chemotaxis (144), neutrophil phagocytosis (145), macrophage effector functions (146), and release of histamine and leukotrienes by basophils and mast cells (142, 147).

Numerous studies support an immunomodulatory role for endogenous opioid peptides as well. Opioid peptides alter antibody production (121, 148), mitogen-stimulated proliferation of lymphocytes (149–152), expression of surface receptors on T-lymphocytes (E-rosette, IL-2 and Ia receptors) (153, 154), production of lymphokines (interferon and T-lymphocyte chemotactic factor) (155–157), NK (158–161) and CTL activity (162), and a number of phagocytic functions (163–166).

# 4   Neuroendocrine mediators of neural–immune modulation

## 4.1   GENERAL EFFECTS OF HYPOX ON IMMUNE FUNCTION

Every hormone secreted or regulated by the pituitary gland has been shown to affect at least some parameters within the immune system. The earliest evidence indicating the importance of the neuroendocrine system in immune regulation comes from clinical studies in patients with neuroendocrine deficiencies, and from studies using laboratory animals in which the pituitary has been removed. One of the most striking changes in HypoX animals is the marked atrophy of the thymus and secondary lymphoid organs. The thymus involutes at a rapid rate in HypoX animals (167), and is associated with decreased turnover of both nucleic acids and phospholipids. Treatment with GH or prolactin reverses thymic involution (167, 168), and enhances turnover of both these substances (169, 170). Rapid involution of the thymus and its low nucleic acid turnover in HypoX and aged animals is completely reversible with syngeneic pituitary grafts. This effect of grafting is reversed by treatment with antibodies directed against prolactin, while replacement therapy with CHAT, FSH, LH, or TSH has no restorative capacity (168). Conversely, administration of ACTH to HypoX animals accelerates further the involution of the thymus, as well as other lymphoid organs (171–175). Similar to the thymus, secondary lymphoid organs from HypoX rats become atrophic and DNA turnover is significantly reduced. These abnormalities are reversible by administration of GH, prolactin, or syngeneic pituitary grafts, and exacerbated by treatment with ACTH (12, 168, 173–175).

Numerous investigators have found minimal effects of HypoX on the primary antibody response. Duquesnoy *et al.* (176) reported that recovery of hemagglutinating antibody formation to antigen challenge with SRBC was defective after sublethal irradiation of adult HypoX rats. Splenocytes explanted from HypoX donors demonstrated a chronic depression of immune responses *in vitro* (177), and this was virtually restored by administration of GH to the HypoX animals prior to culture (which acted to interfere with the immunosuppressive effects of endogenous corticosterone). Long-term HypoX rats, maintained on corticosterone, deoxycorticosterone, and thyroxine with salt supplementation in the drinking water, responded better to immunization with SRBC than age-matched unoperated animals. HypoX suppressed the humoral immune response and abrogated the suppressive effects of intracisternally administered 6-OHDA on antibody response (18). HypoX also blocked the androgen-induced secretion of IgA and the secretory component of tears in male rats.

HypoX animals displayed prolonged skin allograft survival (168, 176), enhanced clearance of injected colloidal carbon, and reduced sensitivity to cutaneously applied 1-chloro2-,4-dinitrobenzene (DNCB). DNCB-sensitized HypoX rats displayed reduced weights of draining lymph nodes, but no change in lymphocyte proliferative responses compared with normal sensitized controls. However, when a range of doses of DNCB was used, HypoX rats demonstrated a more linear dose–response relationship with lymph node weight, and with cellular proliferation than was observed in control rats.

The role of the pituitary in mediating the effects of CNS lesions has also been examined. NK cell numbers were lower in spleens from C57B/6J female mice following HypoX, an effect which was reversible by administration of ovine GH (100 $\mu$g/day i.p. for 10 days) (178). Bilateral electrolytic lesions in the preoptic/anterior hypothalamus in F344 rats resulted in a transient decrease in NK activity. When HypoX was performed prior to lesioning, suppressed NK-cell activity was observed in both lesioned and nonlesioned rats, suggesting that factors released by the pituitary mediate, at least in part, the effects of the electrolytic lesion (7). Preoptic/anterior hypothalamic lesions also reduced proliferative responses of splenocytes to T-cell mitogens, while lesions in the hippocampus enhanced splenic and thymic cellularity and mitogenic responsiveness. These lesion effects on proliferation and cellularity in the spleen were abrogated by HypoX. The effects of ablation of hippocampus (or amygdala) on thymocyte number and function were also abolished by HypoX, but HypoX resulted in greater numbers of thymocytes and suppressed mitogenic activity in hypothalamic-lesioned rats. These findings indicate that the effect of these brain lesions are mediated primarily, but not exclusively, by the pituitary (7).

Extensive studies by Berczi and Nagy (168, 179) found a general immunodeficiency in HypoX rats, including marked suppression of the primary antibody response to immunization with SRBC (T-cell dependent) and with *E. coli* 055:B5 lipopolysaccharide (LPS) (T-cell independent), decreased DTH responses to DNCB, prolonged skin graft survival, and retarded development of adjuvant-induced arthritis following administration of Freund's complete adjuvant. Both IgM and IgG antibodies were affected, and the secondary antibody response to SRBC also was suppressed, but to a lesser degree than the primary response. The effects of HypoX on antibody response were restored to normal levels either by syngeneic pituitary grafts placed under the kidney capsule or by daily subcutaneous injections of GH, prolactin, or human placental lactogen. Similarly, the DTH response to DNCB in HypoX animals was restored by syngeneic pituitary grafts or by administration of GH, prolactin, or human placental lactogen. Restoration of the DTH reaction to DNCB, but not the antibody response to SRBC, was demonstrated in rats transplanted with anterior pituitary tumors MtT/W5 (which secretes GH), MTT/W10 (which secretes GH and prolactin), or MtT/F4 (which secretes ACTH, prolactin, and GH). Treatment with dopaminergic agents such as bromocriptine or pergolide (dopamine (DA) agonist) suppressed the DTH response to DNCB and the primary antibody response to the same degree as HypoX. This effect was mediated through DA-inhibited release of prolactin, since administration significantly decreased serum prolactin levels, and replacement of prolactin or GH (at 5X the dose needed to restore the immunosuppressive effects of HypoX) alleviated the suppressive effects of dopaminergic therapy. Adjuvant-induced arthritis also was attenuated in HypoX and bromocriptine-treated rats.

## 4.2 GROWTH HORMONE

The principal mechanisms for regulation of immune function by GH are through its regulation of growth and maturation of lymphoid organs. Some of the earliest studies demonstrated that administration of this hormone increased the size of lymphatic tissues, particularly the thymus glands, and suggested that GH also affects the activities of lymphocytes and macrophages. Cells of the immune system which possess receptors for GH include thymocytes, transformed lymphocytes, and peripheral blood mononuclear cells (180). Their distribution on such mononuclear cell subsets as NK cells, macrophages, B-cells, and CD4+ and CD8+ cells has yet to be examined.

GH augments unstimulated *in vitro* proliferation of transformed and nomal lymphocytes (181–186). Numerous investigators have reported GH-induced changes in mitogen-stimulated proliferative responses; although the direction of change has not been consistent (182, 184–187). Higher mitogen-induced proliferative responses were found in splenocytes from mice that carry the transgene for rat GH compared with littermate controls (188) despite the fact that IL-2 synthesis did not differ in these two groups of animals. In GH-deficient children, treatment with GH augmented mitogenic responses of peripheral blood mononuclear cells (186, 189).

When administered to hypopituitary animals, GH enhanced a number of immune responses, including antibody synthesis, NK cell activity, CTL responses, and skin graft rejection (190–197). Saxena and colleagues (178) showed that GH, in nanogram concentrations, enhanced CTL activity stimulated with allogeneic cells *in vitro*. In HypoX mice, NK cell killing of virus-infected target cells was markedly reduced. When 100 µg of ovine GH was administered to these animals for 10 days, NK cell activity was elevated to greater than 50 per cent of the cytolytic activity found in sham-operated animals. In rats and humans, NK cell activity declined as a function of age, and was augmented by treatment with GH (188, 198). Similarly, NK cell activity was reduced in children with GH deficiency; however, administration of GH to these children did not enhance cytolytic activity, possibly the result of a developmental defect in NK cells since these cells also failed to respond to the cytokine, interferon $\alpha$.

While GH was not essential for the maturation of granulocytic precursor cells in the bone marrow, addition of recombinant human GH incubated with human marrow mononuclear cells in the presence of granulocyte-macrophage colony-stimulating factor more than doubled the maturation of granulocytic cells (199). This effect appeared to be mediated by GH-stimulated release of insulin-like growth factor I (IGF-I) from bone marrow-derived monocytes since introduction of a monoclonal antibody directed against the IGF-I receptor into the culture abrogated this stimulatory effect of GH. Similarly, the GH-induced maturation of erythrocytes resulted from the stimulation by GH of IGF-I synthesis and release from macrophages. Kelley (200) has proposed that the same mechanism is responsible for fibroblast proliferation in fibrotic lung disease.

GH exerts many of its effects on immune functions through interaction with GH receptors on macrophages. Macrophages incubated with GH acquired morphological characteristics of activated macrophages (201), and GH enhanced the *in vitro* and *in vivo* production of reactive oxygen intermediates such as hydroxyl radicals, singlet oxygen molecules and superoxide anion $(O_2^-)$ and $H_2O_2$ which is important in the killing of ingested bacteria.

It is clear that the role of GH in the modulation of immune function involves an interplay between the neuroendocrine system, the thymus gland, and cells of the immune system. Viral and bacterial infections, and LPS (the major constituent in the outer cell wall of Gram-negative bacteria) increased GH secretion in humans (202, 203), and induced secretion of macrophage-derived cytokines including IL-1 and TNF$\alpha$ (204–207). Laboratory animals may respond differently to LPS and viruses. Kasting and Martin (208) reported that high doses of endotoxin injected into rats initially suppressed plasma GH, followed by a significant rise in GH on day 2 after endotoxin treatment. Persistent viral infections in mice (that is lymphocytic choriemeningitis virus which replicates in GH-producing pituitary cells) reduced plasma GH concentrations and transcripts for pituitary derived GH (209).

GH-stimulated secretion of IL-1 and TNF$\alpha$ from cells of the immune system may enter the blood for interaction with the CNS. Administration of IL-1 into the third ventricle (at concentrations that did not induce fever) elevated circulating levels of GH (210). Similarly, IL-1 (211) and TNF$\alpha$ (212) stimulated GH secretion from pituitary cells *in vitro*. Plasma GH concentrations were also increased in humans with a wide variety of cancers, although the mechanisms underlying this elevation have not been elucidated (213, 214). Elevated plasma levels of GH may be important in the elimination of viral or bacterial infections at local sites of inflammation, by activation of macrophages to produce reactive oxygen intermediates and release IGF-I and TNFα (215). Elimination of the virus or bacteria by GH-primed macrophages would then remove the signal molecules for induction of GH secretion. GH also may counteract the immunosuppressive effects of an IL-1 induced rise in plasma GC levels (172, 216, 217).

In addition to the anterior pituitary as a source of GH, cells of the immune system (thymocytes, T- and B-lymphocytes) have been shown to contain immunoreactive GH and specific mRNA for GH (218, 219). The contribution made by GH released from cells of the immune system in the modulation of immune functions is unknown at the present time. It is likely that this source of GH may promote macrophage activation and killing of bacteria and viruses, as well as stimulate the local production of such cytokines as thymulin in the thymus under normal physiological conditions.

### 4.3 PROLACTIN

Bernton *et al.* (220) showed that suppression of prolactin secretion in mice treated with bromocriptine increased mortality after Listeria challenge, attenuated T-lymphocyte-dependent activation of macrophages (possibly through decreased production of interferon-γ (INFγ)) following inoculation with *Mycobacterium bovis*, and inhibited T-lymphocyte proliferation without altering IL-2 production. These alterations in immune reactivity were blockable by co-administration of ovine prolactin and bromocriptine. Macrophages obtained from inoculated mice treated with bromocriptine still responded normally to exogenous macrophage-activating factor and INFγ. Splenocytes obtained from these same mice failed to proliferate in response to either T- or B-cell mitogens (220), suggesting decreased clonal expansion of antigen-recognizing T- and B-lymphocytes *in vivo*. Diminished IL-2 production or decreased density of IL-2 receptors on the surface of T- and B-cells did not contribute to their impaired proliferation *in vitro*.

Administration of exogenous prolactin or DA antagonists which stimulate secretion of endogenous prolactin enhanced mitogen-stimulated lymphocyte proliferation by 30 to 70 per cent over controls (221). Administration of the DA antagonist haloperidol reversed cyclosporin-induced immunosuppression in rats (218), and increased DTH response to DNCB in mice (222). Haloperidol-induced effects on DTH occurred only when treated during the afferent (sensitization) phase, but not during the effector phase after DNCB rechallenge, indicating an effect on the acquisition of specific cellular immunity and not on inflammatory mechanisms.

Russell and co-workers (223) showed biochemical alterations in lymphoid organs following administration of prolactin. Intact and HypoX rats receiving 22 mg/kg of pituitary-derived prolactin showed marked elevation of ornithine decarboxylase activity (ODC) in spleen and thymus, the rate-limiting enzyme for polyamine biosynthesis important in manufacturing protein, and in cell proliferation. These effects were antagonized by cyclosporine. The doses of prolactin used in this study were superphysiological and were possibly contaminated with small quantities of other pituitary hormones. In support of these findings, Buckley *et al.* (224) demonstrated that membrane translocation of protein kinase C (PKC), a biochemical marker associated with prolactin induction of ODC, was induced in rat liver following treatment with rat prolactin and human GH, but not with rat GH, which is nonlactogenic. HypoX resulted in a twofold increase in basal spleen and thymus ODC activity and greatly potentiated the ODC response to prolactin.

*In vitro* effects of prolactin on immune function thus far have been difficult to characterize for a variety of reasons. Since fetal bovine serum supplements often contain large amounts of prolactin which would obscure any effects of prolactin in physiological concentrations, lymphocytes must be cultured in carefully defined media. While specific prolactin receptors have been demonstrated on human and rat lymphocytes, the density of these receptors is comparatively small (specific binding of 30 pg of prolactin per $10^6$ cells, or about 360 receptors per cell) relative to other organs such as liver, prostate, or breast tissue. Furthermore, prolactin receptors on lymphocytes have been poorly characterized with respect to conditions that will alter their expression on lymphocytes, and their intracellular second messenger system. Lastly, mitogen-stimulated lymphocytes produce a factor with prolactin-like bioactivity and immunoreactivity (225); this ability of lymphocytes to synthesize prolactin-like protein further complicates *in vitro* studies examining the effects of prolactin.

Russell *et al.* (226) hypothesized coupling of PKC as the second messenger system in the stimulation of ODC and mitogenesis in NB-2 cells, a lymphoma T-cell line that expresses high affinity prolactin receptors and is dependent on lactogenic hormones for growth. Murphy and co-worker (227), however, could detect neither an elevation of intracellular calcium nor an activation of PKC following administration of prolactin to mitogen- or antigen-stimulated NB-2 cells in culture. This raises the question of the usefulness of the NB-2 cell line in studying the effects of prolactin *in vitro*, since both these pathways appear to be involved in transduction of early proliferative signals in normal lymphocytes.

Bernton *et al.* (228) were unable to detect reproducible alterations in proliferative response or IL-2 production following application of prolactin to mitogen- or antigen-stimulated lymphocytes in lactogen-free culture conditions. However, addition of antisera directed against pituitary prolactin inhibited DNA synthesis and cellular proliferation (211, 229). This inhibitory activity involved interference of a distal event subsequent to the $G_0$ to $G_1$ transition, and inhibited responses of mononuclear cells to the growth factors IL-4 and GM–CSF (granulocyte–monocyte colony-stimulating factor) as well as IL-2. In serum-free cultures of lymphocytes, antibody to prolactin clearly interacts with a protein expressed by the cells, not with a media constituent or added growth factor.

## 4.4 THE HYPOTHALAMIC (CRH)–PITUITARY (ACTH)–ADRENAL (GC) AXIS

### 4.4.1   CRH

CRH has indirect effects on immune function through regulation of the release of proopiomelanocortin (POMC), which is cleaved enzymatically to form ACTH (as well as $\beta$-endorphin), from the anterior pituitary, and subsequently the release of GC from the adrenal gland. CRH also exerts direct effects on immune function through its binding with CRH receptors on cells of the immune system. Webster and de Souza (230) demonstrated the presence of high-affinity binding sites for CRH on macrophages in the marginal zone of the spleen which have structural and pharmacological characteristics similar to CRH receptors described in the pituitary, brain, and placental tissue (231). Smith *et al.* (232) showed that CRH can induce human peripheral blood lymphocytes to produce proopiomelanocortin (POMC) after *in vitro* stimulation, an effect that is potentiated by the application of arginine-vasopressin. CRH-induced secretion of POMC does not appear to act directly on lymphocytes (of the B subset) (233), but rather through its interaction with monocytes, possibly by inducing the release of IL-1 from these cells, since addition of IL-1 to purified human B-cell lines in culture, in the absence of CRH, results in the production of $\beta$-endorphin by these lymphocytes (233, 234). GC appear to be involved in regulating the production of $\beta$-endorphin by CRH, presumably through down regulating the expression of CRH receptors on monocytes and thus ultimately decreasing IL-1 production (234).

### 4.4.2   *Proopiomelanocortin (POMC)-derived peptides*

Like CRH, ACTH and endorphins can modulate immune function. ACTH indirectly modulates immune reactivity through its ability to stimulate the release of GC from the adrenal gland. ACTH also can interact directly with cells of the immune system by binding to high affinity and low affinity receptors on mononuclear leukocytes that are very similar in structural and pharmacological features to those present on adrenal cells (235). B-cells express approximately 3 times more ACTH receptors than T-cells (236). $ACTH_{1-39}$ applied to lymphocyte cultures can suppress *in vitro* antibody production (121) and macrophage-mediated tumouricidal activity (89), alter B-lymphocyte function (237), and decrease IFNγ production (238).

IgM secretion by a B-cell line was enhanced by exposure to $10^{-12}$–$10^{-10}$ M ACTH *in vitro*, with or without LPS stimulation (239). Furthermore, ACTH may act to increase B-cell proliferation at later stages of B-cell stimulation, in concert with IL-5 (240). However, *in vivo* treatment of adrenalectomized mice with ACTH had no effect on spleen cell antibody production *in vitro* (216). NK cell activity was enhanced in pigs treated with ACTH (241), but ACTH had no effect on NK cell activity when added *in vitro*, suggesting that ACTH acts indirectly to effect NK cell activity, possibly through reduced CRF production. Both ACTH and β-endorphin, as well as other opioid peptides, also modulate immune responses by altering receptors on lymphocytes, including CD2 expression, expression and conformation of CD3, and the affinity of IL-2 receptors for IL-2 (reviewed in ref. 242). Further research using both *in vitro* and *in vivo* techniques is needed to fully elucidate the role of ACTH as an immunomodulator.

Two recent studies showed that αMSH (ACTH 1–13) can have similar actions to ACTH. Mason and Van Epps (243) reported that αMSH was more potent and faster acting than the parent ACTH in inhibiting migration in response to IL-1 and other chemotactic agents. Smith *et al.* (244) demonstrated a similar ability of αMSH over ACTH in preventing spontaneous neutrophil activation. The ability of αMSH to block several functions of IL-1 suggests that it may have an important role in down regulating immune responses (243–245).

The products obtained from β-lipotropin (pituitary derived opioid peptides) include α-endorphin (31 amino acids) and products derived from its N-terminus, including α-endorphin (16 amino acids), δ-endorphin (27 amino acids), and γ-endorphin (17 amino acids). This family of opioid peptides is also an important group of immunomodulators. β-endorphins can alter the proliferative activity of lymphocytes (149, 246), NK cell activity (159, 161, 247), antibody synthesis by B-cells (121, 148), and IFNγ production by T-cells (157, 248). β-endorphin also inhibited production of a T-lymphocyte chemotactic factor by Con A-stimulated human peripheral blood mononuclear cells (156), and may serve as a chemotactic factor itself since increased migration of human T-lymphocytes was demonstrated *in vitro* in the presence of this peptide (249). Enhancement of Con A-stimulated splenocyte proliferation (149, 250, 251), suppression of phytohemagglutinin (PHA)-stimulated human lymphocyte proliferation (150), and inhibition of prostaglandin $E_1$-induced suppression (252) by β-endorphin appear to be mediated through a non-opioid receptor-mediated mechanism. Non-opioid-mediated effects of β-endorphin may be due to C-terminal binding to an as yet unidentified receptor. Whether other effects of β-endorphin are mediated through the interaction of β-endorphin with genuine μ-type opioid receptors or a non-opioid receptor has not been resolved.

The addition of β-endorphin (or ACTH) to freshly cultured lymphocytes for 15–20 minutes altered the response of these cells to mitogenic stimulation, with enhancement or suppression dependent on the concentration of the peptide applied, and on the donor of the blood cells tested. Similar effects were observed when γ-endorphin, but not α-endorphin (smaller fragments of β-endorphin that differ only by one amino acid), was applied to the culture. α-Endorphin generally suppressed proliferative response to Con A (253). This difference may be related to the fact that γ-endorphin, but not α-endorphin, has an α-helical conformation. Activated lymphocytes appear to be extremely sensitive to the proliferative effects of β-endorphin, with conflicting data in the literature indicating both an enhancing (149, 151), and a suppressive (150) effect of this peptide on their mitogen-induced proliferation.

*In vivo*, immuno-enhancing effects of β-endorphin were demonstrated by Kusnecov *et al*. (254). Three hours after infusion of rats with β-endorphin, spleen cell Con A-induced proliferation *in vitro* was enhanced in the absence of altered IL-2 production. This effect was blocked by pretreatment with naloxone, although naloxone treatment alone reduced splenocyte responsiveness to Con A.

Johnson and colleagues (121, 238) first demonstrated that endorphins (and ACTH) can alter the primary antibody response of murine splenocytes *in vitro*. They reported that α-endorphin and ACTH suppressed primary antibody production to SRBC, and that β-endorphin and γ-endorphin had no effect. α-Endorphin-induced suppression of a primary antibody response appears to be mediated via an opiate receptor since the opiate antagonist naloxone reversed the effect. Heijnen *et al*. (148) reported similar suppressive effects of α-endorphin on the primary antibody response of human peripheral blood lymphocytes challenged with ovalbumin, but also found that β-endorphin enhanced the antibody response. While the response to α-endorphin appears to be mediated via opiate receptors, the effects of β-endorphin on the antibody response were mediated via non-opiate receptors. β-Endorphin elicited either enhancement or suppression of the secondary antibody response in human peripheral blood lymphocytes, depending on the donor studied and the magnitude of the primary antibody response (255). In donors with low response to tetanus toxoid the peptide enhanced the secondary antibody response, while in high responding donors, β-endorphin-inhibited the response. Heijnen *et al*. (255) proposed that T-helper cells down regulate in response to the peptide when primary antibody production is optimal.

In response to suboptimal doses of LPS, IL-1 production by bone marrow-derived macrophages was enhanced in the presence of β-endorphin (256), an effect that was blockable by naloxone, although naloxone itself also inhibited IL-1 production.

ACTH and $\beta$-endorphin also are produced and released from cells of the immune system. Human peripheral blood lymphocytes stimulated with LPS, or infected with Newcastle disease virus and unstimulated MAC-1 + murine macrophages, can produce mRNA for ACTH and immunoreactive ACTH (257–261). These findings raise the possibility that localized release of ACTH into the lymphoid tissue may mediate interaction between cells of the immune system at this site. Production of ACTH from these lymphoid cells may be regulated in a similar fashion to pituitary-derived ACTH, since Blalock and colleagues (232) showed that the production and release of ACTH by unstimulated human peripheral blood lymphocytes could be stimulated by CRH and inhibited by dexamethasone.

### 4.4.3 Glucocorticoids (GC)

Possible mechanisms of GC-induced immunosuppression include lysis of lymphocytes, inhibition of lymphocyte function, or changes in lymphocyte distribution (262). However, this depends on species, lymphoid target cell, state of lymphocyte maturation and activation; and location of the lymphocyte population involved (reviewed in refs 263, 264). Increasing plasma GC concentration was correlated with a decrease in splenic weight, a decline in the number of nucleate cells in lymphoid organs, and a lower baseline of Ig-secreting cells (265). Thymic involution and a reduction in the numbers of lymphocytes in the thymus, spleen, and peripheral blood resulted from exogenous administration of GC, particularly at supraphysiological concentrations (262). GC-induced cell death particularly targeted immature T-cells in the thymic cortex, and follicular B-cells, while sparing mature (medullary) T-cells and activated B-cells (266). Infusion of prednisolone redistributed circulating thoracic duct lymphocytes from the blood to the bone marrow, decreased cellular localization of lymph nodes, and impaired lymphocyte crossing of high endothelial venules which is a route of egress into secondary lymphoid sites (267). Dexamethasone decreased lymphocyte outflow from sheep popliteal lymph nodes (268). These findings indicate that GC promote cell death in a small population of T- and B-cells, and induce alterations in lymphocyte circulation and migration through lymphoid tissues.

GC suppressed mitogen- and alloantigen-stimulated T-lymphocyte proliferation *in vitro* (269–271), and inhibited IL-1 production by macrophages (272). Several investigators demonstrated that GC reduced IL-2 production while enhancing IL-4 production from activated T-lymphocytes, both *in vivo* and *in vitro* (273–275). GC have differential effects on T-lymphocyte function depending on the presence of macrophages. When lymphocytes were co-cultured with macrophages, T-helper cell function was protected from GC-mediated suppression (276). Bertoglio and Leroux (277) reported that GC augmented or suppressed [³H]-thymidine incorporation by antigen-specific T-cell clones depending on the proliferative stimulus, and the presence of growth factors such as IL-2 or IL-4. Under certain conditions, GC also potentiated human B-cell differentiation *in vitro* (278, 279). GC effects on macrophage production of cytokines, and on lymphocyte proliferation appear to be mediated through binding with cytoplasmic GC receptors in T- and B-cells and macrophages, indicating that the complex immunosuppressive effects of GC *in vivo* are not mediated solely through cell death and lymphopenia.

The effects of GC on immune function *in vivo* also may be influenced by another product of the adrenal gland, dehydroepiandrosterone (280). Dehydroepiandrosterone is an intermediary metabolite formed in the synthesis of testosterone and oestradiol, and is produced in response to ACTH. This adrenal steroid hormone blocked GC-induced suppression of IL-2 production *in vivo*.

### 4.5 TSH AND THE THYROID HORMONES

Like ACTH, TSH can exert direct effects on the immune system, or act indirectly through TSH-stimulated release of the thyroid hormones, $T_3$ and $T_4$ (thyroxine) from the thyroid gland. In the presence of physiological (nanomolar) concentrations of highly purified TSH *in vitro*, antibody responses by murine splenocytes to both T-dependent and T-independent antigens were enhanced (281, 282). This TSH-mediated potentiation required suboptimal culture conditions (no 2-mercaptoethanol and low concentrations of antigen). In a subsequent study, thyroid releasing hormone (TRH), but not other releasing factors, was shown to stimulate TSH mRNA and immunoreactive TSH production by murine lymphocytes (283). TRH in picomolar concentrations also enhanced antibody production to a T-independent antigen *in vitro*; an effect blocked by anti-TSH antibody. These results suggest that endogenous production of TSH is regulated in a manner similar to pituitary-derived TSH, and that lymphocyte-derived TSH has immunological activity that is an enhancement of murine antibody responses. A human T-lymphoma cell line, MOLT-4, has also been demonstrated to produce immunoreactive TSH, similar in subunit structure, molecular weight, and antigenicity to pituitary-derived TSH (284). Regulation of immunoreactive TSH release by MOLT-4 cells was induced by TRH and inhibited by $T_3$ (triiodothyronine), a regulatory mechanism similar to that of pituitary-derived TSH. TSH receptors have been recently reported on several B-cell lines and LPS-stimulated B-cells (285).

Effects of $T_3$ and $T_4$ (thyroxine) on immune functions were apparent following thyroidectomy. Thyroidectomy in neonatal and adult rats, or thiouracil-induced hypothyroidism in chickens, decreased lymphoid organ weight, reduced numbers of circulating lymphocytes, diminished antibody responses, and decreased mitogen-induced proliferative responses (286–288). $T_3$ and $T_4$ replacement in thyroidectomized animals reversed these effects. In euthyroid animals, $T_3$ or $T_4$ administration enhanced antibody and mitogen responses (286, 287). Administration of $T_4$ to aged mice restored NK cell activity to levels observed in young mice, but had no effect in young mice (289). $T_4$ had no effect on NK cell activity *in vitro*, even in the presence of such NK stimulants as IL-2 or IFNγ. Thus, restoration of immune activity with $T_3$ and $T_4$ may have been achieved indirectly through interaction with non-lymphoid cells.

## 4.6 GONADAL STEROIDS

Several lines of evidence implicate the sex steroids as important regulatory hormones of the immune system (reviewed in refs. 290, 291). It is well documented that sexual dimorphism exists within the immune system. Females have higher levels of serum IgG, $IgG_1$, IgM, and IgA than males in several species (292). Antibody responses to T-independent and T-dependent antigens are greater in magnitude and longer lasting in females than in males (293, 294). Furthermore, a higher incidence of autoimmune diseases, such as systemic lupus erythrematosus (SLE), rheumatoid arthritis, and autoallergic thyroiditis occurs in females (295, 296). Studies of immunoresponsiveness during pregnancy suggest that humoral immunity is enhanced and cell-mediated immunity is depressed.

### 4.6.1 Oestrogen

Oestrogen receptors have been demonstrated on human and rodent thymocytes (297–303), rodent peritoneal macrophages (304), chick bursa (305), and rodent and human suppressor/cytotoxic T-cells (306, 307). Through interaction with these receptors oestrogen influences cellular and humoral mediated immune functions, as well as reticuloendothelial activity.

The oestrogenic hormones, in general, are the most potent stimulators of reticuloendothelial cell activity. While testosterone had little or no effect on the rate of phagocytosis of circulating colloidal carbon injected into mice, oestrogen promoted phagocytosis and clearance (308). During the oestrous cycle of female rodents, there appears to be peak periods of reticuloendothelial activity during the follicular phase of the cycle and during the luteal phase when endometrial degeneration occurs (309). Similarly, during pregnancy two peak periods of phagocytic activity were observed, one at the time of implantation and the other approaching the end of pregnancy, prior to parturition. After ovariectomy, reticuloendothelial cell activity declines. Interaction of oestrogen with its receptor on macrophages results in the production of a number of proteins, including IL-1 and IL-6 (310). Oestradiol also increases the number of myelomonocytic colonies developing from stem cells *in vitro*, a possible explanation for the elevation in monocyte numbers found in pregnancy and in the luteal phase of the menstrual cycle (311).

Gonadal steroids have also been shown to effect cell mediated immune responses. One of the earliest reported influences of sex hormones on the immune system was the observation that gonadectomy induced thymic hyper-trophy, particularly in female animals (294, 312–316). Administration of exogenous steroids can reverse this effect. Stimson and Crilly (317) demon-strated that oestrogen, at physiological concentrations, can elicit secretion of thymic hormones from cultured thymic epithelial cells. High doses of oestrogen suppress DNA synthesis in the thymus and in thymic-dependent tissues (313, 318), and possibly, in high enough doses, may be thymolytic. These thymolytic effects are independent of adrenal function since oestrogen-induced thymic involution occurs in the absence of an adrenal gland (319).

The effects of oestrogen upon mitogenic activity and normal functioning of cellular immunity are similar to those of corticosteroids. Oestrogen in low concentrations simulates mitosis in immunocompetent cells, but at high con-centrations is inhibitory (320). Administration of oestrogen at high concentra-tions decreased mitogen induced proliferation of peripheral blood lymphocytes and blocked DNA synthesis in T-lymphocytes (319–322).

Oestrogen appears to have differential effects on the onset and progression of autoimmune-linked disorders. The patients with SLE disorders in steroid metabolism have increased 16α-hydroxyoestrone; a strongly oestrogenic agent which may act to inhibit suppressor cell activity and consequent autoantibody production in a similar way to oestradiol in SLE. This hypothesis is supported by the higher incidence and increased severity of SLE under conditions of elevated oestrogen; that is during the luteal phase of the menstrual cycle (323). However, oral contraceptives have not been convincingly demonstrated to precipitate or potentiate SLE symptoms (324–328). Tamoxifen, a competitive oestrogen antagonist, was not shown to be beneficial for patients with SLE in clinical trials (329), while cytoproterone acetate, an antigonadotrophic agent, apparently reduced the severity of the disease and plasma oestradiol levels (but not testosterone concentration), suggesting a possible role for oestrogen in the attenuation of SLE.

In contrast to SLE, rheumatoid arthritis in women is often less severe during periods of elevated circulating oestrogen content, including pregnancy (330), the luteal phase of the menstrual cycle (331, 332), and, in some cases, during the use of oral contraceptives (333). The discrepancy in the role of oestrogen in the precipitation and progression of autoimmune diseases may result from important differences in the triggering phase of a disease compared to the chronic phase. For example, humoral immunity may play a more important role in the development of SLE, while cell-mediated immunity may be more important in the development of rheumatoid arthritis. There is some evidence in the literature to support this notion. Oestrogen inhibits secretion of rheumatoid factor from polyclonal activated splenocytes *in vitro*, possibly through interaction with receptors on suppressor cytotoxic T-cells (334).

High doses of oestrogen have also been observed to retard rejection of skin grafts (335, 336) and inhibit DTH. Chronic administration of oestrogen results in decreased NK cell activity in splenocyte cultures from both male and female mice (337). Removal of the ovaries of female mice and the testes of male mice, however, does not alter NK cell activity. Administration of a single dose of oestradiol (2.5 µg) from 1 day prior to antigen challenge until 3.5 days after the challenge increased splenic PFC (320). This effect presumably is mediated, at least in part, by a direct effect on lymphocytes, since oestrogen effects are seen as late as 3.5 days after challenge (and antigen processing and presentation to lymphocytes). Furthermore, application of physiological concentrations of oestrogen *in vitro* alters proliferation of antibody-secreting cells after antigen processing.

Oestrogen elevates serum immunoglobulin concentrations (320, 338, 339) and IgA and IgG content in rat uterine tissue during phases of the oestrous cycle (that is proestrus) when oestrogen is maximal (340). Oestrogen-induced increases in serum Ig levels result from an inhibition of Ig decay (341). Elevation of immunoglobulin content in uterine tissue does not occur with administration of other steroids, including progesterone, cortisol, and dihydrotestosterone. Suppressive effects of oestrogen on immunoglobulin production have been reported, an effect that appears to be mediated by the thymus (342, 343).

### 4.6.2  Androgens

Administration of testosterone can enhance the susceptibility to infection (344), reduce skin test reactivity to *Candida albicans* of passively transferred lymphocytes (345), inhibit the development and/or retard progression of some autoimmune-related diseases, such as autoallergic thyroiditis in males, adjuvant-induced arthritis (346), and SLE in (NZB X NZW)F1 mice (NZBW). The attenuating effects of androgens on the development of autoimmune disease in NZBW mice is, at least in part, dependent on the presence of the thymus (347).

Testosterone contributes to the thymic atrophy that occurs at puberty. The enhancing effect of androgens on cortical thymocyte cell loss associated with thymic atrophy may involve interactions of testosterone with androgen receptors on thymic epithelium (348–351), possibly through the stimulated release of immunoregulatory factors from these cells. Androgen receptors have yet to be demonstrated on lymphocytes. Sullivan and Wira (231) have reported androgen receptors in the Bursa of Fabricius. In this organ, androgens may reduce stem cell differentiation toward the B-cell lineage (352, 353).

At physiological concentrations, androgen stimulates the production of thymic hormones from the thymic epithelium (317, 354) which are possibly involved in maturation and differentiation of lymphocytes *in vivo*. Additionally, studies examining the effects of supernatants from thymic epithelial culture on immune cell activity *in vitro* suggest that products produced by these cells also modulate the functions of mature lymphocytes (317).

### 4.6.3   Progestogens

Progesterone, at the physiological concentrations achieved during pregnancy, inhibited mitogen-induced proliferation of T-lymphocytes (355–357), suppressed mixed leukocyte reaction (358), enhanced suppressor T-cell activity (359), and had little or no effect on secretion of thymic hormones from the thymic epithelium (317) or on thymic involution (317). IL-2 was shown by Scambia and colleagues to reverse the effects of progesterone on mitogen-induced T-cell proliferation. Administration of progesterone improved skin graft survival in rodents (360, 361). In breast cancer patients treated with methoxyprogesterone acetate, a synthetic progestogen, the number of circulating CD4+ cells in the peripheral blood was reduced, perhaps resulting from interaction of this drug with GC receptors.

Kaiser *et al.* (362) have suggested that some of progesterone's effects are mediated through interaction with GC receptors present on thymocytes. Strahle and colleague (243) have shown that both GC receptors and progesterone receptors bind to the same elements within DNA. High affinity receptors specific for progesterone have been demonstrated in the rat thymic epithelium (240, 241). Chick bursa (239) and thymus (236) also possess progesterone receptors.

### 4.7   MELATONIN

The pineal gland modulates immune response through its circadian synthesis and release of melatonin. Mice raised for 3–4 generations under constant lighting conditions, inhibiting the dark-dependent synthesis of melatonin (235), resulted in cellular depletion of the thymic cortex, atrophy of the splenic red and white pulp, and inability to mount humoral immune responses to T-dependent antigens (231). Pharmacological intervention to block the synthesis of melatonin reduced the antibody response to SRBC and lowered the autologous mixed-lymphocyte reaction, whilst leaving transplantation immunity unaffected (231). These effects were reversible by exogenous administration of melatonin. Similar findings were observed in surgically pinealectomized animals (230).

Exogenous administration of melatonin in the evening, but not the morning, enhanced the primary antibody response to SRBC as measured in a PFC assay (226, 227), but had no effect on the primary antibody response to T-independent antigens (224). Melatonin treatment in mice at the time of primary antigenic challenge did not alter the CTL response to vaccinia virus or SRBC. However, upon re-expose to the antigen, the secondary response was significantly higher than in saline-treated control mice (224, 363). Exposure of various strains of mice to melatonin at a range of concentrations and for various periods of time had no significant effect on NK cell activity or natural CTL activity. These findings suggest that the immuno-enhancing effect of melatonin in normal mice is dependent on the presence of T-dependent antigens.

Maestroni and colleagues (363) have suggested that melatonin plays a role in preparing the animal to better handle environmental stressors. Thymic atrophy and immunosuppression of secondary antibody response to T-dependent antigen induced by administration of GC or acute restraint stress was blocked by administration of melatonin (1 μg/mouse/day) (221). These effects of melatonin appear not to directly antagonize the effects of GC. The mechanisms through which melatonin exerts its effect on immune responses is not entirely clear. Maestroni and co-workers have evidence to suggest that it may involve the stimulated release of opioid peptides by activated immuno-competent cells and/or that melatonin may influence the binding affinity of opioid receptors for their ligand.

Several investigators have reported the presence of opioid receptors on murine and human activated lymphocytes, and that these cells are capable of synthesizing opioid peptides (126, 163, 364). Furthermore, Maestroni and Conti (363) have shown that physiological concentrations of melatonin stimulate activated T-helper lymphocytes to synthesize and release opioid peptides, which in turn can enhance the immune response in normal mice, counteract the effects of acute stress, and selectively displace radiolabelled-naloxone from mouse brain membrane preparations.

# 5   Summary and conclusions: implications and neural–immune interactions in health and illness

This chapter has summarized the rapidly emerging literature supporting bidirectional communication between the nervous and immune systems. We have only just begun to identify the signal molecules involved, routes of communication, and mechanisms of interactions which link these parts of the body. Future research is needed to elucidate fully the mechanisms of interaction between these systems under normal physiological conditions across the lifespan of an individual, and during stressful life events and disease states. Based on the literature reviewed in this chapter, clearly both the nervous and immune systems are altered in the development and course of many pathological conditions. Future research should be directed towards identifying the neural–immune and/or immune–neural signalling involved in the aetiology of specific disease states, and contributing factors that are important in increasing and decreasing susceptibility of the host to these diseases. These questions will only be answered through an integrative approach involving behavioural, pharmacological, neurological, and immunological hypothesis testing. Through this multidisciplinary research effort, we anticipate the development of novel multifaceted and individualized therapeutic interventions prophylactically for the prevention of illness and for the treatment of such diseases as cancer and autoimmune disorders.

# 6   References

1.  Felten, D. L., Cohen, N., Ader, R., Felten, S. Y., Carlson, S. L., and Roszman, T. L. (1991). Central neural circuits involved in neural–immune interactions. In *Psychoneuroimmunology*, (2nd edn), (eds R. Ader, D. L. Felten, and N. Cohen), pp. 1–26. Academic Press, New York.
2.  Brooks, W. H., Cross, R. J., Roszman, T. L., and Markesbery, W. R. (1982). Neuroimmunomodulation: Neural anatomical basis for impairment and facilitation. *Ann. Neurol.*, **12**, 56–61.
3.  Katayama, M., Kobayashi, S., Kuramoto, N., and Yokoyama, M. M. (1987). Effects of hypothalamic lesions on lymphocyte subsets in mice. *Ann. N. Y. Acad. Sci.*, **496**, 366–376.
4.  Cross, R. J., Markesbery, W. R., Brooks, W. H., and Roszman, T. L. (1980). Hypothalamic–immune interactions. I. The acute effect of anterior hypothalamic lesions on the immune response. *Brain Res.*, **196**, 79–87.
5.  Cross, R. J., Brooks, W. H., Roszman, T. L., and Markesbery, W. R. (1982). Hypothalamic–immune interactions. Effect of hypophysectomy on neuroimmunomodulation. *J. Neurol. Sci.*, **53**, 557–566.
6.  Roszman, T. L., Cross, R. J., Brooks, W. H., and Markesbery, W. R. (1982). Hypothalamic–immune interactions II. The effect of hypothalamic lesions on the ability of adherent spleen cells to limit lymphocyte blastogenesis. *Immunol.*, **45**, 737–742.
7.  Cross, R. J., Markesbery, W. R., Brooks, W. H., and Roszman, T. L. (1984). Hypothalamic–immune interactions: Neuromodulation of natural killer activity by lesioning of the anterior hypothalamus. *Immunol.*, **51**, 399–405.
8.  Cross, R. J., Brooks, W. H., Roszman, T. L., and Markesbery, W. R. (1984). Neuromodulation of lymphocyte reactivity in aged rats. *Neurobiol. Aging*, **5**, 89–92.
9.  Tyrey, L. and Nalbandov, A. V. (1972). Influence of anterior hypothalamic lesions on circulating antibody titers in the rat. *Am. J. Physiol.*, **222**, 179–185.
10. Sobue, H., Minagawa, M., Inoue, K., Ueki, K., Tanaka, R., and Aoki, T. (1981). Immune response influencing regions in the rat hypothalamus. In

*Manipulation of Host Defense Mechanisms*, (eds T. Aoki, I. Urushizaki, and E. Tsubura). Excerpta Medica, New York.

11. Stein, M., Schleiffer, S. J., and Keller, S. E. (1981). Hypothalamic influences on immune responses. In *Psychoneuroimmunology*, (ed. R. Ader), pp. 429–447. Academic Press, New York.

12. Dann, J. A., Wachtel, S. S., and Rubin, A. L. (1979). Possible involvement of the central nervous system in graft rejection. *Transplantation*, **27**, 223–226.

13. Korneva, E. A., Klimenko, V. M., and Shkhinek, E. K. (1985). *Neurohumoral Maintenance of Immune Homeostasis*. University of Chicago Press, Chicago.

14. Besedovsky, H., Sorkin, E., Felix, D., and Haas, H. (1977). Hypothalamic changes during the immune response. *Eur. J. Immunol.*, **7**, 323–325.

15. Nance, D. M., Rayson, D., and Carr, R. I. (1987). The effects of lesions in the lateral septal and hippocampal areas on the humoral immune response of adult female rats. *Brain Behav. Immun.*, **1**, 292–305.

16. Masek, K., Kadlecova, O., and Petrovicky, P. (1983). The effect of brain stem lesions on the immune response. In *Advances in Immunopharmacology*, (eds J. W. Hadden, L. Chedid, P. Dukor, F. Spreafico and D. Willoughby), pp. 443–450. Pergamon Press, New York.

17. Isakovic, K. and Jankovic, B. D. (1973). Neuro-endocrine correlates of immune response. II. Changes in the lymphatic organs of brain-lesioned rats. *Int. Arch Allergy*, **45**, 373–384.

18. Cross, R. J., Brooks, W. H., and Roszman, T. L. (1987). Modulation of T-suppressor cell activity by central nervous system catecholamine depletion. *J. Neurosci. Res.*, **18**, 75–81.

19. Besedovsky, H. O., del Rey, A., Sorkin, E., Da Prada, M., Burri, R., and Honegger, C. (1983). The immune response evokes changes in brain noradrenergic neurons. *Science*, **221**, 564–565.

20. Dunn, A. J. (1988). Systemic interleukin-1 administration stimulates hypothalamic norepinephrine metabolism paralleling the increased plasma corticosterone. *Life Sci.*, **43**, 429–435.

21. Kahiersh, A., del Rey, A., Honegger, G., and Besedovsky, H. D. (1988). Interleukin-1 induces changes in norepinephrine metabolism in the rat brain. *Brain Behav. Immun.*, **2**, 267–274.

22. Besedovsky, H. O., Sorkin, E., Keller, M., and Müller, J. (1975). Changes in blood hormone levels during the immune response. *Proc. Soc. Exp. Biol. Med.*, **150**, 466–470.

23. Kadlecova, O., Masek, K., Seifert, J., and Petrovicky, P. (1987). The involvement of some brain structures in the effects of immunomodulators. *Ann. N. Y. Acad. Sci.*, **496**, 394–398.

24. Renoux, G., Biziere, K., Renoux, M., Bardos, P., and Degenne, D. (1987). Consequences of bilateral brain neocortical ablation on imuthiol-induced immunostimulation in mice. *Ann. N. Y. Acad. Sci.*, **496**, 346–353.

25. Renoux, G., Biziere, K., Renoux, M., Guillaumin, J. M., and Degenne, D. (1983). A balanced brain asymmetry modulates T cell-mediated events. *J. Neuroimmunol.*, **5**, 227–238.

26. Renoux, G., Renoux, M., Biziere, K., Guillaumin, J. M., Bardos, P., and Degenne, D. (1984). Involvement of brain neocortex and liver in the regulation

of T-cells: The mode of action of sodium diethyldithiocarbamate (Imuthiol). *Immunopharm.*, **7**, 89–100.

27.  Recnoux, G. and Biziere, K. (1991). Neocortex lateralization of immune function and of the activities of imuthiol, a T-cell specific immunopotentiator. In *Psychoneuroimmunology*, (2nd ed), (eds R. Ader, D. L. Felten, and N. Cohen), pp. 127–147. Academic Press, New York.

28.  Newlands, G. F. J., Huntley, J. F., and Miller, H. R. P. (1984). Concomitant detection of mucosal mast cells and eosinophils in the intestines of normal and Nippostrongylus-immune rats. A re-evaluation of histochemical and immunocytochemical techniques. *Histochemistry*, **81**, 585–589.

29.  Ackerman, K. D., Felten, S. Y., Bellinger, D. L., and Felten, D. L. (1987). Noradrenergic sympathetic innervation of the spleen: III. Development of innervation in the rat spleen. *J. Neurosci. Res.*, **18**, 49–54.

30.  Felten, S. Y. and Felten, D. L. (1991). The innervation of lymphoid organs. In *Psychoneuroimmunology*, (2nd edn), (eds R. Ader, D. L. Felten, and N. Cohen), pp. 27–69. Academic Press, New York.

31.  Ackerman, K. D., Bellinger, D. L., Felten, S. Y., and Felten, D. L. (1991). Ontogeny and senescence of noradrenergic innervation of the rodent thymus and spleen. In *Psychoneuroimmunology*, (2nd edn), (eds. R. Ader, D. L. Felten, and N. Cohen), pp. 72–125. Academic Press, New York.

32.  Ackerman, K. D., Felten, S. Y., Bellinger, D. L., Livnat, S., and Felten, D. L. (1987). Noradrenergic sympathetic innervation of spleen and lymph nodes in relation to specific cellular compartments. *Prog. Immunol.*, **6**, 588–600.

33.  Ackerman, K. D., Felten, S. Y., Dijkstra, C. D., Livnat, S., and Felten, D. L. (1989). Parallel development of noradrenergic innervation and cellular compartmentation in the rat spleen. *Exp. Neurol.*, **103**, 239–255.

34.  Bellinger, D. L., Felten, S. Y., Collier, T. J., and Felten, D. L. (1987). Noradrenergic sympathetic innervation of the spleen: IV. Morphometric analysis in adult and aged F344 rats. *J. Neurosci. Res.*, **18**, 55–63.

35.  Bellinger, D. L., Felten, S. Y., Lorton, D., and Felten, D. L. (1989). Origin of noradrenergic innervation of the spleen in rats. *Brain Behav. Immun.*, **3**, 291–311.

36.  Bulloch, K. and Pomerantz, W. (1984). Autonomic nervous system innervation of thymic related lymphoid tissue in wild-type and nude mice. *J. Comp. Neurol.*, **228**, 57–68.

37.  Calvo, W. (1968). The innervation of the bone marrow in laboratory animals. *Am. J. Anat.*, **123**, 315–328.

38.  Calvo, W. and Forteza-Vila, J. (1969). On the development of bone marrow innervation in new-born rats as studied with silver impregnation and electron microscopy. *Am. J. Anat.*, **126**, 355–359.

39.  Felten, D. L., Ackerman, K. D., Wiegand, S. J., and Felten, S. Y. (1987). Noradrenergic sympathetic innervation of the spleen: I. Nerve fibers associate with lymphocytes and macrophages in specific compartments of the splenic white pulp. *J. Neurosci. Res.*, **18**, 28–36.

40.  Felten, D. L., Felten, S. Y., Bellinger, D. L., Carlson, S. L., Ackerman, K. D., Madden, K. S. *et al.* (1987). Noradrenergic sympathetic neural interactions with the immune system: structure and function. *Immunol. Rev.*, **100**, 225–260.

41. Felten, D. L., Felten, S. Y., Carlson, S. L., Olschowka, J. A., and Livnat, S. (1985). Noradrenergic and peptidergic innervation of lymphoid tissue. *J. Immunol.*, **135**, 755s–765s.

42. Felten, D. L., Overhage, J. M., Felten, S. Y., and Schmedtje, J. F. (1981). Noradrenergic sympathetic innervation of lymphoid tissue in the rabbit appendix: further evidence for a link between the nervous and immune systems. *Brain Res. Bull.*, **7**, 595–612.

43. Felten, D. L., Livnat, S., Felten, S. Y., Carlson, S. L., Bellinger, D. L., and Yeh, P. (1984). Sympathetic innervation of lymph nodes in mice. *Brain Res. Bull.*, **13**, 693–699.

44. Felten, S. Y., Bellinger, D. L., Collier, T. J., Coleman, P. D., and Felten, D. L. (1987). Decreased sympathetic innervation of spleen in aged Fischer 344 rats. *Neurobiol. Aging*, **8**, 159–165.

45. Felten, S. Y. and Felten, D. L. (1989). Are lymphocytes targets of noradrenergic innervation? In *Frontiers of Stress Research*, (eds H. Weina, D. Helhammer, R. Murison and I. Florin), pp. 56–71. Hans Huber Publishing, Toronto.

46. Felten, S. Y. and Olschowka, J. A. (1987). Noradrenergic sympathetic innervation of the spleen: II. Tyrosine hydroxylase (TH)-positive nerve terminals form synaptic-like contacts on lymphocytes in the splenic white pulp. *J. Neurosci. Res.*, **18**, 37–48.

47. Giron, L. T., Crutcher, K. A., and Davis, J. N. (1980). Lymph nodes—a possible site for sympathetic neuronal regulation of immune responses. *Ann. Neurol.*, **8**, 520–525.

48. Livnat, S., Felten, S. Y., Carlson, S. L., Bellinger, D. L., and Felten, D. L. (1985). Involvement of peripheral and central catecholamine systems in neural-immune interactions. *J. Neuroimmunol.*, **10**, 5–30.

49. Singh, U. (1984). Sympathetic innervation of fetal mouse thymus. *Eur. J. Immunol.*, **14**, 757–759.

50. Walcott, B. and McLean, J. R. (1985). Catecholamine-containing neurons and lymphoid cells in a lacrimal gland of the pigeon. *Brain Res.*, **328**, 129–137.

51. Williams, J. M. and Felten, D. L. (1981). Sympathetic innervation of murine thymus and spleen: A comparative histofluorescence study. *Anat. Rec.*, **199**, 531–542.

52. Williams, J. M., Peterson, R. G., Shea, P. A., Schmedtje, J. F., Bauer, D. C., and Felten, D. L. (1981). Sympathetic innervation of murine thymus and spleen: Evidence for a functional link between the nervous link between the nervous and immune systems. *Brain Res. Bull.*, **6**, 81–94.

53. Felten, S. Y., Housel, J., and Felten, D. L. (1986). Use of *in vivo* dialysis for evaluation of splenic norepinephrine and serotonin. *Soc. Neurosci. Abstr.*, **12**, 1065.

54. von Euler, U. S. (1946). The presence of a substance with sympathin E properties in spleen extracts. *Acta Physiol. Scand.*, **11**, 168.

55. Bidart, J. M., Motte, Ph., Assicot, M., Bohuon, C., and Bellett, D. (1983). Catechol-O-methyltransferase activity and aminergic binding sites distribution in human peripheral blood lymphocyte subpopulations. *Clin. Immunol. Immunopathol.*, **26**, 1–9.

56. Bishopric, N. H., Cohen, H. J., and Lefkowitz, R. J. (1980). Beta adrenergic receptors in lymphocyte subpopulations. *J. Allergy Clin. Immunol.*, **65**, 29–33.

57. Hadden, J. W., Hadden, E. M., and Middleton, E., Jr. (1970). Lymphocyte blast transformation. I. Demonstration of adrenergic receptors in human peripheral lymphocytes. *Cell. Immunol.*, **1**, 583–595.

58. Landmann, R., Bittiger, H., and Bühler, F. R. (1981). High affinity beta-2-adrenergic receptors in mononuclear leucocytes: Similar density in young and old subjects. *Life Sci.*, **29**, 1761–1771.

59. Landmann, R., Burgisser, E., West, M., and Buhler, F. R. (1985). Beta adrenergic receptors are different in subpopulations of human circulating lymphocytes. *J. Recept. Res.*, **4**, 37–50.

60. Loveland, B. E., Jarrott, B., and McKenzie, I. F. C. (1981). The detection of beta adrenoceptors on murine lymphocytes. *Int. J. Immunopharm.*, **3**, 45–55.

61. Miles, K., Atweh, S., Otten, G., Arnason, B. G. W., and Chelmicka-Schorr, E. (1984). Beta-adrenergic receptors on splenic lymphocytes from axotomized mice. *Int. J. Immunopharm.*, **6**, 171–177.

62. Motulsky, H. J., Cunningham, E. M. S., Deblasi, A., and Insel, P. A. (1986). Desensitization and redistribution of $\beta$-adrenergic receptors on human mononuclear leukocytes. *Am. J. Physiol.*, **250**, E583–E590.

63. Pochet, R., Delespesse, G., Gausset, P. W., and Collet, H. (1979). Distribution of beta-adrenergic receptors on human lymphocyte subpopulations. *Clin. Exp. Immunol.*, **38**, 578–584.

64. Pochet, R. and Delesppesse, G. (1983). $\beta$-Adrenoreceptors display different efficiency on lymphocyte subpopulations. *Biochem. Pharmacol.*, **32**, 1651–1655.

65. Williams, L. T., Snyderman, R., and Lefkowitz, R. J. (1976). Identification of $\beta$-adrenergic receptors in human lymphocytes by [$^3$H]-alprenolol binding. *J. Clin. Invest.*, **57**, 149–155.

66. Hall, N. R., McGillis, J. P., Spangelo, B. L., Henly, D. L., Chrousos, G. P., Schulte, H. M. *et al.* (1985). Thymic hormone effects on the brain and neuroendocrine circuits. In *Neural Modulation of Immunity*, (eds R. Guillemin, M. Cohn, and T. Melnechuk), pp. 179–196. Raven Press, New York.

67. Ernström, U. and Sandberg, G. (1973). Effects of adrenergic alpha- and beta-receptor stimulation on the release of lymphocytes and granulocytes from the spleen. *Scand. J. Haematol.*, **11**, 275–286.

68. Ernström, U. and Sandberg, G. (1974). Stimulation of lymphocyte release from the spleen by theophylline and isoproterenol. *Acta Physiol. Scand.*, **90**, 202–209.

69. Ernström, U. and Söder, O. (1975). Influence of adrenaline on the dissemination of antibody-producing cells from the spleen. *Clin. Exp. Immunol.*, **21**, 131–140.

70. Singh, U. (1979). Effect of catecholamines on lymphopoiesis in fetal mouse thymic explants. *Eur. J. Immunol.*, **14**, 757–759.

71. Singh, U. and Owen, J. J. T. (1976). Studies on the maturation of thymus stem cells. The effects of catecholamines, histamine, and peptide hormones on the expression of T alloantigens. *Eur. J. Immunol.*, **6**, 59–62.

72. Webber, R. H., DeFelice, R., Ferguson, R. J., and Powell, J. P. (1970). Bone marrow response to stimulation of the sympathetic trunks in rats. *Acta Anat.*, **77**, 92–97.

73. Titinchi, S. and Clark, B. (1984). Alpha$_2$-adrenoceptors in human lymphocytes: Direct characterization by [$^3$3H]yohimbine binding. *Biochem. Biophys. Res. Commun.*, **121**, 1–7.

74. Spengler, R. N., Allen, R. M., Remick, D. G., Strieter, R. M., and Kunkel, S. L. (1990). Stimulation of alpha-adrenergic receptor augments the production of macrophage-derived tumor necrosis factor. *J. Immunol.*, **145**, 1430–1434.

75. Besedovsky, H. O., del Rey, A., Sorkin, E., Da Prada, M., and Keller, H. H. (1979). Immunoregulation mediated by the sympathetic nervous system. *Cell. Immunol.*, **48**, 346–355.

76. Hall, N. R., McClure, J. E., Hu, S.-K., Tare, N. S., Seals, C. M., and Goldstein, A. L. (1982). Effects of 6-hydroxydopamine upon primary and secondary thymus dependent immune responses. *Immunopharm.*, **5**, 39–48.

77. Kasahara, K., Tanaka, S., Ito, R., and Hamashima, Y. (1977). Suppression of the primary immune response by chemical sympathectomy. *Res. Commun. Chem. Pthl. Pharmacol.*, **16**, 687–694.

78. Goodwin, J. S., Messner, R. P., and Williams, R. C., Jr. (1979). Inhibitors of T-cell mitogenesis: Effect of mitogen dose. *Cell. Immunol.*, **45**, 303–308.

79. Johnson, D. L., Ashmore, R. C., and Gordon, M. A. (1981). Effects of beta-adrenergic agents on the murine lymphocyte response to mitogen stimulation. *J. Immunopharmacol.*, **3**, 205–219.

80. Watson, J. (1975). The influence of intracellular levels of cyclic nucleotides on cell proliferation and the induction of antibody synthesis. *J. Exp. Med.*, **141**, 97–111.

81. Beckner, S. K. and Farrar, W. L. (1988). Potentiation of lymphokine-activated killer cells differentiation and lymphocyte proliferation by stimulation of protein kinase C or inhibition of adenylate cyclase. *J. Immunol.*, **140**, 208–214.

82. Strom, T. B., Carpenter, C. B., Garovoy, M. R., Austen, K. F., Merrill, J. P., and Kaliner, M. (1973). The modulating influence of cyclic nucleotides upon lymphocyte-mediated cytotoxicity. *J. Exp. Med.*, **138**, 381–393.

83. Didier, M., Aussel, C., Ferrua, B., and Fehlmann, M. (1987). Regulation of interleukin 2 synthesis by cAMP in human T-cells. *J. Immunol.*, **139**, 1179–1184.

84. Melmon, K. L., Bourne, H. R., Weinstein, Y., Shearer, G. M., Kram, J., and Bauminger, S. (1974). Hemolytic plaque formation by leukocytes *in vitro*. Control by vasoactive hormones. *J. Clin. Invest.*, **53**, 13–21.

85. Watson, J., Epstein, R., and Cohn, M. (1973). Cyclic nucleotides as intracellular mediators of the expression of antigen-sensitive cells. *Nature*, **246**, 405–409.

86. Sanders, V. M. and Munson, A. E. (1984). Beta adrenoceptor mediation of the enhancing effect of norepinephrine on the murine primary antibody response *in vitro*. *J. Pharm. Exp. Ther.*, **230**, 183–192.

87. Sanders, V. M. and Munson, A. E. (1984). Kinetics of the enhancing effect produced by norepinephrine and terbutaline on the murine primary antibody response *in vitro*. *J. Pharm. Exp. Ther.*, **231**, 527–531.

88. Sanders, V. M. and Munson, A. E. (1985). Norepinephrine and the antibody response. *Pharmacol. Rev.*, **37**, 229–248.

89. Koff, W. C. and Dunegan, M. A. (1985). Modulation of macrophage-mediated

tumoricidal activity by neuropeptides and neurohormones. *J. Immunol.*, 135, 350–354.

90.  Koff, W. C. and Dunegan, M. A. (1986). Neuroendocrine hormones suppress macrophage-mediated lysis of herpes simplex virus-infected cells. *J. Immunol.*, 136, 705–709.

91.  Lappin, D. and Whaley, K. (1979). Adrenergic receptors on monocytes modulate complement component synthesis. *J. Histochem. Cytochem.*, 27, 936.

92.  Hellstrand, K., Hermodsson, S., and Strannegård, Ö. (1985). Evidence for a β-adrenoceptor-mediated regulation of human natural killer cells. *J. Immunol.*, 134, 4095–4099.

93.  Katz, P., Zaytoun, A. M., and Fauci, A. S. (1982). Mechanisms of human cell-mediated cytotoxicity. I. Modulation of natural killer cell activity by cyclic nucleotides. *J. Immunol.*, 129, 287–296.

94.  Livnat, S., Eisen, J., Felten, D. L., Felten, S. Y., Irwin, J., Madden, K. S. *et al.* (1988). Behavioural and sympathetic neural modulation of immune function. In *Progress in Catecholamine Research, Part A: Basic Aspects and Peripheral Mechanisms*, (eds A. Dahlstrom, R. M. Belmaker, and M. Sandler), pp. 539–546. Alan R. Liss, New York.

95.  Depelchin, A. and Letesson, J. J. (1981). Adrenaline influence on the immune response. I. Accelerating or suppressor effects according to the time of application. *Immunol. Lett.*, 3, 199–205.

96.  Crary, B., Borysenko, M., Sutherland, D. C., Kutz, I., Borysenko, J. Z., and Benson, H. (1983). Decreases in mitogen responsiveness of mononuclear cells from peripheral blood after epinephrine administration in humans. *J. Immunol.*, 130, 694–697.

97.  Crary, B., Hauser, S. L., Borysenko, M., Kutz, I., Hoban, C., Ault, K. A. *et al.* (1983). Epinephrine-induced changes in the distribution of lymphocyte subsets in peripheral blood of humans. *J. Immunol.*, 131, 1178–1181.

98.  Gader, A. M. A. (1974). The effects of β-adrenergic blockage on the responses of leukocyte counts to intravenous epinephrine in man. *Scand. J. Haematol.*, 13, 11–16.

99.  Livnat, S., Madden, K. S., Felten, D. L., and Felten, S. Y. (1987). Regulation of the immune system by sympathetic neural mechanisms. *Prog. Neuropsychopharmacol. & Biol. Psychiat.*, 11, 145–152.

100.  Madden, K. S. and Livnat, S. (1991). Catecholaminergic influences on immune reactivity. In *Psychoneuroimmunology*, (2nd edn), (eds. R. Ader, D. L. Felten, and N. Cohen), pp. 283–310. Academic Press, New York.

101.  Madden, K. S., Felten, S. Y., Felten, D. L., and Livnat, S. (1989). Sympathetic neural modulation of the immune system. I. Depression of T-cell immunity *in vivo* and *in vitro* following chemical sympathectomy. *Brain Behav. Immun.*, 3, 72–89.

102.  Bellinger, D. L., Earnest, D. J., Gallagher, M., and Felten, D. L. (1992). Presence and availability of VIP in primary and secondary lymphoid organs. *Soc. Neurosci. Abstr.*, 18, 1009.

103.  Lorton, D., Bellinger, D. L., Felten, S. Y., and Felten, D. L. (1989). Substance P (SP) and calcitonin gene-related peptide (CGRP) innervation of the rat spleen. *Soc. Neurosci. Abstr.*, 15, 714.

104. Lorton, D., Bellinger, D. L., Felten, S. Y., and Felten, D. L. (1990). Substance P innervation of the rat thymus. *Peptides*, 11, 1269–1275.

105. Lorton, D., Bellinger, D. L., Felten, S. Y., and Felten, D. L. (1991). Substance P innervation of spleen in rats: nerve fibers associate with lymphocytes and macrophages in specific compartments of the spleen. *Brain Behav. Immun.*, 5, 29–40.

106. Felten, D. L., Bellinger, D. L., and Felten, S. Y. (1989). Age-related alterations in the distribution of neuropeptide Y (NPY)-positive nerve fibers in the rat spleen. *Soc. Neurosci. Abstr.*, 15, 714.

107. Olschowka, J. A., Felten, S. Y., Bellinger, D. L., Lorton, D., and Felten, D. L. (1988). NPY-positive nerve terminals contact lymphocytes in the periarteriolar lymphatic sheath of the rat splenic white pulp. *Soc. Neurosci. Abstr.*, 14, 1280.

108. Romano, T. A., Olschowka, J. A., Felten, S. Y., and Felten, D. L. (1989). Neuropeptide-Y involvement in neural-immune interactions in the rat spleen. *Soc. Neurosci. Abstr.*, 15, 714.

109. O'Dorisio, M. S. (1988). Neuropeptide modulation of the immune response in gut associated lymphoid issue. *Intern. J. Neurosci.*, 38, 189–198.

110. O'Dorisio, M. S., Hermina, N. S., O'Dorisio, T. M., and Balcerzak, S. P. (1981). Vasoactive intestinal polypeptide modulation of lymphocyte adenylate cyclase. *J. Immunol.*, 127, 2551–2554.

111. O'Dorisio, M. S., Wood, C. L., and O'Dorisio, T. M. (1985). Vasoactive intestinal peptide and neuropeptide modulation of the immune response. *J. Immunol.*, 135, 792s–796s.

112. Bellinger, D. L., Lorton, D., Romano, T., Olschowka, J. A., Felten, S. Y., and Felten, D. L. (1990). Neuropeptide innervation of lymphoid organs. *Ann. N. Y. Acad. Sci.*, 594, 17–33.

113. Blalock, J. E., Harbour-McMenamin, D., and Smith, E. M. (1985). Peptide hormones shared by the neuroendocrine and immunologic systems. *J. Immunol.*, 135, 858s–861s.

114. Goetzl, E. J., Turck, C., and Sreedharan, S. (1991). Production and recognition of neuropeptides by cells of the immune system. In *Psychoneuroimmunology*, (2nd edn), (eds R. Ader, D. L. Felten, and Cohen), pp. 263–282. Academic Press, New York.

115. Beed, E. A., O'Dorisio, M. S., O'Dorisio, T. M., and Gaginella, T. S. (1983). Demonstration of a functional receptor for vasoactive intestinal polypeptide on Molt 4b lymphoblasts. *Regulatory Peptides*, 6, 1–12.

116. Hanley, M. R., Lee, C. M., Jones, L. M., and Michel, R. H. (1980). Similar effects of substance P and related peptides on salivation and on phosphatidlinositol turnover in rat salivary glands. *Mol. Pharmacol.*, 18, 78–83.

117. Payan, D. G., McGillis, J. P., and Organist, M. L. (1986). Characterization of the lymphocyte substance P receptor. *J. Biol. Chem.*, 261, 14321–14329.

118. Payan, D. G., Brewster, D. R., and Goetzl, E. J. (1983). Specific stimulation of human T-lymphocytes by substance P. *J. Immunol.*, 131, 1613–1615.

119. Goetzl, E. J., Chernov, T., Renold, F., and Payan, D. G. (1985). Neuropeptide regulation of the expression of immediate hypersensitivity. *J. Immunol.*, 135, 802S–805S.

120. Lopker, A., Abood, L. G., Hoss, W., and Lionetti, F. J. (1980). Stereoselective

muscarinic acetylcholine and opiate receptors in human phagocytic leukocytes. *Biochem. Pharmacol.*, **29**, 1361–1365.

121. Johnson, H. M., Smith, E. M., Torres, B. A., and Blalock, J. E. (1982). Regulation of the *in vitro* antibody response by neuroendocrine hormones. *Proc. Natl. Acad. Sci. (USA)*, **79**, 4171–4174.

122. Mehrishi, J. N. and Mills, I. H. (1983). Opiate receptors on lymphocytes and platelets in man. *Clin. Immunol. Immunopathol.*, **27**, 240–249.

123. Hazum, E., Chang, K.-J., and Cuatrecasas, P. (1979). Specific nonopiate receptors for β-endorphin. *Science*, **205**, 1033–1035.

124. Ansiello, C. M. and Roda, L. G. (1984). Leu-enkephalin binding to cultured human T-lymphocytes. *Cell Biol. Int. Rep.*, **8**, 353–362.

125. Schweigerer, L., Schmidt, W., Teschemacher, H., and Gramsch, C. (1985). β-Endorphin: Surface binding and internalization in thymoma cells. *Proc. Natl. Acad. Sci. (USA)*, **82**, 5751–5755.

126. Falke, N.E. and Fischer, E. G. (1986). Opiate receptor mediated internalization of 125-I-β-End in human polymorphonuclear leukocytes. *Cell Biol. Int. Rep.*, **19**, 429–435.

127. Ottaway, C. A. and Greenberg, G. R. (1984). Interaction of vasoactive intestinal peptide with mouse lymphocytes: Specific binding and the modulation of mitogen responses. *J. Immunol.*, **132**, 417–423.

128. Stanisz, A. M., Befus, D., and Bienenstock, J. (1986). Differential effects of vasoactive intestinal peptide, substance P, and somatostatin on immunoglobulin synthesis and proliferations by lymphocytes from Peyer's patches, mesenteric lymph nodes, and spleen. *J. Immunol.*, **136**, 152–156.

129. Rola-Pleszczynski, M., Bulduc, D., and St. Pierre, A. (1985). The effects of VIP on human NK cell function. *J. Immunol.*, **135**, 2659–2673.

130. Ottaway, C. A. (1984). *In vitro* alteration of receptors for vasoactive intestinal peptide changes the *in vivo* localization of mouse T-cells. *J. Exp. Med.*, **160**, 1054–1069.

131. Ottaway, C. A., Lewis, D. L., and Asa, S. L. (1987). Vasoactive intestinal peptide-containing nerves in Peyer's patches. *Brain Behav. Immun.*, **1**, 148–158.

132. Moore, T. C. (1984). Modification of lymphocyte traffic by vasoactive neurotransmitter substances. *Immunol.*, **52**, 511–518.

133. Moore, T. C. and Lachmann, P. J. (1982). Cyclic AMP reduces and cyclic GMP increases the traffic of lymphocytes through peripheral lymph nodes of sheep *in vivo*. *Immunol.*, **47**, 423–428.

134. Payan, D. G., Levine, J. D., and Goetzl, E. J. (1984). Modulation of immunity and hypersensitivity by sensory neuropeptides. *J. Immunol.*, **132**, 1601–1604.

135. Foreman, J. C. and Jordan, C. C. (1983). Histamine release and vascular changes induced by neuropeptides. *Agents and Actions*, **13**, 105–111.

136. Lofstrom, B., Pernow, B., and Wahren, J. (1985). Vasodilating action of substance P in human forearm. *Acta Physiol. Scand.*, **63**, 311–315.

137. Lundbert, J. M., Saria, A., Brodin, E., Rosell, S., and Folkars, K. (1983). A substance P antagonist inhibits vagally-induced increase in vascular permeability and bronchial smooth muscle contraction in the guinea pig. *Proc. Natl. Acad. Sci. (USA)*, **80**, 1120–1124.

138. Foreman, J. C. and Piotrowski, W. (1984). Peptides and histamine release. *J. Allergy Clin. Immunol.*, **74**, 127–131.

139. Foreman, J. C., Jordan, C. C., and Piotrowski, W. (1982). Interaction of neurotensin with the substance P receptor mediating histamine release from rat mast cells and the flare in human skin. *Br. J. Pharmacol.*, **77**, 531–539.

140. Pawlikowski, M., Stepien, H., Kunert-Radek, J., and Schally, A. V. (1985). Effect of somatostatin on the proliferation of mouse spleen lymphocytes *in vitro*. *Biochem. Biophys. Res. Commun.*, **129**, 52–55.

141. Stanisz, A. M., Scicchitano, R., Payan, D. G., and Bienenstock, J. (1987). *In vitro* studies of immunoregulation of substance P and somatostatin. *Ann. N. Y. Acad. Sci.*, **496**, 217–225.

142. Payan, D. G., Hess, C. A., and Goetzl, E. J. (1984). Inhibition by somatostatin of the proliferation of T-lymphocytes and Molt-4 lymphoblasts. *Cell Immunol.*, **84**, 433–438.

143. Theoharides, T. C. and Douglas, W. W. (1981). Mast cell histamine secretion in response to somatostatin analogues: Structural considerations. *Eur. J. Pharmacol.*, **73**, 131–136.

144. Ruff, M. R., Wahl, S. M., and Pert, C. B. (1985). Substance P receptor-mediated chemotaxis of human monocytes. *Peptides*, **6**, 107–111

145. Bar-Shavit, Z., Goldman, R., Stabinsky, Y., Gottleib, F., Fridkin, M., Teichberg, V., and Blumberg, S. (1980). Enhancement of phagocytosis—a newly found activity of substance P residing in its N-terminal tetrapeptide sequence. *Biochem. Bioshys. Res. Commun.*, **94**, 1445–1451.

146. Hartung, H.-P., Wolfers, K., and Toyka, K. V. (1986). Substance P: Binding properties and studies on cellular responses in guinea pig macrophages. *J. Immunol.*, **136**, 3856–3863.

147. Shanahan, F., Denburg, J. A., Fox, J., Bienenstock, J., and Befus, D. (1985). Mast cell heterogeneity: Effects of neuroenteric peptides on histamine release. *J. Immunol.*, **135**, 1331–1337.

148. Heijnen, C. J., Bevers, C., Kavelaars, A., and Ballieux, R. E. (1986). Effect of alpha-endorphin on the anligen-induced primary antibody response of human blood B-cells *in vitro*. *J. Immunol.*, **136**, 213–216.

149. Gilman, S. C., Schwartz, J. M., Milner, R. J., Bloom, F. E., and Feldman, J. D. (1982). β-Endorphin enhances lymphocyte proliferative responses. *Proc. Natl. Acad. Sci. (USA)*, **79**, 4226–4230.

150. McCain, H. W., Lamster, I. B., Bozzone, J. M., and Grbic, J. T. (1982). β-endorphin modulates human immune activity via non-opiate receptor mechanisms. *Life Sci.*, **31**, 1619–1624.

151. Plotnikoff, N. P. and Miller, G. C. (1983). Enkephalins as immunomodulators. *Int. J. Immunopharm.*, **5**, 437–441.

152. Wybran, J. (1986). Enkephalins as molecules of lymphocyte activation and modifiers of the biological response. In *Enkephalins and Endorphins*, (eds N. P. Plotnikoff, R. E. Faith, A. J. Murgo, and R. A. Good), pp. 253–282. Plenum Press, New York.

153. Wybran, J., Appelboom, T., Famaey, J.-P., and Govaerts, A. (1979). Suggestive evidence for receptors for morphine and methionine-enkephalin on normal human blood T-lymphocytes. *J. Immunol.*, **123**, 1068–1070.

154. Miller, G. C., Murgo, A. J., and Plotnikoff, N. P. (1984). Enkephalins: Enhancement of active T-cell rosettes from normal volunteers. *Clin. Immunol. Immunopathol.*, **31**, 132–137.

155. Mandler, R. N., Biddison, W. E., Mandler, R., and Serrate, S. A. (1986). β-endorphin augments the cytolytic activity and interferon production of natural killer cells. *J. Immunol.*, **136**, 934–939.

156. Brown, S. L. and Van Epps, D. E. (1985). Suppression of T-lymphocyte chemotactic factor production by the opioid peptides β-endorphin and met-enkephalin. *J. Immunol.*, **134**, 3384–3390.

157. Brown, S. L. and Van Epps, D. E. (1986). Opioid peptides modulate production of interferon gamma by human mononuclear cells. *Cell. Immunol.*, **103**, 19–26.

158. Shavit, Y., Lewis, J. W., Terman, G. W., Gale, R. P., and Liebeskind, J. C. (1984). Opioid peptides mediate the suppressive effect of stress on natural killer cell cytotoxicity. *Science*, **223**, 188–190.

159. Kay, N., Allen, J., and Morley, J. E. (1984). Endorphins stimulate normal human peripheral blood lymphocyte natural killer activity. *Life Sci.*, **35**, 53–59.

160. Faith, R. E., Liang, H. J., Murgo, A. J., and Plotnikoff, N. P. (1984). Neuro-immunomodulation with enkephalins: Enhancement of human natural killer (NK) cell activity *in vitro*. *Clin. Immunol. Immunopathol.*, **31**, 412–418.

161. Mathews, P. M., Froelich, C. J., Sibbitt, W. L., Jr., and Bankhurst, A. D. (1983). Enhancement of natural cytotoxicity by β-endorphin. *J. Immunol.*, **130**, 1658–1662.

162. Carr, D. J. J. and Klimpel, G. R. (1986). Enhancement of the generation of cytotoxic T-cells by endogenous opiates. *J. Neuroimmunol.*, **12**, 75–87.

163. Sibinga, N. E. S. and Goldstein, A. (1988). Opioid peptides and opioid receptors in cells of the immune system. *Ann. Rev. Immunol.*, **6**, 219–249.

164. Simpkins, C. O., Dickey, C. A., and Fink, M. P. (1984). Human neutrophil migration is enhanced by beta-endorphin. *Life Sci.*, **34**, 2251–2255.

165. Foris, G., Medgyesi, E., Gyimesi, E., and Hauck, E. (1984). Met-enkephalin induced alterations of macrophage functions. *Mol. Immunol.*, **21**, 747–750.

166. Miller, G. C., Murgo, A. J., and Plotnikoff, N. P. (1982). The influence of leucine and methionine enkephalin on immune mechanisms. *Int. J. Immunopharmacol.*, **4**, 367.

167. Marx, W., Simpson, M. E., Reinhardt, W. O., and Evans, H. M. (1942). Response to growth hormone of hypophysectomized rats when restricted to food intake of controls. *Am. J. Physiol.*, **135**, 614–618.

168. Berczi, I. and Nagy, E. (1991). Effect of hypophysectomy on immune function. In *Psychoneuroimmunology*, (2nd edn), (eds. R. Ader, D. L. Felten, and N. Cohen), pp. 339–375. Academic Press, New York.

169. Fraenkel-Conrat, J. and Li, C. H. (1949). Hormonal effects on the nucleic acid and phospholipid turnover of rat liver and thymus. *Endocrinology*, **44**, 487–491.

170. Li, C. H. and Evans, H. M. (1948). The biochemistry of pituitary growth hormone. In *Recent Progress in Hormone Research*, (ed. G. Pincus), pp. 3–44. Academic Press, New York.

171. Asling, C. W., Reinhardt, W. O., and Li, C. H. (1951). Effects of adreno-corticotropic hormone on body growth, visceral proportions, and white blood cell counts of normal and hypophysectomized male rats. *Endocrinology*, **48**, 534–547.

172. Chatterton, R. T., Jr., Murray, C. L., and Hellman, L. (1973). Endocrine effects on leukocytopoiesis in the rat. I. Evidence for growth hormone secretion as the leukocytopoietic stimulus following acute cortisol-induced lymphopenia. *Endocrinology*, **92**, 755–787.

173. Enerback, L., Lundin, P. M., and Mellgren, J. (1961). Pituitary hormones elaborated during stress. Action on lymphoid tissues, serum proteins and antibody titres. *Acta Pathol. Microbiol. Immunol. Scand., Suppl.*, **144**, 141–144.

174. Feldman, J. D. (1951). Endocrine control of lymphoid tissue. *Anat. Rec.*, **110**, 17–39.

175. Pandian, M. R. and Talwar, G. P. (1971). Effect of growth hormone on the metabolism of thymus and on the immune response against sheep erythrocytes. *J. Exp. Med.*, **134**, 1095–1113.

176. Duquesnoy, R. J., Mariani, T., and Good, R. A. (1969). Effect of hypophysectomy on immunological recovery after sublethal irradiation of adult rats. *Proc. Soc. Exp. Biol. Med.*, **131**, 1076–1178.

177. Gisler, R. H., Bussard, A. E., Mazié, J. C., and Hess, R. (1971). Hormonal regulation of the immune response. I. Induction of an immune response *in vitro* with lymphoid cells from mice exposed to acute systemic stress. *Cell. Immunol.*, **2**, 634–645.

178. Saxena, Q. B., Saxena, R. K., and Adler, W. H. (1982). Regulation of natural killer activity *in vivo*. III. Effect of hypophysectomy and growth hormone treatment on the natural killer activity of the mouse spleen cell population. *Int. Arch. Allergy Appl. Immun.*, **67**, 169–174.

179. Berczi, I. and Nagy, E. (1987). The effect of prolactin and growth hormone on hemolymphopoietic tissue and immune function. In *Hormones and Immunity*, (eds I. Berczi and K. Kovacs), pp. 145–171. MTP Press, Lancaster.

180. Kiess, W., and Butenandt, O. (1985). Specific growth hormone receptors on human peripheral mononuclear cells: Reexpression, identification, and characterization. *J. Clin. Endocrinol. Metab.*, **60**, 740–746.

181. Desai, L. S., Lazarus, H., Li, C. H., and Foley, G. E. (1973). Human leukemic cells: Effects of human growth hormone. *Exp. Cell. Res.*, **81**, 330–332.

182. Mercola, K. E., Cline, M. J., and Colde, D. W. (1981). Growth hormone stimulation of normal and leukemic human T-lymphocyte proliferation *in vitro*. *Blood*, **58**, 337–340.

183. Rogers, P. C., Komp, D., Rogol, A., and Sabio, H. (1977). Possible effects of growth hormone on development of acute lymphoblastic leukemia. *Lancet*, **2**, 434–435.

184. Astaldi, A., Jr., Yalcin, B., Meardi, G., Burgio, G. R., Merolla, R., and Astaldi, G. (1973). Effects of growth hormone on lymphocyte transformation in cell culture. *Blut*, **26**, 74–81.

185. Kiess, W., Holtmann, H., Butenandt, O., and Eife, R. (1983). Modulation of lymphoproliferation by human growth hormone. *Eur. J. Pediatr.*, **140**, 47–50.

186. Rapaport, R., Oleske, J., Adhieh, H., Skuza, K., Holland, B. K., Passannante, M. R. *et al.* (1987). Effects of human growth hormone on immune functions: In vitro studies on cells of normal and growth hormone-deficient children. *Life Sci.*, **41**, 2319–2324.

187. Vanderschueren-Lodeweyckx, M., Staf, B., Van Den Berghe, H., Eggermont, E., and Eeckels, R. (1973). Growth hormone and lymphocyte transformation. *Lancet*, **1**, 441.

188. Davila, D. R., Brief, S., Simon, J., Hammer, R. E., Brinster, R. L., and Kelley, K. W. (1987). Role of growth hormone in regulating T-dependent immune events in aged, nude, and transgenic rodents. *J. Neurosci. Res.*, **18**, 108–116.

189. Abbassi, V. and Bellanti, J. A. (1985). Humoral and cell-mediated immunity in growth hormone-deficient children: Effect of therapy with human growth hormone. *Pediat. Res.*, **19**, 299–301.

190. Baroni, C. D., Fabris, N., and Bertoli, G. (1969). Effects of hormones on development and function of lymphoid tissues. Synergistic action of thyroxin and somatotrophic hormone in pituitary dwarf mice. *Immunol.*, **17**, 303–314.

191. Comsa, J., Leonhardt, H., and Schwarz, J. A. (1975). Influence of the thymus-corticotropin-growth hormone interaction on the rejection of skin allografts in the rat. *Ann. N. Y. Acad. Sci.*, **249**, 387–401.

192. Comsa, J., Schwarz, J. A., and Neu, H. (1974). Interaction between thymic hormone and hypophyseal growth hormone on production of precipitating antibodies in the rat. *Immunol. Commun.*, **3**, 11–18.

193. Fabris, N., Pierpaoli, W., and Sorkin, E. (1971). Hormones and the immunological capacity. IV. Restorative effects of developmental hormones or of lymphocytes on the immunodeficiency syndrome of the dwarf mouse. *Clin. Exp. Immunol.*, **9**, 227–240.

194. Fabris, N., Pierpaoli, W., and Sorkin, E. (1971). Hormones and the immunological capacity. III. The immunodeficiency disease of the hypopituitary Snell-Bagg dwarf mouse. *Clin. Exp. Immunol.*, **9**, 209–225.

195. Marsh, J. A., Gause, W. C., Sandhu, S., and Scanes, C. G. (1984). Enhanced growth and immune development in dwarf chickens treated with mammalian growth hormone and thyroxine. *Proc. Soc. Exp. Biol. Med.*, **175**, 351–360.

196. Nagy, E., Berczi, I., and Friesen, H. G. (1983). Regulation of immunity in rats by lactogenic and growth hormones. *Acta Endocrinol.*, **102**, 351–357.

197. Nagy, E., Friesen, H. G., Sehon, A. H., and Berczi, I. (1985). Immunomodulation in rats by transplantable anterior pituitary tumors. *Endocrinology*, **116**, 1117–1122.

198. Crist, D. M., Peake, G. T., MacKinnon, L. T., Sibbit, W. L., Jr., and Kraner, J. C. (1987). Exogenous growth hormone treatment alters body composition and increases natural killer cell activity in women with impaired endogenous growth hormone secretion. *Metabolism*, **36**, 1115–1117.

199. Merchav, S., Tatarsky, I., and Hochberg, Z. (1988). Enhancement of human granulopoiesis in vitro by biosynthetic insulin-like growth factor I/somatomedin C and human growth hormone. *J. Clin. Invest.*, **81**, 791–797.

200. Nielsch, U. and Keen, P. (1987). Effects of neonatal 6-hydroxydopamine administration on different substance P-sensory neurones. *Eur. J. Pharmacol.*, **138**, 193–197.

201. Edwards, C. K., III, Ghiasuddin, S. M., Schepper, J. M., Yunger, L. M., and Kelley, K. W. (1988). A newly defined property of somatotropin: Priming of macrophages for production of superoxide anion. *Science*, **239**, 769–771.

202. Bunner, D. L., Morris, E., and Smallridge, R. C. (1984). Circadian growth hormone and prolactin blood concentration during a self-limited viral infection and artificial hyperthermia in man. *Metabolism*, **33**, 337–341.

203. Frohman, L. A., Horton, E. S., and Lebovitz, H. E. (1967). Growth hormone releasing action of a Pseudomonas endotoxin (Piromen). *Metabolism*, **16**, 57–67.

204. Besedovsky, H., del Rey, A. E., Sorkin, E., and Dinarello, C. A. (1986). Immunoregulatory feedback between interleukin-1 and glucocorticoid hormones. *Science*, **233**, 652–654.

205. Beutler, B. and Cerami, A. (1988). Cachetin (tumor necrosis factor): A macrophage hormone governing cellular metabolism and inflammatory response. *Endocrin. Rev.*, **9**, 57–66.

206. Dinarello, C. A. (1988). Biology of interleukin 1. *FASEB J.*, **2**, 108–115.

207. Lorence, R. M., Rood, P. A., and Kelley, K. W. (1988). Newcastle disease virus as an antineoplastic agent: Induction of tumor necrosis factor-a and augmentation of its cytotoxicity. *J. Natl. Cancer Inst.*, **80**, 1305–1312.

208. Kasting, N. W. and Martin, J. B. (1982). Altered release of growth hormone and thyrotropin induced by endotoxin in the rat. *Am. J. Physiol.*, **243**, 332–337.

209. Valsamakis, A., Riviere, Y., and Oldstone, B. A. (1987). Perturbation of differentiated functions in vivo during persistent viral infection. III. Decreased growth hormone mRNA. *Virology*, **156**, 214–220.

210. Rettori, V., Jurcovicova, J., and McCann, S. M. (1987). Control action of interleukin-1 in altering the release of TSH, growth hormone, and prolactin in the male rat. *J. Neurosci. Res.*, **18**, 179–183.

211. Bernton, E. W., Beach, J. E., Holaday, J. W., Smallridge, R. C., and Fein, H. G. (1987). Release of multiple hormones by a direct action of interleukin-1 on pituitary cells. *Science*, **238**, 519–521.

212. Milenkovic, L., Rettori, V., Snyder, G. D., Beutler, B., and McCann, S. M. (1989). Cachectin alters anterior pituitary hormone release by a direct action in vitro. *Proc. Natl. Acad. Sci. (USA)*, **86**, 2418–2422.

213. Andrews, G. S. (1983). Growth hormone and malignancy. *J. Clin. Pathol.*, **36**, 935–937.

214. Kamijo, K., Saito, A., Yachi, A., and Wada, T. (1980). Growth hormone response to thyrotropin-releasing hormone in cancer patients. *Endocrinol. Japan.*, **27**, 451–455.

215. Edwards, C. K., Lorence, R. M., Dunham, D. M., Yunger, L. M., and Kelley, K. W. (1989). Peritoneal macrophages from hypophysectomized rats treated in vivo with interferon-a or growth hormone are primed to release tumor necrosis factor-α. *Proc. 7th International Cong. Immunol.*, **93**, 618.

216. Gisler, R. H. and Schenkel-Hulliger, L. (1971). Hormonal regulation of the immune response. II. Influence of pituitary and adrenal activity on immune responsiveness *in vitro*. *Cell. Immunol.*, **2**, 646–657.

217. Hayashida, T. and Li, C. H. (1957). The influence of adrenocorticotropic and growth hormones on antibody formation. *J. Exp. Med.*, **105**, 93–98.

218. Hiestand, P. C., Mekler, P., Nordmann, R., Grieder, A., and Permmongkol, C. (1986). Prolactin as a modulator of lymphocyte responsiveness provides a possible mechanism of action for cyclosporine. *Proc. Natl. Acad. Sci. (USA)*, **83**, 2599–2603.

219. Weigent, D. A., Baxter, J. B., Wear, W. E., Smith, L. R., Bost, K. L., and Blalock, J. E. (1988). Production of immunoreactive growth hormone by mononuclear leukocytes. *FASEB J.*, **2**, 2812–2818.

220. Bernton, E. W., Meltzer, M. T., and Holaday, J. W. (1988). Suppression of macrophage activation and T-lymphocyte function in hypoprolactinemic mice. *Science*, **239**, 401–404.

221. Maestroni, G. J. M., Conti, A., and Pierpaoli, W. (1988). Role of the pineal gland in immunity: III. Melatonin antagonizes the immunosuppressive effect of acute stress via an opiatergic mechanism. *Immunol.*, **63**, 465–469.

222. Shaskan, E. G. and Lovett, E. J., III (1980). Effects of haloperidol, a dopamine receptor antagonist on a delayed type hypersensitivity reduction to 1-chloro 2-, 4-dinitrobenzene in mice. *Res. Commun. Psychol. Psych. Behav.*, **5**, 241.

223. Russell, D. H. and Larson, D. F. (1985). Prolactin-induced polyamine biosynthesis in spleen and thymus: Specific inhibition by cyclosporine. *Immunopharm.*, **9**, 165–174.

224. Maestroni, G. J. M., Conti, A., and Pierpaoli, W. (1988). Pineal melatonin, its fundamental immunoregulatory role in aging and cancer. *Ann. N. Y. Acad. Sci.*, **521**, 140–148.

225. Montgomery, D., Zukoski, C., Shah, G., Buckley, A., Pacholczyk, T., and Russell, D. (1987). Con A stimulated murine splenocytes produce a factor with prolactin-like bioactivity and immunoreactivity. *Biochem. Biophys. Res. Commun.*, **145**, 692–698.

226. Maestroni, G. J. M., Conti, A., and Pierpaoli, W. (1986). Role of the pineal immunity. Circadian synthesis and release of melatonin modulates the antibody response and antagonizes the immunosuppressive effect of corticosterone. *J. Neuroimmunol.*, **13**, 19–30.

227. Maestroni, G. J. M., Conti, A., and Pierpaoli, W. (1987). The pineal gland and the circadian, opiatergic, immunoregulatory role of melatonin. *Ann. N. Y. Acad. Sci.*, **496**, 67–77.

228. Bernton, E. W., Bryant, H. U., and Holaday, J. W. (1991). Prolactin and immune function. In *Psychoneuroimmunology*, (2nd edn), (eds R. Ader, D. L. Felten, and N. Cohen), pp. 403–428. Academic Press, New York.

229. Hartman, D., Holaday, J. W., and Bernton, E. W. (1989). Inhibition of lymphocyte proliferation by antibodies to PRL. *FASEB J.*, **3**, 2194–2202.

230. Becker, J., Veit, G., Handgretinger, R., Attanasio, A., Bruchett, G., Trenner, I., Niethammer, D., and Gupta, D. (1988). Circadian variations in the immunomodulatory role of the pineal gland. *Neuroendocrinol. Lett.*, **10**, 65–80.

231. Maestroni, G. J. M. and Pierpaoli, W. (1981). Pharmacologic control of the hormonally mediated immune response. In *Psychoneuroimmunology*, (ed. R. Ader), pp. 405–425. Academic Press, New York.

232. Smith, E. M., Morrill, A. C., Meyer III, W. J., and Blalock, J. E. (1986). Corticotropin releasing factor induction of leukocyte-derived immunoreactive ACTH and endorphins. *Nature*, **321**, 881–882.

233. Kavelaars, A., Ballieux, R. E., and Heijnen, C. J. (1989). The role of

interleukin-1 in the CRH- and AVP-induced secretion of ir-β-endorphin by human peripheral blood mononuclear cells. *J. Immunol.*, **142**, 2338–2342.

234. Kavelaars, A., Ballieux, R. E., and Heijnen, C. J. (1990). β-endorphin secretion by human peripheral blood mononuclear cells: regulation by glucocorticoids. *Life Sci.*, **46**, 1233–1240.

235. Ebadi, M. (1984). Regulation of the synthesis of melatonin and its significance to neuroendocrinology. In *The Pineal Gland*, (ed. R. J. Reiter), pp. 1–39. Raven Press, New York.

236. Naray, A. (1981). Progesterone receptor in chick thymus. *Biochem. Biophys. Res. Commun.*, **98**, 866–874.

237. Alvarez-Mon, M., Kehrl, J. H., and Fauci, A. S. (1985). A potential role for adrenocorticotropin in regulating human B-lymphocyte functions. *J. Immunol.*, **135**, 3823–3826.

238. Johnson, H. M., Torres, B. A., Smith, E. M., Dion, L. D., and Blalock, J. E. (1984). Regulation of lymphokine (gamma-interferon) production by corticotropin. *J. Immunol.*, **132**, 246–250.

239. Ylikomi, T., Gasc, J. M., Tuohimaa, P., and Baulieu, E. E. (1987). Ontogeny of estrogen-sensitive mesenchymal cells in the bursa of Fabricius of the chick embryo. An immunohistochemical study on progesterone receptor. *Develop.*, **101**, 61–66.

240. Sakabe, K., Seiki, K., and Fujii, H. (1986). Histochemical localisation of progestin receptor in the rat thymus. *Thymus*, **8**, 97–107.

241. Pearce, P. T., Khalid, P. A. K., and Funder, J. W. (1983). Progesterone receptors in rat thymus. *Endocrinology*, **13**, 1287–1291.

242. Heijnen, C. J., Kavelaars, A., and Ballieux, R. E. (1991). CRH and POMC-derived peptides in the modulation of immune function. In *Psychoneuroimmunology*, (2nd edn) (eds R. Ader, D. L. Felton, and N. Cohen), pp. 429–446. Academic Press, New York.

243. Strahle, U., Boshart, M., Klock, G., Stewart, F., and Schutz, G. (1989). Glucocorticoid' and progesterone' specific effects are determined by differential expression of the respective hormone receptors. *Nature*, **339**, 629–632.

244. Smith, E. M., Hughes, T. K. Jr., Hashemi, F., and Stefano, G. B. (1992). Immunosuppressive effects of corticotropin and melanotropin and their possible significance in human immunodeficiency virus infection. *Proc. Natl. Acad. Sci.*, **89**, 782–786.

245. Sundar, S. K., Cierpial, M. A., Kamaraju, L. S., Long, S., Hsieh, S., Lorenz, C. *et al.* (1991). Human immunodeficiency virus glycoprotein (gp120) infused into rat brain induces interleukin 1 to elevate pituitary-adrenal activity and decrease peripheral cellular immune responses. *Proc. Natl. Acad. Sci.*, **88**, 11246–11250.

246. Fontana, L., Fattorossi, A., D'Amelio, R., Migliorati, A., and Perricone, R. (1987). Modulation of human concanavalin A-induced lymphocyte proliferative response by physiological concentrations of β-endorphin. *Immunopharm.*, **13**, 111–115.

247. Froehich, C. J. and Bankhurst, A. D. (1984). The effect of β-endorphin on natural cytotoxicity and antibody dependent cellular cytotoxicity. *Life Sci.*, **35**, 261–265.

248. Van Epps, D. E. and Saland, L. (1984). Beta-endorphin and met-enkephalin

stimulate human peripheral blood mononuclear cell chemotaxis. *J. Immunol.*, **132**, 3046–3053.

249. Heagy, W., Laurence, M., Cohen, E., and Finberg, R. (1990). Neurohormones regulate T-cell function. *J. Exp. Med.*, **171**, 1625–1633.

250. Gilmore, W. and Weiner, L. P. (1989). The opioid specificity of beta-endorphin enhancement of murine lymphocyte proliferation. *Immunopharm.*, **17**, 19–30.

251. Van Den Bergh, P., Rozing, J., and Nagelkerken, L. (1991). Two opposing modes of action of β-endorphin on lymphocyte function. *Immunol.*, **72**, 537–543.

252. Hemmick, L. M. and Bidlack, J. M. (1990). β-Endorphin stimulates rat T-lymphocyte proliferation. *J. Neuroimmunol.*, **29**, 239–248.

253. Heijnen, C. J., Zijlstra, J., Kavelaars, A., Croiset, G., and Ballieux, R. E. (1987). Modulation of the immune response by POMC-derived peptides. I. Influence on proliferation of human lymphocytes. *Brain Behav. Immun.*, **1**, 284–291.

254. Kusnecov, A. W., Husband, A. J., King, M. G., Pang, G., and Smith, R. (1987). *In vivo* effects of β-endorphin on lymphocyte proliferation and interleukin 2 production. *Brain Behav. Immun.*, **1**, 88–97.

255. Heijnen, C. J., Kavelaars, A., and Ballieux, R. E. (1991). Corticotropin-releasing hormone and proopiomelanocortin-derived peptides in the modulation of immune function. In *Psychoneuroimmunology*, (2nd edn), (eds R. Ader, D. L. Felten, and N. Cohen), pp. 429–446. Academic Press, New York.

256. Apte, R. N., Oppenheim, J. J., and Durum, S. K. (1989). β-endorphin regulates interleukin 1 production and release by murine bone marrow macrophages. *Int. Immun.*, **1**, 465–470.

257. Smith, E. M. and Blalock, J. E. (1981). Human lymphocyte production of corticotropin and endorphin-like substances: Association with leukocyte interferon. *Proc. Natl. Acad. Sci. (USA)*, **78**, 7530–7534.

258. Lolait, S. J., Lim, A. T. W., Toh, B. H., and Funder, J. W. (1984). Immunoreactive β-endorphin in a subpopulation of mouse spleen macrophages. *J. Clin. Invest.*, **73**, 277–280.

259. Westly, H. J., Kleiss, A. J., Kelley, K. W., Wong, P. K. Y., and Yuen, P.-H. (1986). Newcastle disease virus-infected splenocytes express the proopiomelanocortin gene. *J. Exp. Med.*, **163**, 1589–1594.

260. Blalock, J. E. (1984). The immune system as a sensory organ. *J. Immunol.*, **132**, 1067–1070.

261. Harbour-McMenamin, D., Smith, E. M., and Blalock, J. E. (1985). Bacterial lipopolysaccharide induction of leukocyte-derived corticotropin and endorphins. *Infect. Immun.*, **48**, 813–817.

262. Dracott, B. N. and Smith, C. E. T. (1979). Hydrocortisone and the antibody response in mice. I. Correlations between serum cortisol levels and cell numbers in thymus, spleen, marrow and lymph nodes. *Immunol.*, **38**, 429–435.

263. Munck, A. and Guyre, P. M. (1991). Glucocorticoids and immune function. In *Psychoneuroimmunology*, (2nd edn), (eds R. Ader, D. L. Felten, and N. Cohen), pp. 447–493. Academic Press, New York.

264. Munck, A., Guyre, P. M., and Holbrook, N.J. (1984). Physiological functions

of glucocorticoids in stress and their relation to pharmacological actions. *Endocrin. Rev.*, **5**, 25–44.

265. del Rey, A., Besedovsky, H., and Sorkin, E. (1984). Endogenous blood levels of corticosterone control the immunologic cell mass and B-cell activity in mice. *J. Immunol.*, **133**, 572–575.

266. Cohen, J. J. and Duke, R. C. (1984). Glucocorticoid activation of a calcium-dependent endonuclease in thymocyte nuclei leads to cell death. *J. Immunol.*, **132**, 38–42.

267. Cox, J. H. and Ford, W. L. (1982). The migration of lymphocytes across specialized vascular endothelium. IV. Prednisolone acts at several points on the recirculation pathways of lymphocytes. *Cell. Immunol.*, **66**, 407–422.

268. Hall, J. G. (1986). Sulphated polysaccharides, corticosteroids and lymphocyte recirculation. *Immunol.*, **57**, 275–279.

269. Smith, K. A., Crabtree, G. R., Kennedy, S. J., and Munck, A. U. (1977). Glucocorticoid receptors and glucocorticoid sensitivity of mitogen stimulated and unstimulated human lymphocytes. *Nature*, **267**, 523–525.

270. Cupps, T. R. and Fauci, A. S. (1982). Corticosteroid-mediated immunoregulation in man. *Immunol. Rev.*, **65**, 133–155.

271. Werb, Z., Foley, R., and Munck, A. (1978). Interaction of glucocorticoids with macrophages. Identification of glucocorticoid receptors in monocytes and macrophages. *J. Exp. Med.*, **147**, 1684–1694.

272. Snyder, D. S. and Unanue, E. R. (1982). Corticosteroids inhibit macrophage Ia expression and interleukin 1 production. *J. Immunol.*, **129**, 1803–1805.

273. Gillis, S., Crabtree, G. R., and Smith, K. A. (1979). Glucocorticosteroid-induced inhibition of T-cell growth factor production. I. The effect on mitogen-induced lymphocyte proliferation. *J. Immunol.*, **123**, 1624–1631.

274. Pinkston, P., Saltini, C., Muller-Quernheim, J., and Crystal, R. G. (1987). Corticosteroid therapy suppresses spontaneous interleukin 2 release and spontaneous proliferation of lung T-lymphocytes of patients with active pulmonary sarcoidosis. *J. Immunol.*, **139**, 755–760.

275. Daynes, R. A. and Araneo, B. A. (1989). Contrasting effects of glucocorticoids on the capacity of T-cells to produce the growth factors interleukin 2 and interleukin 4. *Eur. J. Immunol.*, **19**, 2319–2325.

276. Bradley, L. M. and Mishell, R. I. (1981). Differential effects of glucocorticosteroids on the functions of helper and suppressor T-lymphocytes. *Proc. Natl. Acad. Sci. (USA)*, **78**, 3155–3159.

277. Bertoglio, J. H. and Leroux, E. (1988). Differential effects of glucocorticoids on the proliferation of a murine helper and a cytolytic T-cell clone in response to IL-2 and IL-4. *J. Immunol.*, **141**, 1191–1196.

278. Emilie, D., Karray, S., Crevon, M.-C., Vazquez, A., and Galanaud, P. (1987). B-cell differentiation and interleukin 2 (IL2): Corticosteroids interact with monocytes to enhance the effect of IL2. *Eur. J. Immunol.*, **17**, 791–795.

279. Orson, F. M., Grayson, J., Pike, S., De Seau, V., and Blaese, R. M. (1983). T-cell-replacing factor for glucocorticosteroid-induced immunoglobulin production. *J. Exp. Med.*, **158**, 1473–1482.

280. Daynes, R. A., Dudley, J. J., and Araneo, B. A. (1990). Regulation of murine

lymphokine production in vivo. II. Dehydroepiandrosterone is a natural enhancer of interleukin 2 synthesis by helper T-cells. *Eur. J. Immunol.*, **20**, 793–802.

281. Blalock, J. E., Johnson, H. M., Smith, E. M., and Torres, B. A. (1984). Enhancement of the in vitro antibody response by thyrotropin. *Biochem. Biophys. Res. Commun.*, **125**, 30–34.

282. Kruger, T. E. and Blalock, J. E. (1986). Cellular requirements for thyrotropin enhancement of in vitro antibody production. *J. Immunol.*, **137**, 197–200.

283. Kruger, T. E., Smith, L. R., Harbour, D. V., and Blalock, J. E. (1989). Thyrotropin: An endogenous regulator of the in vitro immune response. *J. Immunol.*, **142**, 744–747.

284. Harbour, D. V., Kruger, T. E., Coppenhaver, D., Smith, E. M., and Meyer, W. J. III (1989). Differential expression and regulation of thyrotropin (TSH) in T-cell lines. *Mol. Cell. Endocrinol.*, **64**, 229–241.

285. Harbour, D. V., Leon, S., Keating, C., and Hughes, T. K. (1990). Thyrotropin modulates B-cell function through specific bioactive receptors. *Prog. Neuro-EndocrinImmunology*, **3**, 266–276.

286. Fabris, N. (1973). Immunodepression in thyroid-deprived animals. *Clin. Exp. Immunol.*, **15**, 601–611.

287. Chatterjee, S. and Chandel, A. S. (1983). Immunomodulatory role of thyroid hormones: in vivo effect of thyroid hormones on the blastogenic response of lymphoid tissues. *Acta Endocrinol.*, **103**, 95–100.

288. Scott, T. and Glick, B. (1987). Organ weights, T-cell proliferation, and graft vs host capabilities of hypothyroidic chickens. *Gen. Comp. Endocrinol.*, **67**, 270–276.

289. Provinciali, M., Muzzioli, M., DiStefano, G., and Fabris, N. (1991). Recovery of spleen cell natural killer activity by thyroid hormone treatment in old mice. *Nat. Immun. Cell. Growth Regul.*, **10**, 226–236.

290. Lahita, R. G. (1990). Sex hormones and the immune system-part 1. Human data. *Bailliere's Clin. Rheu.*, **4**, 1–12.

291. Ansar Ahmed, S., Dauphinee, M. J., Montoya, A. I., and Talal, N. (1989). Sex hormones, immune responses, and autoimmune diseases. *J. Immunol.*, **142**, 2647–2653.

292. Butterworth, M., McClellan, B., and Allansmith, M. (1967). Influence of sex on immunoglobulin levels. *Nature*, **214**, 1224–1225.

293. Terres, G., Morrison, S. L., and Habicht, G. S. (1968). A quantitative difference in the immune response between male and female mice. *Proc. Soc. Exp. Biol. Med.*, **127**, 664–667.

294. Eidinger, D. and Garrett, T. J. (1972). Studies of the regulatory effects of the sex hormones on antibody formation and stem cell differentiation. *J. Exp. Med.*, **136**, 1098–1116.

295. Masi, A. T. and Kaslow, R. A. (1978). Sex effects in SLE: A clue to pathogenesis. *Arthritis Rheum.*, **21**, 480–484.

296. Duvic, M., Steinberg, A. D., and Klassen, L. W. (1978). Effect of the anti-estrogen, nafoxidine, on NZB/W autoimmune disease. *Arthritis Rheum.*, **21**, 414–417.

297. Barr, I. G., Pyke, K. W., Pearce, P., Toh, P.-H., and Funder, J. W. (1984).

Thymic sensitivity to sex hormones develops post-natally; an in vivo and an in vitro study. *J. Immunol.*, **132**, 1095–1099.

298. Brodie, J. Y., Hunter, I. C., Stimson, W. H., and Green, B. (1980). Specific oestradiol binding in cytosols from the thymus glands from normal and hormone-treated male rats. *Thymus*, **1**, 337–345.

299. Malacarne, P., Piffanelli, A., Indelli, M., Fumero, S., Mondino, A., Gion-chiglia, E. *et al.* (1980). Estradiol binding in rat thymus cells. *Horm. Res.*, **12**, 224–232.

300. Reichman, M. E. and Villee, C. A. (1978). Estradiol binding by rat thymus cytosol. *Biochemistry*, **9**, 637–641.

301. Detlefson, M. A., Smith, B. C., and Pickerman, H. W. (1978). A high affinity and low capacity receptor for estradiol in normal and anaemic mouse spleen cytosols. *Biochem. Biophys. Res. Commun.*, **76**, 1151–1158.

302. Nilsson, B., Carlsson, S., Damer, M.-G., Lindholm, G., Sodergard, R., and Schoultz, B. von. (1984). Specific binding of 17β-estradiol in human thymus. *Am. J. Obstet. Gynecol.*, **149**, 544–547.

303. Ranelletti, R. O., Carmignani, M., Marchetti, P., Natoli, C., and Jacobelli, S. (1984). Estrogen binding by neoplastic human thymus cytosol. *Eur. J. Cancer*, **16**, 951–955.

304. Stimson, W. H. (1983). Serum proteins, steroids and the maternal immune response. In *Immunology of Reproduction*, (eds T. G. Wegman and T. J. Gill), pp. 281–301. Oxford University Press.

305. Sullivan, D. A. and Wira, C. R. (1979). Sex hormone and glucococorticoid receptors in the bursa of Fabricius of immature chicks. *J. Immunol.*, **122**, 2617–2623.

306. Cohen, J. H. M., Danel, L., Cordier, G., Saez, S., and Revillard, J.-P. (1983). Sex steroid receptors in peripheral T-cells. Absence of androgen receptor and restriction of oestrogen receptor to OKT8 positive cells. *J. Immunol.*, **131**, 2767–2771.

307. Stimson, W. H. (1988). Oestrogen and human T-lymphocytes: Presence of specific receptors in the T-suppressor/cytotoxic subset. *Scand. J. Immunol.*, **28**, 345–350.

308. Nicol, T. D., Bilbey, D. L. J., Charles, L. M., Cordingley, J. L., and Vernon-Roberts, B. (1964). Oestrogen: The natural stimulant of body defense. *J. Endocrin.*, **30**, 277–291.

309. Nicol, T. and Vernon-Roberts, B. (1965). The influence of the estrus cycle, pregnancy, and ovariectomy on RES activity. *J. Reticuloendothel. Soc.*, **2**, 15–29.

310. Gulshan, S., McCruden, A. B., and Stimson, W. H. (1990). Estrogen receptors in macrophages. *Scand. J. Immunol.*, **31**, 691–697.

311. Maoz, H., Kaiser, N., Halimi, M., Barak, V., Haimovitz, A., Weinstein, D. *et al.* (1985). The effect of oestradiol on human myelomoncytic cells. I. Enhancement of colony formation. *J. Reprod. Immunol.*, **7**, 325–335.

312. Castro, J. E. and Hamilton, D. N. H. (1972). Adrenalectomy and orchidectomy as immunopotentiating procedures. *Transplantation.* **13**, 615–616.

313. Dougherty, T. F. (1952). Effect of hormones on lymphatic tissue. *Physiol. Rev.*, **32**, 379–401.

314. Frey-Wettstein, M. and Craddock, C. G. (1970). Testosterone induced depletion of thymus and marrow lymphocytes as related to lymphopoiesis and hematopoiesis. *Blood*, **35**, 257–271.

315. Gregoire, C. (1945). Sur le mechanisme de l'hypertorphie thymique declanchee par la castration. *Arch. int. Pharmacodyn.*, **67**, 45–77.

316. Hammer, J. A. (1929). Die menschenthymus in Gezundheit und Krankheit. II. Das Organ unter anomale Verhaltnisse. *Z. mikrosk. -anat. Forsch.*, **16** (Suppl.),

317. Stimson, W. H. and Crilly, P. J. (1981). Effects of steroids on the secretion of immunoregulatory factors by thymic epithelial cell cultures. *Immunol.*, **44**, 401–407.

318. Batchelor, J. R. and Chapman, B. A. (1965). The influence of sex upon the antibody response to an incompatible tumour. *Immunol.*, **9**, 553–564.

319. Schacher, J., Browne, J. S. L., and Seyle, H. (1937). Effect of various steroids on thymus in the adrenalectomized rat. *Proc. Soc. Exp. Biol. Med.*, **36**, 488–491.

320. Kenny, J. F., Pangburn, P. C., and Trail, G. (1976). Effect of estradiol on immune competence: in vivo and in vitro studies. *Infect. Immun.*, **13**, 448–456.

321. Albin, R. J. (1976). Possible suppression of host resistance by estrogen therapy for prostatic cancer. *Can. Med. Assoc. J.*, **115**, 1082–1084.

322. Ablin, R. J., Guinan, P. D., Bruns, G. R., Al Sheik, H. L., Sadoughi, N., and Bush, I. M. (1976). Evaluation of cellular immunologic responsiveness in the clinical management of patients with prostatic cancer. *Urol. Int.*, **31**, 383–400.

323. Steinberg, A. D. and Steinberg, B. J. (1985). Lupus disease activity associated with the menstrual cycle. *J. Rheumatol.*, **12**, 816–817.

324. Chapel, T. A. and Burns, R. E. (1971). Oral contraceptives and exacerbation of lupus erythematous. *Am. J. Obstet. Gynecol.*, **110**, 366–369.

325. Jungers, P., Dougados, M., Pelissier, C., Kuttenn, F., Tron, F., Lesavre, P. *et al.* (1982). Influence de la contraception hormonal sur l'evolutivitée des nephropathies lupiques. *La Nouvelle Presse Medicale*, **11**, 3765–3768.

326. Jungers, P., Dougados, M., Pelissier, C., Kuttenn, F., Tron, F., Lesavre, P. *et al.* (1982). Influence of oral contraceptive therapy on the activity of SLE. *Arthritis Rheum.*, **25**, 618–623.

327. Garovich, M., Agudelo, C., and Pisko, E. (1980). Oral contraceptives and systemic lupus erythematosus. *Arthritis Rheum.*, **23**, 1396–1398.

328. Travers, R. L. and Hughes, G. R. V. (1978). Oral contraceptive therapy and SLE. *J. Rheumatol.*, **5**, 448–451.

329. Sturgess, A. D., Evans, D. T. P., MacKay, I. R., and Riglar, A. (1984). Effect of the oestrogen antagonist tamoxifen in disease indices in SLE. *Clin. Lab. Immunol.*, **13**, 11–14.

330. Lawrence, J. S. (1970). Rheumatoid arthritis: Nature of nurture? *Ann. Rheum. Dis.*, **29**, 357–379.

331. Latman, N. S. (1983). Relation of menstrual cycle phase to symptoms of rheumatoid arthritis. *Am. J. Med.*, **74**, 957–960.

332. Rudge, S. R., Kuwanko, I. C., and Druy, P. L. (1983). Menstrual cyclicity of finger joint size and grip strength in patients with rheumatoid arthritis. *Ann. Rheum. Dis.*, **42**, 425–430.

333. Blais, J. A. and Demers, R. (1962). The use of norethynodrel in the treatment or rheumatoid arthritis. *Arthritis Rheum.*, 5, 284.

334. McCruden, A. B. and Stimson, W. H. (1991). Sex hormones and immune function. In *Psychoneuroimmunolog*, (2nd edn) (eds R. Ader, D. L. Felten, and N. Cohen), pp. 475–493. Academic Press, New York.

335. Heslop, R. W., Krohn, P. L., and Sparrow, F. M. (1954). The effect of pregnancy on the survival of skin homografts in rabbits. *J. Endocrin.*, 10, 325–332.

336. Waltman, S. R., Burde, R. M., and Berrios, J. (1971). Prevention of corneal homografts rejection by estrogens. *Transplantation*, 11, 194–196.

337. Seaman, W. E., Blackman, M. A., Gindhart, T. D., Roubinian, J. R., Loeb, J. M., and Talal, N. (1978). β-Estradiol reduces natural killer cells in mice. *J. Immunol.*, 121, 2193–2198.

338. Broome, A. W. J. and Lamming, G. E. (1959). Studies on the relationship between ovarian hormones and uterine infection. III. The role of the antibody system in uterine defense. *J. Endocrin.*, 18, 229–235.

339. Tsao, S. N. (1941). Bactericidal property of blood serum of male rabbits treated with urinary estrogens. *Proc. Soc. Exp. Biol. Med.*, 48, 38–41.

340. Wira, C. R. and Sandoe, C. P. (1977). Sex steroid hormone regulation of IgA and IgG in rat uterine secretions. *Nature*, 268, 534–535.

341. Feigen, G. A., Fraser, R. C., and Peterson, N. S. (1978). Sex hormone and the immune response. II. Pertubation of antibody production by estradiol 17β1. *Int. Arch. Allergy Appl. Immunol.*, 57, 488–497.

342. Thompson, J. S., Severson, C. D., and Reilly, R. W. (1969). Autoradiographic study of the effect of estradiol and irradiation on nucleic acid metabolism of the thymus and lymph node of mice. *Radiat. Res.*, 40, 46–62.

343. Von Haam, E. and Rosenfeld, I. (1942). The effect of the various sex hormones upon experimental pneumococcus infections in mice. *J. Infect. Dis.*, 70, 243–247.

344. Lewine, H. B. and Madin, S. H. (1962). Enhancement of experimental coccidiomycosis in mice with testosterone and estradiol. *Sabouraudia*, 2, 47–52.

345. Rifkind, D., Frey, J. A., and Davis, J. R. (1973). Influence of gonadal factors on skin reactivity of CFW mice to Candida albicans. *Infect. Immun.*, 7, 322–328.

346. Kappas, A., Jones, H. E. S., and Roitt, I. M. (1963). Effects of steroid sex hormones on immunological phenomena. *Nature*, 198, 902–904.

347. Roubinian, J. R., Talal, N., Greenspan, J. S., Goodman, J. R., and Siiteri, P. K. (1978). Effect of castration and sex hormone treatment on survival, anti-nucleic acid antibodies and glomerulonephritis in NZB/NZW F1 mice. *J. Exp. Med.*, 147, 1568–1583.

348. Grossman, C. J., Nathan, P., Talyor, B. B., and Sholiton, L. J. (1979). Rat dihydrotestosteroned receptor: Preparation, location and physiochemical properties. *Steroids*, 34, 539–553.

349. McCruden, A. B. and Stimson, W. H. (1980). Androgen and other sex steroid cytosol receptors in the rat thymus. *J. Endocrin.*, 85, 47–48.

350. Raveche, E. S., Vigersky, R. A., Rice, M. K., and Steinberg, A. D. (1980). Murine thymic androgen receptors. *J. Immunopharmacol.*, 2, 425–434.

351. Sasson, S. and Mayer, M. (1981). Effect of androgen steroids on rat thymus and thymocytes in suspension. *J. Steroid Biochem.*, **14**, 509–517.

352. Kotani, M., Nawa, Y., and Fujii, H. (1974). Inhibition by testosterone of immune reactivity and of lymphoid regeneration in irradiated and marrow reconstituted mice. *Experientia*, **30**, 1343–1345.

353. Kotani, M., Nawa, Y., and Fujii, H. (1975). Histological observations of inhibitory effects of testosterone on lymphoid regeneration in the thymus independent areas of mice. *Arch. Histol. Jap.*, **38**, 117–120

354. Stimson, W. H., Crilly, P. J., and McCruden, A. B. (1980). Effect of sex steroids on the synthesis of immunoregulatory factors by thymic epithelial cell cultures. *IRCS Med. Sci.*, **8**, 263–264.

355. Wyle, F. A. and Kent, J. R. (1977). Immunosuppression by sex hormones. The effect upon PHA and PPD stimulated lymphocytes. *Clin. Exp. Immunol.*, **27**, 407–415.

356. Tomoda, Y., Fuma, M., Mina, T., Saiki, N., and Ishraka, N. (1976). Cell mediated immunity in pregnancy. *Gynecol. Invest.*, **37**, 280–292.

357. Scambia, G., Panici, P. B., Maccio, A., Castelli, P., Serri, F., Mantovani, G. *et al.* (1988). Effects of antiestrogen and progestin on immune functions in breast cancer. *Cancer*, **61**, 2214–2218.

358. Shiff, R. I., Mercier, D., and Buckley, R. H. (1975). Inability of gestational hormones to account for the inhibitory effects of pregnancy plasmas on lymphocyte responses *in vitro*. *Cell. Immunol.*, **20**, 69–80.

359. Holdstock, G., Chastenay, B. F., and Krawitt, E. L. (1982). Effects of testosterone, estradiol and progesterone on immune reaction. *Clin. Exp. Immunol.*, **47**, 449–456.

360. Kincl, F. A. and Ciaccio, L. A. (1980). Suppression of the immune response by progesterone. *Endocrinol. Exp.*, **14**, 27–33.

361. Sekiya, S., Kamiyama, M., and Takamizawa, H. (1975). In vivo and in vitro tests of inhibitory effect of progesterone on cell-mediated immunity in rats bearing a syngeneic uterine adenocarcinoma. *J. Natl. Cancer Inst.*, **54**, 769–771.

362. Kaiser, N., Mayer, M., Milholland, R. J., and Rosen, F. (1979). Studies of the antiglucocorticoid action of progesterone in rat thymocytes: Early *in vitro* effects. *J. Steroid Biochem.*, **10**, 379–386.

363. Maestroni, G. J. M. and Conti, A. (1991). Role of the pineal neurohormone melatonin in the psycho-neuroendocrine-immune network. In *Psychoneuroimmunology*, (2nd edn), (eds R. Ader, D. L. Felten, and N. Cohen), pp. 465–513. Academic Press, New York.

364. Plotnikoff, N. P., Faith, R. E., Murgo, A. J., and Good, R. A. (1986). *Enkephalins and Endorphins: Stress and the Immune System*. Plenum Press, New York.

# 3

# Control logic, nutrition of cells, and mechanisms in psychoimmunology

## E. A. NEWSHOLME AND M. HOLDEN

## 1  Introduction

There is considerable evidence in support of the possibility that psychological stress can interfere with the function of the immune system and hence the predisposition to a variety of serious illnesses, including cancer (1, 2). It is generally assumed that, if indeed such stress does influence the immune system, it must do so via a direct interaction between the brain and the immune system (see chapter 2 of this volume). However, the interaction between the brain and the immune system may not be direct: it may well involve other tissues, either directly or indirectly. A further problem arises in that giving a new field an exciting name—psychoimmunology—provides an implication that the subject is well understood and can be discussed in terms of testable hypotheses. So far, in general in this field, hypotheses have lacked scientific substance—that is they are too general or too complex to test. In this chapter, a theoretical and experimental framework is provided for a testable hypothesis which links the brain, the muscle, adipose tissue, and the immune system. In order to understand the theoretical basis of the hypothesis, some relevant aspects of metabolic control logic will be described.

## 1.1 THE STRUCTURE OF A BIOCHEMICAL PROCESS

It is sometimes difficult to appreciate that a string of reactions in a diagram in a biochemical text can have both a thermodynamic and a kinetic structure. This structure is, however, essential not only to establish a steady state but also to understand how it is controlled and the role of the process *in vivo*. Failure to do this has led, and is still leading, to misinterpretations of the physiological functions of biochemical processes and this, sadly, can lead to a failure to understand the pathology arising from an abnormality in the biochemistry and, therefore, failure to treat patients satisfactorily. This will be illustrated below for the process of glutamine utilization by immune cells.

### 1.1.1 *Near-equilibrium, non-equilibrium, and flux-generating reactions*

Reactions in a biochemical process, whether it is a classical metabolic pathway or a recently proposed signal transduction system, can be divided into two classes: those that are very close to equilibrium (near-equilibrium) and those that are far-removed from equilibrium (non-equilibrium).

A reaction in a biochemical process is non-equilibrium if the activity of the enzyme that catalyses the reaction is low in comparison with the activities of other enzymes in the pathway, so that the concentration of substrate(s) of the reaction is maintained high whereas that of the product is maintained low. Consequently, the rate of the reverse component $(v_r)$ of the reaction is very much less than the rate of the forward component $(v_f)$. In the following example, the rate in the forward direction (A to B) is 1000-fold greater than the rate in the reverse direction (B to A).

$$S \longrightarrow A \underset{0.01}{\overset{10.01}{\rightleftarrows}} B \longrightarrow P$$

Hence the reaction is non-equilibrium.

A reaction is near-equilibrium if the catalytic activity of the enzyme is high in relation to the activities of other enzymes in the pathway, so that the rates of the forward and the reverse components of the reaction are much greater than the overall flux. In the following example, the difference between the forward and reverse components is only 10 per cent and the rate of the forward component is 10-fold greater than the flux.

$$S \longrightarrow A \underset{90}{\overset{100}{\rightleftarrows}} B \longrightarrow P$$

Note that, in both examples, the flux is the same, 10 units, and the numbers represent actual rates that can occur in a reaction in a living cell. The methods to establish the equilibrium nature of a reaction together with further discussion of this subject are provided elsewhere (3, 4).

One particular type of non-equilibrium reaction can be of particular importance in understanding flux. If an enzyme catalyses a non-equilibrium reaction in a biochemical process and approaches saturation with its pathway-substrate (that substrate which represents the flow of matter through the pathway), so that the catalytic rate is almost independent of the substrate concentration, then the reaction is known as the flux-generating step for the process. In other words, in the steady state, this reaction initiates a flux to which *all* other reactions in the pathway *must* adjust. (Such a reaction must approach saturation with its pathway-substrate; otherwise, as the reaction proceeds the substrate concentration would decrease and this would decrease the rate of the reaction and hence the flux through the biochemical process; a steady state would then be impossible.) One important development from the concept of flux-generating step is that it provides a physiologically useful definition of a metabolic pathway or a biochemical process. A pathway or process is defined as a *series of reactions initiated by a flux-generating step and which ends with the loss of end-product to a metabolic sink (storage form), to the environment or it ends in a reaction that precedes another flux-generating step* (3).

The significance of this definition and its relation to the immune system should become clear in the discussion provided below.

### 1.1.2 Control of the transmission of a flux

In the following hypothetical linear pathway, the flux (J) is generated at reaction $E_1$ (the flux-generating step which is denoted by the sign $\rightarrow\!\!\!\!\!\not\rightarrow$).

This flux is transmitted along the pathway by the response of the subsequent reactions to the metabolic intermediates A, B, and C, so

$$S \xrightarrow{\quad} A \overset{\overset{X}{\oplus}}{\xrightarrow{\quad}} B \longrightarrow C \longrightarrow (J)$$
$$\quad E_1 \qquad E_2 \qquad E_3 \qquad E_4$$

these metabolites link all the component reactions of the pathway and help to produce the overall steady-state flux. The role of the metabolic intermediates can best be explained by reference to the effect of an activation of one of the component reactions. Thus compound X stimulates enzyme $E_2$ so that, if the concentration of X were increased, the activity of this enzyme would increase. However, this would result in a decrease in the concentration of substrate A, which would lower the activity of enzyme $E_2$. The decrease in the concentration of A will continue until the activity of $E_2$ reaches its original activity, so that the overall steady-state flux will *not* change. The only difference would be a lowered concentration of A; hence the increase in activity of $E_2$ is only transient. This shows that, in this example, the concentration of A is determined by the flux, and this is determined by the activity of the enzyme that catalyses the flux-generating step, $E_1$, together with the kinetic properties of enzyme $E_2$. Similarly, the concentrations of B and C are determined by the flux and the kinetic properties of $E_3$ and $E_4$, respectively. Intermediates in a biochemical process whose concentrations are determined by the flux (and which, therefore, help to maintain the steady-state flux) are termed internal effectors for that flux. From this definition it should be clear that *totally* internal effectors cannot change the flux through a linear biochemical process, unless their concentration is artificially elevated.

In relation to regulation of flux, this situation changes completely if the compound A is an allosteric inhibitor of enzyme $E_1$. In this case reaction $E_2$ *can* communicate with enzyme $E_1$, which catalyses the flux-generating step. Hence changes in X that affect $E_2$ can now affect $E_1$ and hence can alter the flux. An important question to ask for any biochemical process is as follows: is there a feedback link within the process to provide for such a communication? This simple point of control-logic is very important for understanding the hypothesis of immunosuppression in stress.

### 1.2  USE OF MAXIMUM ACTIVITIES OF ENZYMES AS QUANTITATIVE INDICES OF MAXIMUM FLUX THROUGH METABOLIC PATHWAYS

The advantage of a near-equilibrium reaction, in a metabolic pathway *in vivo*, is that the reaction may be very sensitive to small changes in concentrations of substrate, product, cosubstrate, or coproduct. Consequently, large changes in flux can be transmitted through such a reaction without any requirement for complex regulatory properties. In general, this means that the activity of the enzyme *in vitro* can be measured relatively easily in crude extracts of the tissue; this ease of assay has, unfortunately, been used by some investigators as the only criterion for the selection of an enzyme whose *in vitro* activity can provide an indication of the maximum flux through a metabolic pathway or biochemical process. This cannot be done with such enzymes! Metabolic-control logic tells us that these enzymes possess maximum catalytic activities well in excess of the maximum flux through the pathway (see above) and hence their activities *in vitro* cannot be used to provide any useful quantitative information.

Enzymes that catalyse non-equilibrium reactions in a metabolic pathway provide directionality in that pathway and are usually subject to allosteric control (see above). Indeed the control mechanisms may be complex. This means that knowledge of such control mechanisms must be available *before* a satisfactory assay for measurement of the *maximum in vitro* activity can be developed; hence, knowledge of metabolic control is necessary to enable the maximal activity of the enzyme to be assayed in extracts of the tissue *in vitro*; knowledge of which activators to add the assay system and which inhibitors to omit from the assay medium is very important.

If the maximum *in vitro* catalytic activity of such an enzyme can be measured, this information may be used to provide quantitative information about the maximum flux through the pathway. It is, however, necessary to demonstrate experimentally that the maximum activities of such enzymes *in vitro* are indeed similar to the maximum flux through the pathway at least in some conditions or in some tissues. This is done by comparison of the *in vitro* enzyme activity with the measured or calculated maximum flux through the pathway (3, 5).

### 1.3 ENZYMES, FUELS, AND FUNCTIONS

The maximal catalytic activities of a number of *key* enzymes (that catalyse non-equilibrium reactions) in a number of various tissues or cells have been measured to provide information on fuels and function.

Systematic studies in the 1970s on the maximum activities of key enzymes of carbohydrate and fatty metabolism in muscle have provided information on the types of fuels utilized by different muscles from various animals across the animal kingdom and their maximum contribution to ATP formation to support contractile activity (3, 5, 6). This work has led to a better understanding of fuel utilization and function of muscle and, in addition, to a novel mechanism for central fatigue. The latter may have significance under conditions of stress (7, 8).

A similar 'key enzyme activity' approach to the study of fuel utilization was applied to some immune cells (lymphocytes and macrophages); it provided, *for the first time*, evidence that these cells could use glutamine at a high rate for energy formation and, indeed, that this fuel could be quantitatively more important than glucose (8, 9, 10). Until this work, it had been considered that glucose was the major, if not the only, fuel to be used by lymphocytes. Despite the undoubted importance of these cells in defence of the body and in repair after injury, it was surprising that, until this recent work, almost nothing was known about the fuels that these cells require to carry out their functions, the rates of utilization or fates of the fuels, and whether the fuel selection relates to their specific cell biology.

The results of studies in key enzyme activity provided the stimulus for the measurement of rates of utilization of this fuel by the lymphocytes and by macrophages under different conditions, including culture for 96 hours: this demonstrated that, as predicted by the enzyme activities, the rates of utilization of glutamine are indeed high (11). The fact that these enzyme activities are high in lymphocytes removed from lymph nodes or the peripheral circulation suggests that the rate of glutamine utilization *in vivo* is similar to that measured *in vitro*. Furthermore, of the glutamine (and glucose) utilized by these cells, very little is oxidized via acetyl-CoA and the classic Krebs cycle: glutamine is converted almost totally into glutamate, aspartate, and lactate. Hence, the oxidation of glutamine is only partial and, in an analogous manner to the terminology used to describe the partial oxidation of glucose by these cells, the partial oxidation of glutamine has been termed glutaminolysis.

To demonstrate unequivocably that rates of utilization of glucose and glutamine by these cells are indeed high, a comparison with another tissue is instructive: the rate of utilization of glutamine by *resting* lymphocytes is almost 20 per cent of the rate of glucose utilized by a maximally active perfused rat heart.

### 1.4  A NOVEL ROLE FOR THE HIGH RATE OF GLUTAMINE UTILIZATION BY IMMUNE CELLS: BRANCHED-POINT-SENSITIVITY

The question arises as to the function of this cellular nutrition: why is the rate of glutaminolysis so high in these cells? The importance of this process in other cells has been considered: since glutamine and aspartate provide both nitrogen and carbon for *de novo* synthesis of important macromolecules (for example purine and pyrimidine nucleotides for DNA and RNA) it has been proposed that this is the role of glutaminolysis in such cells. However, knowledge of the rate of glutamine utilization by lymphocytes and the rate of synthesis of pyrimidine nucleotides shows that the rate of glutaminolysis is markedly in excess (perhaps 100-fold) of that of its use in pyrimidine nucleotide synthesis (12). An alternative suggestion was that the high rate of glutaminolysis provides energy for these cells. However, if energy generation *per se* was the major reason for the high rates, it would be expected that much more of the carbon skeleton of glutamine would be converted to acetyl-CoA for complete oxidation via the Krebs cycle (that is that glutamine oxidation rather than glutaminolysis would occur) and this is not so.

On the basis of metabolic-control-logic, it has been suggested that the high rate of glutaminolysis (and also, importantly, that of glycolysis), provide ideal conditions for sensitive control of changes in the rate of the use of the intermediates of this pathway for biosynthesis precisely at the time required by the cell (for example glutamine for purine and pyrimidine nucleotide synthesis; aspartate for pyrimidine synthesis) (13, 14). This principle in metabolic control is known as branched-point-sensitivity. High rates of glutaminolysis (and also glycolysis) can thus be seen as part of a mechanism of control to permit synthesis of macromolecules when required without any need for extracellular signals to make more glutamine (or glucose) available. This will be important for proliferation of lymphocytes which can occur at any time in response to an immune challenge. Similarly, it will be important for those cells that require, at specific times, high rates of mRNA synthesis (for example macrophages).

The pathway for glutamine utilization by these cells *in vivo* uses glutamine from the bloodstream. The importance of the concentration of glutamine in the blood for lymphocyte function can be analysed both theoretically and experimentally. Studies on glutamine utilization by isolated lymphocytes or macrophages demonstrate that this pathway of glutamine utilization is not saturated with external glutamine. Hence the utilization of glutamine by these cells, which appears to be so important for their function, will be affected by the plasma concentration. Since glutamine is produced elsewhere in the body, the plasma glutamine can be considered, according to metabolic-control-logic, to be an internal regulator of the pathway of glutaminolysis in lymphocytes and macrophages (see above). An important prediction from this is that if the plasma glutamine concentration is decreased below the physiological level, the rate of utilization of glutamine will be decreased and so will the proliferation of lymphocytes and the function of macrophages; this will impair the function of the immune system as a whole. This prediction has been tested *in vitro*: thus both rat and human lymphocytes in culture stimulated to proliferate respond less well as the concentration of glutamine in the culture medium is decreased, and phagocytosis by macrophages is similarly decreased (12, 15).

The important point to emerge from this discussion is that glutamine must be used at a *high* rate by the cells of the immune system even when they are quiescent. The immune response to invasion by a microorganism must be rapid: hence, the rate of glutamine utilization must always be high to provide optimal conditions for an immediate response to an immune challenge at *any* time. Although this high rate of utilization, even at times when it is not required, might seem wasteful it should be noted that the function of these cells is *essential* for the survival of the animal, as has been dramatically emphasized recently by the effects of HIV infection on the immune system and consequently patient survival.

This then raises the questions, what is the source of this glutamine, and what is the flux-generating step for the provision of plasma glutamine and therefore for glutaminolysis in immune cells?

## 2   Muscle and the provision of glutamine for the immune system

Although it can be considered that glutamine present in the blood is made 'available' from dietary protein via digestion, this is *not* the case. Most, if not all, of the glutamine absorbed into the epithelial cells of the intestine is metabolized within these cells. Hence the blood glutamine level must be maintained by tissues that can synthesize glutamine—mainly liver and muscle, and it seems that skeletal muscle plays an important if not a major role (16). This has considerable implications for modern medicine.

It has been known for many years that surgery, trauma, sepsis, or burns result in negative nitrogen balance and this is due largely to an increased net rate of skeletal muscle breakdown. The reason for the increased net rate of protein degradation has been discussed for many years and several suggestions have been put forward; for example it provides amino acids for protein synthesis which will be required for repair processes, for acute phase protein synthesis, and for the cells of the immune system. It also provides amino acids that act as precursors for hepatic gluconeogenesis. On the basis of above discussions, one further hypothesis can be put forward. Increased rates of protein degradation will provide branched-chain and other amino acids that will donate their nitrogen for the synthesis of glutamine in the muscle. Indeed this may be the reason for the very high rates of degradation—to satisfy the very high demands for glutamine. Hence protein degradation in muscle can be considered to be part of the process that provides branched-point-sensitivity to maintain the *essential* function of some cells of the immune system (17).

Skeletal muscle not only synthesizes glutamine but it stores a large amount: the concentration may be approximately 20 mM in man. Since the process of glutamine transport across the muscle cell membrane from inside to outside is non-equilibrium and since it is close to saturation with the intracellular glutamine, this transport process appears to be the flux-generating step for release of glutamine, and, therefore, for the maintenance of the plasma level and its *utilization* by the immune cells. Consequently under physiological conditions, the outward transport of glutamine (and not synthesis) from muscle controls the rate of uptake by and, therefore, the function of the immune cells. Since this process is of considerable importance in defence of the body, it is not surprising that the rate of release appears to be influenced by a number of hormones, metabolites, or changes in physiological conditions (18).

The two pieces of information provided above suggest that muscle can be considered to be part of the immune system in that the overall metabolic pathway which provides glutamine for the immune cells starts in muscle. That is, muscle contains the flux-generating step for a process that is essential for proper function of the immune cells. However, there is no evidence of a direct feedback communication link in this glutamine pathway from immune cells to skeletal muscle (see above). Therefore, failure of muscle to provide enough glutamine could result in a lowering of the plasma glutamine level and hence an impairment in the function of the immune system.

Can the extension of the immune system, to include muscle, provide an indirect link between brain and the immune cells and hence for an additional or alternative explanation for the role of stress in causing immunosuppression and therefore increasing the risk of cancer?

## 3 Glutamine, immune cells, and cancer

A systematic study of the activities of key enzymes in neoplastic cells has been carried out. The activity of glutaminase is high and, in most cases, greater than that of hexokinase so that glutamine may be more important than glucose as a fuel in these cells (19). In general, the activities of glutaminase in tumour cells are approximately similar to those in immune cells.

The presence of considerable activities of glutaminase in the neoplastic cells is consistent with the proposal that high rates of glutaminolysis provide optimal conditions for precise regulation of changes in the rate of the biosynthetic processes which use intermediates of glutaminolysis—that is, branched-point-sensitivity for purine and pyrimidine nucleotide synthesis in these cells. If this is the case, there may well be competition between tumour cells and immune cells for glutamine and hence for 'proliferation'. It may also be the case that although tumour cells do not, in general, have a higher activity of the key enzyme of this pathway, the enzyme in tumour cells may have a lower $K_M$ value for glutamine so that tumour cells will be able to compete more effectively for the limited glutamine that is available to both types of cell. One could speculate that the demand for glutamine by the tumour is so great that when glutamine concentrations are decreased not only in the plasma but also in the vicinity of the growing tumour, immune function (for example lymphocyte killer activity, macrophage phagocytosis, and secretion of cytokines) in this local area may be markedly inhibited. This may, in part, result in the tumour's ability to grow largely unhindered by the normal defence mechanism of the body.

It has been shown, in tumour-bearing animals, that although the rate of glutamine release by muscle increases, the plasma level of glutamine decreases. Indeed the demand by the tumour for glutamine and, therefore, for protein degradation (see above) may be such as to be a possible cause of cancer cachexia (18, 19). It is possible to speculate that the role of the increased rate of protein breakdown in skeletal muscle that occurs in this condition may be primarily to supply amino acid precursors for the synthesis and release of glutamine which is required by the tumour. In this case, the tumour will act as a 'sink' for muscle-derived glutamine, and this may be so great that cachexia develops. This may eventually limit the ability of muscle to provide glutamine at previous rates and the plasma concentration may decrease even further.

It is, therefore, possible to suggest that if stress has a similar effect on lowering the plasma glutamine level this might encourage tumour growth at the expense of immune function. The next question is how stress may influence muscle function, especially in relation to glutamine release. To answer this, it is necessary to move the biochemical discussions laterally, to discuss brain 5-hydroxytryptamine and central fatigue.

## 4   Plasma tryptophan, brain 5-hydroxytryptamine, and central fatigue

One important role of some amino acids is that they act as precursors for certain brain neurotransmitters — in particular, the monoamines. One of these amino acids is tryptophan, which is converted in the brain to the neurotransmitter 5-hydroxytryptamine (5-HT).

There is some evidence to support the view that, if the concentration of a neurotransmitter in the brain is decreased, this may limit the rate of neuronal firing in some parts of the brain, especially if the rate of neuronal firing is high. And there is evidence to support the view that an increase in the level of 5-HT in the brain can result in tiredness and sleep. It has been suggested, as a working hypothesis, that an increase in the concentration of this neurotransmitter in certain areas of the brain might maintain a high rate of neuronal firing in a specific part of the brain which results in an increase in the sensitivity to fatigue. This would be described as central fatigue. The metabolic-control-logic underlying the hypothesis is as follows.

It is generally considered that none of the reactions in the pathway for formation of 5-HT in the brain approach saturation with pathway substrate, that is there is no flux-generating step in this pathway. The reactions include: transport of tryptophan across the blood–brain barrier, transport of tryptophan across the nerve cell membrane, and those catalysed by tryptophan 5-mono-oxygenase and aromatic amino acid decarboxylase. Hence, an increase in the plasma concentration of tryptophan (an internal regulator) could lead to an increase in the rate of formation and hence an increase in the concentration of 5-HT in the brain (20, 21). In addition, tryptophan is the only amino acid in the bloodstream that binds to albumin so that plasma tryptophan occurs in both bound and free forms. Since it is likely that the free rather than the total concentration controls the rate of uptake by the brain, the free concentration rather than the total concentration of tryptophan will control the rate of entry into the brain. The proportion of tryptophan bound to albumin can be decreased (that is the free concentration can be increased) by increasing the plasma concentration of long-chain fatty acids, which are also bound to albumin. Since the plasma fatty acid concentration can be increased as a result of physical activity, and also by stress, this would be expected to increase the free plasma concentration of tryptophan and the brain concentration of 5-HT. This might result in central fatigue.

Support for this hypothesis has been based on experiments which make use of the fact that tryptophan entry into brain suffers competition from the entry of branched-chain amino acids. Hence, it is likely to be the concentration ratio of free tryptopban/branched-chain amino acids in the blood that influences the 5-HT level in the brain. This ratio can be modified, simply, by ingestion of branched-chain amino acids which raise their plasma level and hence lowers the plasma concentration ratio of free tryptopban/branched-chain amino acids. This has been shown to influence physical and mental performance in some athletes (22, 23).

The important question here is how this may relate to the release of glutamine by muscle. It is suggested that the answer is via the sympathetic nervous system. From the brain stem, 5-HT neurons project to the hypothalamus which is considered to be the major centre for autonomic, endocrine, and neuronal integration. A chronic increase in the stimulation of the sympathetic system might cause a decrease in the rate of release of glutamine from skeletal muscle. Thus, it has been shown that whereas an acute increase in adrenaline has no effect on glutamine release, chronic elevation of the plasma adrenaline level in the rat decreases the rate of glutamine release from muscle (18). Consistent with this, exposure of rats to the cold for 48 hours decreases their rate of glutamine release from muscle (18). Furthermore, a prolonged bout of exercise or daily intense exercise-training results in a decrease in the rate of glutamine release by muscle and a decrease in the plasma glutamine level and hence immune cell function (24).

Hence an effect of stress on mobilization of fatty acids from adipose tissue, or an effect of stress on the binding of tryptophan by albumin, could lead to an increase in plasma concentration ratio of free tryptophan/branched-chain amino acids, and hence in the level of brain 5-HT. The latter via the sympathetic system could affect glutamine release by muscle and this could have detrimental effects on immune cell function. Although the hypothesis is complicated, each component part is testable and by using old-fashioned biochemical techniques.

## 5   Glucocorticoid hormones, 5-hydroxytryptamine, and stress

Stress results in adaptation within the body which improves the ability of the body to respond to the change in conditions. However this adaptation appears to be finite — both in extent and in time. Selye (25) proposed that the body possesses a certain amount of 'adaptational energy' to allow the body to adapt to changed conditions, and that when this energy runs out, illness results. What is the biochemical basis of this 'adaptational energy'?

The suggestion that the increase in the blood level of glucocorticoids could impair immune function may occur via direct effects on the immune cells, or on muscle glutamine release (18) but also via effects on the brain.

Two types of glucocorticoid receptors exist in the brain, Type I or corticosterone receptors (CR) and Type II or glucocorticoid receptors (GR). These two types of receptors participate in different responses to corticosterone (26). The CR receptors respond to the normal diurnal variations in corticosterone levels, and are considered to be responsible for increased appetite and exploratory activity at the beginning of the waking period. The GR receptors are considered to be involved in the adaptation that occurs in response to the raised levels of glucocorticoids as a result of exposure to stress. One effect of GR receptor-stimulation is a decrease in the number or affinity of 5-HT receptors in the brain, in an attempt to oppose the stress-induced elevation of brain 5-HT level (see above). Thus, in this case, corticosterone could be seen to be attempting to protect the body from some of the effects of stress.

It is possible that prolonged exposure to stress and, therefore, a more chronic increase in the glucocorticoid level could lead to down-regulation of the GR receptors. This might then result in a restoration of the 5-HT receptors to normal numbers or normal sensitivity. This action would allow 5-HT receptors to mediate the full response to the elevated levels of 5-HT, one of which may be central fatigue and another may be a decreased rate of glutamine release from muscle and hence decreased plasma glutamine levels and, therefore, as indicated above, impaired immune function.

It is hypothesized, therefore, that the immunosuppression observed in stress is due to prolonged exposure to the elevated corticosterone levels, which may affect the immune system indirectly via a decrease in the number of GR receptors in the brain and the consequent effect on muscle. Consequently, the normal adaptation in response to stress will occur until the GR receptors are down-regulated. This will be equivalent to the start of 'exhaustion' of the adaptational energy which will also depend upon the time necessary to restore the 'activity' of the brain 5-HT receptors to normal. This, via effects on the rate of muscle glutamine release, could lead to a markedly increased risk of disease, including the development of cancer.

# 6 References

1. Klitzman, S., House, J. S., Israel, E., and Mero, R. P. (1990). Works stress, non work stress and health. *J. Behav. Med.*, **13**, 221–243.
2. Khansari, D. N., Murgo, A. J., and Faith, R. E. (1990). Effects of stress on the immune system. *Immunology Today*, **11** (5), 170–175.
3. Newsholme, E. A. and Leech, A. R. (1983*b*). *Biochemistry for the medical sciences*. Wiley Chichester.
4. Newsholme, E. A. and Start, C. (1973). *Regulation in Metabolism*. Wiley, Chichester.
5. Newsholme, E. A., Crabtree, B., and Zammit, V. A. (1980). Use of enzyme activities as indices of maximum rates of fuel utilisation. *Ciba Found. Symp. 1980*, **73**, 245–258.
6. Blomstrand, E., Ekblom, B., and Newsholme. E. A (1986). Maximal activities of key glycolytic and oxidative enzymes in muscle from differently trained individuals. *J. Physiol.*, **381**, 111–119.
7. Newsholme, E. A., Blomstrand, E., and Ekblom, B. (1992). Physical and mental fatigue: metabolic mechanisms and importance of plasma amino acids. *Br. Med. Bull.*, **48**, 477–495.
8. Ardawi, M. S. M. and Newsholme, E. A. (1979). Glutamine metabolism in lymphocytes of the rat. *Blochem. J.*, **212**, 835–842.
9. Ardawi, M. S. M. and Newsholme, E. A. (1985). Metabolism in lymphocytes and its importance to the immune response. *Essays Biochem.*, **21**, 1–44.
10. Newsholme, P., Gordon, S., and Newsholme, E. A. (1987). Rates of utilization and fates of glucose, glutamine, pyruvate, fatty acids and ketone bodies by mouse macrophages. *Biochem. J.*, **242**, 631–636.
11. Newsholme, E. A. and Newsholme, P. (1989). Rates of utilisation of glucose, glutamine and oleate and formation of end-products by mouse peritoneal macrophages in culture. *Biochem. J.*, **261**, 211–218.
12. Szondy, Z. and Newsholme, E. A. (1989). The effect of glutamine concentration on the activity of carbamyl-phosphate synthase II and on the incorporation of [$^3$H]thymidine into DNA in rat mesenteric lymphocytes stimulated by phyto-haemagglutinin. *Biochem. J.*, **261**, 979–983.
13. Newsholme, E. A., Crabtree, B., and Ardawi, M. S. M. (1985). The role of high rates of glycolysis and glutamine utilisation in rapidly-dividing cells. *Biosci. Rep.*, **4**, 393–400.
14. Newsholme, E. A., Crabtree, B., and Ardawi, M. S. M. (1985). Glutamine metabolism in lymphocytes, its biochemical, physiological and clinical importance. *Q.J. Exp. Physiol.*, **70**, 473–489.
15. Parry-Billings, M., Evans, J., Calder, P. C., and Newsholme, E. A. (1990). Immunosuppression following major burns: could glutamine play a role. *Lancet*, **336**, 523–525.
16. Ardawi, M. S. M. (1988). Skeletal muscle glutamine production in thermally injured rats. *Clin. Sci.*, **74**, 165–172.
17. Newsholme, E. A., Newsholme, P., Curi, R., Challoner, E., and Ardawi,

M. S. M. (1988). A role for muscle in the immune system and its importance in surgery, trauma, sepsis and burns. *Nutrition*, **4**, 261–268.

18. Parry-Billings, M. (1989). Studies on glutamine release by skeletal muscle. D. Phil. thesis. Oxford University.

19. Parry-Billings, M., Leighton, B., Dimitriadis, G. D., Colquhoun, A., and Newsholme, E. A. (1991). The effect of tumour bearing on skeletal muscle glutamine metabolism. *Int. J. Biochem.*, **23**, 933–937.

20. Blomstrand, E., Perrett, D., Parry-Billings, M., and Newsholme, E. A. (1989). Effect of sustained exercise on plasma amino acid concentrations and on 5-hydroxytryptamine metabolism in six different brain regions in the rat. *Acta Physiol. Scand.*, **136**, 473–481.

21. Blomstrand, E., Celsing, F., and Newsholme, E. A. (1988). Changes in concentration of aromatic and branched-chain amino acids during sustained exercise in man and their possible role in fatigue. *Acta Physiol. Scand.*, **133**, 115–121.

22. Blomstrand, E., Hassmen, P., and Newsholme, E. A. (1991). Administration of branched-chain amino acids during sustained exercise—effects on performance and on the plasma concentrations of some amino acids. *Eur. J. Appl. Physiol.*, **63**, 83–88.

23. Blomstrand, E., Hassmen, P., and Newsholme, E. A. (1991). Effect of branched-chain amino acid supplementation on mental performance. *Acta Physiol. Scand.*, **143**, 225–226.

24. Parry-Billings, M., Budgett, R., Koutedakis, Y., Blomstrand, E., Brooks, S., and Williams, C. *et al.* (1992). Plasma amino acid concentrations in the overtraining syndrome: possible effects on the immune system. *Med. Sci. Sports Exerc.*, **24**, 1353–1358.

25. Selye, H. (1974). *The Stress of Life*, pp. 25–29. J. B. Lippincot & Co., Philadelphia.

26. McEwan, B. S. (1987). Glucocorticoid-biogenic amine interaction in relation to mood and behaviour. *Biochem. Pharmacol.*, **36**, 1755–1763.

# PART II
# Mind and body in cancer treatment

# 4

# Psychotherapy, stress, and survival in breast cancer

## C. CLASSEN, K. S. HERMANSON, AND D. SPIEGEL

# 1   Introduction

Breast cancer is a profoundly stressful disease, posing both physical and psychological threats to the patient. The diagnosis radically alters an individual's life. She faces the possibility of a foreshortened future, with 50 per cent long-term mortality from the disease. The anxiety and fear this engenders takes its toll, both on her and those around her. In addition, she may begin a regimen of treatment with serious side-effects, such as the loss of a breast, infertility, impaired sexual functioning, hair loss, and a lack of energy. Given the multifaceted nature of this stressor, most breast cancer patients are likely to benefit from psychotherapeutic interventions.

There is a growing literature showing that psychotherapeutic interventions have an important place in the management of breast cancer. There are important differences in the types of interventions, some emphasizing mutual support and emotional expression, others education and behavioural change. Some occur in groups, others in individual settings. There is a growing array of evidence that such interventions positively affect various aspects of the quality of life, as well as reducing symptoms of the disease and its treatment. More recently, several studies have provided evidence of an effect of psychotherapy on survival time, provoking interest in psychophysiological mechanisms mediating such an effect. Research examining the relation between stress and both endocrine and immune function provides some clues to possible mechanisms. These psychotherapeutic approaches pose a challenge to the traditional twentieth century reductionist approaches to medical care, which focus on attacking the disease rather than helping the person with the disease to better cope with it. In this chapter we will review the literature on the various types of psychotherapeutic intervention available for breast cancer patients, their effects on psychosocial and physical outcome, and the possible mechanisms underlying these lines with special emphasis on the immune system (the reader is also referred to the chapters in Part III of this volume for more information on the latter).

The body of evidence reviewed below leaves little question as to the positive impact that psychosocial interventions have in reducing distress and improving the quality of life of cancer patients. There is less evidence regarding their potential impact on the survival time of cancer patients. Questions regarding the impact of psychosocial interventions on immunological variables and survival time in cancer patients will be addressed, along with recommendations for future research and implications for the practice of oncology.

Although the aim of this chapter is to discuss the benefits of psychotherapy on women with breast cancer, very few studies focus solely on breast cancer patients. Consequently, most of the studies discussed below include patients with different types of cancer, including breast cancer. See Table 1 for a summary of these studies.

## 2   Impact of psychosocial interventions on quality of life

### 2.1 PSYCHOSOCIAL ADJUSTMENT

Several studies have examined the effect of psychotherapeutic interventions on psychosocial adjustment in cancer patients (1–10). Some have demonstrated strong positive effects (1–3 , 7–8). One study examined the impact of two forms of psychosocial interventions, group and individual, in comparison with a control group (1) . They found that at the one- to two-week follow-up all subjects were significantly less depressed and anxious than at baseline. At six-month follow-up, however, the participants in the two intervention groups were significantly less depressed and anxious than the control group subjects. Similar positive effects of psychosocial treatment were found in another study where newly diagnosed patients in the treatment condition demonstrated less fatigue and confusion, more vigour, and less frustration, depression, anxiety, and apathy than patients in the control condition (2). Interestingly, subjects receiving the treatment condition show less denial and no reduction in hopelessness when compared with control subjects. This suggests that facing the reality of a cancer diagnosis, in combination with psychosocial skills to deal with intense emotion, results in decreased mood disturbance and no increase in feelings of futility or hopelessness.

In another study, 'emotional symptom scores' were assessed for patients undergoing radiation therapy (3). These scores included items of depression, pessimism, hopelessness, somatic preoccupation and worry, social isolation and withdrawal, insomnia, anxiety, and agitation. All patients demonstrated improvement over time, but in contrast to the control group, patients in the psychosocial intervention group demonstrated significantly lower emotional symptom scores from the end of the intervention to the final follow-up assessment.

Other studies have demonstrated more variable effects of psychosocial

**Table 1** Psychotherapeutic intervention reviewed

| Reference | Number of participants | Type of cancer | Type of intervention | Number of sessions | Psychosocial outcome |
|---|---|---|---|---|---|
| Cain et al. 1986 (1)* | 80 women (21 = individual tx; 28 = group tx; 31 = control) | Gynaecological cancer: endometrial, ovarian, vaginal, and vulvar | (1) thematic individual tx; (2) thematic group tx. | 8 weekly sessions (both tx conditions) | Decreased anxiety, depression and improved adjustment for all pts w/time; lower anxiety for those receiving individual tx than for those in other conditions |
| Capone et al. (6) 1980 | 97 women (56 = tx; 41 = control) | Gynaecological cancer: cervical, endometrial, ovarian, vulvar, vaginal | Individual counselling during hospitalization | Minimum of 4 sessions (no other information available) | No difference in mood disturbance; non-significant difference in return to work (2:1 ratio between groups); improved sexual functioning in the tx condition |
| Christensen 1983 (4)* | 20 couples (10 = tx; 10 = control) | Post-mastectomy breast cancer patients and their spouses | Individual couples therapy: structured communication and problem-solving skills | 4 weekly sessions | Better sexual satisfaction for women and spouses in tx condition; decreased depression for women in tx; no difference between groups in self-esteem, anxiety, or alienation; better psychosocial adjustment for couples in tx. |
| Edgar et al. (48) 1992# | 205 patients (103 = early tx; 102 = late tx) | Mixed cancer: breast (48%), lung, colon, head/neck, other | Individual behavioural skills training conducted by oncology nurse | 5, 1-hour sessions | Late tx condition reports decreased depression, anxiety, and intrusive thoughts, and increased sense of control compared to early tx condition at 8 month follow-up; differences in intrusive thoughts persist at 12 month follow-up. |

| | | | | | |
|---|---|---|---|---|---|
| Fawzy *et al.* 1990*a* (8)* and 1990*b* (78)* | 66 patients (38 = tx; 28 = control) | Malignant melanoma | Structured group intervention: health education, stress management, problem-solving, psychosocial support, coping skills | 6 weekly, 1.5-hour sessions | At 6 week follow-up, increased vigor in tx group compared with control; at 6 months, decreased depression, fatigue, confusion, and mood disturbance in tx group; at both time points, tx group demonstrates more active coping |
| Ferlic *et al.* 1979 (15)+ | 60 patients (30 = tx; 30 = control) | Mixed cancer: no further descriptions | Structured, thematic, educational group intervention | 6, 1.5-hour sessions meeting 3 times a week for two weeks | Post-intervention, tx group shows improved hospital adjustment, better knowledge of disease, improved positive self-concept and better death perception than controls; both tx and controls demonstrated decreased self-concept at 6-month follow-up |
| Forester *et al.* 1985 (3)* | 100 patients (48 = tx; 52 = control) | Mixed cancer: lung, prostate, uterine, bladder, cervical | Unstructured, 'supportive', individual therapy | 10 weekly, 30-minute sessions | Both conditions show better physical and psychosocial adjustment w/time, but tx condition shows more; long-term psychosocial adjustment is better for those patients who know their diagnosis. |

**Table 1** (*continued*)

| Reference | Number of participants | Type of cancer | Type of intervention | Number of sessions | Psychosocial outcome |
|---|---|---|---|---|---|
| Gellert *et al.* (32) 1993 | 136 women (34 = tx; 102 = 'comparison' subjects) | Breast cancer | Programme combining peer support, family therapy, individual counselling, positive mental imagery | On-going, weekly, 1.5-hour sessions (peer groups, only); other is unspecified | Non-significant difference in survival time as a function of participation in the ECaP program |
| Gordon *et al.* 1980 (10)[++] | 308 patients (157 = tx; 151 = control) | Mixed cancer: breast (32%), lung, melanoma | Individual therapy: education, counselling, and consultation aspects | As needed for 6 months; available to in-patients and out-patients | No difference in # of psychosocial problems reported as a function of condition; lower anxiety and depression for breast and lung cancer pts in tx condition; greater physical activity for all pts in tx condition. |
| Heinrich and Coscarelli-Schag (5) 1985 | 51 patients and 25 spouses (26 = tx w/12 spouses; 25 = control w/13 spouses | Mixed cancer: lung, colorectal, prostate, breast (27%) | Structured, 'stress and activity management' group interventions | 6 weekly, 2-hour sessions (spouses and patients combined) | all pts (not spouses) show increased knowledge of disease and improved psychosocial adjustment w/time; higher increase in knowledge for couples in tx than for those in control; no difference in activity level as a function of time or tx condition; pts in tx condition report greater sexual satisfaction |

| Study | Sample | Cancer type | Intervention | Sessions | Findings |
|---|---|---|---|---|---|
| Jacobs *et al.* 1983 (16)* | 81 patients in two studies: 1) 21 = tx, 26 = control; 2) 16 = tx, 18 = control | Hodgkin's disease | (1) educational mailings; (2) unstructured, peer support group | 8 weekly, 1.5-hour sessions (peer support condition only) | (1) increased knowledge of disease, decreased anxiety and tx problems, improved depression, and fewer life disruptions for those in this tx condition; decreased social competency for those in tx condition. (2) all pts show improved depression, interpersonal problems, anxiety, personal habits, and tx problems w/time; those in tx condition show decreased physical activity |
| Linn *et al.* 1982 (9)* | 120 men (62 = tx; 58 = control) | Mixed cancer: lung, colon, stomach, pancreas, prostate, bladder, other | Unstructured, individual therapy (based on a Kubler-Ross model) | Not reported | At 3 months, those in tx condition show decreased depression and alienation, increased life satisfaction and self-esteem; all findings persist at 6, 9 and 12 months except depression; no significant difference in survival time as a function of tx condition |
| Lyles *et al.* 1982 (29)* | 50 patients (18 = relaxation condition; 14 = therapist-present control; 18 = other 'control') | Mixed cancer: breast (28%), lung, ovarian, testicular, lymphoma, Hodgkin's disease, other | (1) training in relaxation skills; (2) therapist sits w/pt during chemo; (3) pt alone, instructed to 'relax' | 3 training sessions (relaxation condition only) | (1) pts in this condition show decreased pulse, systolic blood pressure, anxiety, depression, and nausea by contrast to other conditions (2) pts in this condition show less anxiety than the control pts, more nausea than other conditions, but less intensity of nausea than the control condition |

**Table 1** *(continued)*

| Reference | Number of participants | Type of cancer | Type of intervention | Number of sessions | Psychosocial outcome |
|---|---|---|---|---|---|
| Morgenstern *et al.* 1994 (30) | 136 women (34 = tx; 102 = 'comparison' subjects) | Breast cancer | Programme combining peer support, family therapy, individual counselling, positive mental imagery | On-going, weekly, 1.5-hour sessions (peer groups, only); other is unspecified | Trend suggesting increased survival for ECaP pts (Gellert *et al.*) was non-significant due to selection bias |
| Morrow and Morrell 1982 (28)* | 60 patients (20 = systematic desensitization; 20 = counselling; 20 = control) | Mixed cancer: breast (48%), hematologic, lung, other | (1) desensitization training with progressive muscle relaxation; (2) Rogerian, unstructured counselling; (3) control | 2, 1-hour sessions (each condition) | Pts receiving systematic desensitization show decreased anticipatory nausea, decreased severity and duration of nausea, decreased anticipatory vomiting, decreased severity of vomiting, and higher expectations of psychosocial tx success than pts in other conditions; no differences in duration of anticipatory vomiting |
| Spiegel *et al.* 1981 (7)* and 1989 (31)* | 86 patients (50 = tx; 36 = control) | Metastatic breast cancer | Unstructured, supportive-expressive group therapy | Weekly, 1.5-hour sessions on-going for one year | Pts in tx condition show increased survival time, decreased mood disturbance, decreased maladaptive coping, and decreased phobic responses in contrast to controls |

| Study | Sample | Diagnosis | Intervention | Schedule | Results |
|---|---|---|---|---|---|
| Spiegel and Bloom 1983 (27)* | 58 women (34 = tx; 24 = control) | Metastatic breast cancer | Unstructured, supportive–expressive group therapy with or without self-hypnosis training | Weekly, 1.5-hour sessions on-going for one year | Pts receiving tx w/hypnosis show best ability to control pain sensation, those receiving tx w/o hypnosis control pain sensation better than those in control group; no differences in pain frequency or duration as a function of tx condition; for control group, increased pain duration correlates with increased tension/anxiety, depression, fatigue; for both tx groups, decreased pain sensation correlates with decreased mood disturbance |
| Spiegel and Glafkides 1983 (26) | 34 women (all assigned to tx condition as part of larger study) | Metastatic breast cancer | Unstructured, supportive–expressive group therapy | Weekly, 1.5-hour sessions on-going for one year | Physical deterioration of fellow group members affects content of group sessions, but does not affect group mood |
| Telch and Telch 1986 (42)** | 41 patients with marked distress (27 = tx; 14 = control) | Mixed cancer: breast (36%), Hodgkin's disease, lymphoma, other | (1) structured, behavioural, coping skills group; (2) unstructured, supportive group; (3) control | 6 weekly, 1.5-hour sessions | Pts in the coping skills condition show decreased mood disturbance, increased self-efficacy, but fewer disease-specific problems; pts in support condition show no change in mood disturbance or self-efficacy, fewer disease-specific problems; pts in control condition show increased mood disturbance, decreased self-efficacy, no change in disease-specific problems |

**Table 1** (*continued*)

| Reference | Number of participants | Type of cancer | Type of intervention | Number of sessions | Psychosocial outcome |
|---|---|---|---|---|---|
| Worden and Weisman 1984 (2)* | 117 patients with initial distress (59 = tx; 58 = control) | Mixed cancer: breast, colon, lung, melanoma, Hodgkin's disease, gynaecological cancers | (1) unstructured individual therapy; (2) individual structured coping skills therapy; (3) control | 4 weekly sessions (each condition) | In contrast to controls, pts in tx conditions show decreased distress, no difference in # of problems reported but greater resolution of problems; no difference in rated effectiveness of two txs |

\* Indicates a design including a randomized control group.
\# Indicates random assignment to two treatment conditions with no control group.
\+ No statement of random assignment.
\+\+ Non-equivalent control group design with multiple time series.
\*\* Patients grouped together by order of recruitment, then groups were randomly assigned to intervention conditions.
tx, treatment.

interventions (4–6, 10). Women with breast cancer involved in a couples intervention schedule following mastectomy had lower adjusted mean scores on the Beck Depression Inventory compared with control group members, but did not differ on the State-Trait Anxiety Inventory (4).

Two studies demonstrated better psychosocial adjustment over time for all patients enrolled in their studies irrespective of treatment condition, with neither study demonstrating an effect of psychosocial intervention on measures such as adjustment to illness or mood state (5, 6). The lack of effect on mood and psychosocial adjustment in these studies may be due to the treatment offered to the treatment groups. In one study (5) the treatment was provided in a class format that focused on education of patients and spouses. The intervention was not intended to address issues of support or emotional expression. Knowledge of the disease is helpful but does not necessarily achieve a sense of personal control and emotional adjustment to a diagnosis of cancer. In the second study (6) an attempt was made to address issues of personal importance to the patients. However, individuals in the treatment group were seen only four times during the course of their hospitalizations to treat the cancer and its side-effects. Given the brevity of this intervention, compounded by the fact that many patients were probably very ill during the intervention sessions, it was unlikely that the treatment goals could be accomplished.

## 2.2 COPING PATTERNS

Lazarus and Folkman (11) have studied the interaction between stress, the appraisal of an event as threatening or distressing, and effective coping patterns. Other research has theorized that coping skills and the ability to resolve problems may be related to adjustment among cancer patients. One study found that perceptions of the stressfulness of cancer-related problems were related to coping patterns employed (12). Coping by rallying one's social support was associated with decreased emotional distress while forms of escape-avoidance coping led to increased emotional distress. In another study, two interventions were compared for patients with newly diagnosed cancer who were expected to be at high risk of distress (2). Both interventions focused on problem-solving. The first intervention involved therapist-directed facilitation of problem-related issues and affect; the second taught patients specific problem-solving methods. By contrast with the no-treatment control, the intervention groups reported the same number of problems at follow-up but demonstrated significantly better problem-resolution skills and significantly less distress than did control group members. Another study measured maladaptive coping behaviors used by study participants such as smoking, drinking, or overeating in response to stress (7). At one-year evaluation, women receiving a supportive–expressive group intervention demonstrated significantly fewer maladaptive coping behaviors than did women in the control group.

Similar coping behaviors were found among those participating in a study of group interventions for melanoma patients (8). Patients were assessed on the Psychological Adjustment to Illness–Coping Inventory which measures an individual's behavioural and cognitive responses to stress. Analyses revealed that immediately following the completion of the intervention, the intervention group demonstrated significantly greater use of active-behavioural and active-cognitive coping responses than the control group. These findings remained significant at the six-month follow-up evaluation.

These studies suggest that the addition of efficacious coping skills may be one of the mechanisms by which psychosocial interventions assist cancer patients in reducing their levels of stress. Whether these skills are actively taught (2) or learned via exposure to others' strategies (7), psychosocial interventions appear to provide an environment which encourages the development and maintenance of such skills.

## 2.3 DAILY ACTIVITIES

Activities of daily living are often altered for cancer patients. This may occur for a number of reasons; they may feel ill and lacking in energy, their time may be diverted to treatment-related efforts, or they may retreat from the world because of distress, feelings of isolation, or being overwhelmed by the new demands placed on them. Consequently, reductions in daily activities may reflect that an individual is experiencing some distress. Additionally, reductions in daily activities may lead to increased distress as individuals are again reminded of changes in health status.

Psychosocial interventions may address some of the impediments to active living. In one study, participants completed a 'modified activities of daily living checklist' (10). Participants receiving the treatment condition reported significantly more active lifestyles than those in the control condition at the three-month follow-up. Furthermore, while not statistically significant, at the six month follow-up, twice as many of the breast cancer and melanoma patients in the intervention condition had returned to work than in the control group. Similar findings were reported in an intervention study of gynaecological oncology patients (6). Members of the intervention group returned to work by the three month assessment at twice the rate of the control group members. However, due to small group sizes these results were not statistically significant. In another study with gynaencological oncology patients, those who received a structured, psychosocial intervention, either in an individual or a group format, demonstrated significantly greater participation in leisure activities than control group members at a six month follow-up evaluation (1). Nonetheless, others have found no effect of psychosocial treatment on the level of daily activities at a two-month follow-up assessment (5). While mixed, these studies suggest that daily activity patterns might be responsive to interventions that assist cancer patients in adjusting to emotional factors.

## 2.4 CONTROL AND SELF-EFFICACY

Patients often report a sense of loss of personal control following a diagnosis of cancer. Regaining a sense of control may be instrumental in psychosocial adjustment. Women given a choice regarding their medical treatment have been shown to have fewer symptoms of depression than their counterparts who received no treatment options (13). While in reality, some events are not under a patient's control, the sense of overwhelming helplessness that some patients feel can extend to situations where patients should feel able to assert their wishes. This is another area that potentially could be amenable to change via psychosocial treatment. In a study with advanced stage cancer patients, participation in individual counselling, which focused on decreasing denial while sustaining hope, led to increases in an internal locus of control for those patients surviving to the follow-up assessments (9). Similar results were not seen in control group participants.

## 2.5 SELF-IMAGE

Self-esteem can suffer as patients surrender former roles and identities to the demands of their illness. Debilitation secondary to the disease and its treat-ment, and diminishing roles disrupt usual reinforcers of self-esteem. Patients' perceptions of their bodies are often distorted as a result of surgery and treat-ment side-effects. This can be especially salient for breast cancer patients, whose sense of sexuality is often radically altered by surgery and treatment side-effects (14).

Two studies with late stage cancer patients have shown improvements in self-esteem and self-concept as a result of individual counselling (9) and group counselling (5). In a study of newly diagnosed patients, individual counselling was found to help stave off the decline of self-concept, such as was found in the control group (6). Others hypothesized an increase in self-esteem for treat-ment group participants but found no effect of treatment relative to control (4, 7). These studies provide mixed results regarding the impact of psycho-social intervention on self-concept or self-esteem of cancer patients. Further study is required to know how we can assist cancer patients in adjusting to a loss of prior roles without a concomitant diminution of self-esteem.

## 2.6 SEXUAL RELATIONS

Issues of altered sexual relations may not occur for all cancer patients, but for women with breast or gynaecological cancers sexual functioning may be linked to self-esteem, emotional distress, and adjustment. Three studies have explored the impact of psychosocial interventions on sexual functioning and satisfaction.

In one study, a problem-solving and communication-focused intervention was given to couples in which the woman had recently undergone a mastectomy (4). After controlling for pretreatment scores, husbands and wives participating in the treatment condition reported greater sexual satisfaction than those in the control group. In another study, emotion-focused individual counselling with an additional sexual rehabilitation component was offered to women with gynaecological cancers during their hospitalizations (6). At three-, six-, and twelve-month follow-ups, significantly more women in the treatment condition had resumed their prior levels of sexual activity than those in the control condition. In a similar patient population, women who received either individual or group intervention reported significantly better sexual functioning than women in the control condition by a six-month follow-up assessment (1).

## 2.7 DOCTOR–PATIENT RELATIONSHIPS

Emotional distress can strain interpersonal relationships. Following a diagnosis of cancer, it is important that individuals develop a good working relationship with their oncologist. This relationship is critical because the oncologist is the source of important information for the patient. It can also be stressful because the information patients receive from their oncologists may be unpleasant or frightening. On the other hand, oncologists may fear causing their patients undue distress and may gauge their behaviour in accord with patients' reactions. Open communication, however, and accurate knowledge of the disease seem to improve patients' perceptions of their health care providers. Psychological interventions containing an educational component have been shown to improve participant's knowledge of their illnesses and their satisfaction with health care providers (1, 15). Furthermore, in contrast to controls who demonstrated no increase in their knowledge of disease, groups receiving educational interventions are less depressed and anxious (1, 16) and have fewer treatment problems (16).

In a study of the long-term impact of knowledge of diagnosis, patients with clear knowledge of their cancer had the most initial distress, but less distress over time (3). In contrast, patients stating no knowledge of their diagnoses (11 of which had not received their diagnoses according to their physicians) had the least initial distress, but the most distress with time. Interestingly, those who suspected but were unsure of their diagnoses had decreased distress over time if they were in the psychosocial treatment condition but increased distress over time if they were in the control group. This clearly indicates the need for open communication between patients and their physicians regarding difficult topics. It also demonstrates the utility of psychosocial interventions in assisting doctor–patient communication and adjustment to difficult information.

## 2.8 ALIENATION VERSUS SUPPORT

Although in most group intervention studies some effect of a supportive environment has been posited, the sense of support or connectedness felt by group participants is typically not examined. It is believed that support group members can relate to each other in special ways, countering the social isolation they can experience after a cancer diagnosis (17, 18) Being part of a group affords cancer patients a sense of community which is necessary for successful coping, and provides opportunities to learn from others. In a recent review it was concluded that cancer patients seek interactions with other patients who have either overcome their illness or are adjusting well (19).

The importance of support from family members has been clearly demonstrated (20–23). Patients' perceptions of emotional support from family members were significantly positively correlated with outlook on life, psychological functioning, and a sense of well-being (20). Patients' perceptions of family support were also negatively related to patients' maladaptive coping responses, such as increased alcohol consumption, increased smoking, or poor nutritional habits (21). Social support has been shown to be the strongest predictor of coping response, thereby influencing women's adjustment to the stress of dealing with breast cancer (22). And, marital harmony is related to lower levels of anxiety, depression, and anger in cancer patients (24).

For women with metastatic breast cancer, certain family environment factors have predicted psychosocial adjustment (23). High family expressiveness, open and shared problem-solving, low family conflict, and reduced moral–religious family orientation predicted lower mood disturbance in patients over a one-year period, and better psychosocial adjustment. Breast cancer patients reporting the highest levels of family cohesion have shown the best adjustment to their illness (25).

Other researchers have explored the sense of alienation that many cancer patients feel, and examined whether psychosocial interventions might eliminate it. Although a couples counselling intervention appeared to have no effect on alienation scores (4), a significant and lasting decrease in alienation occurred for patients receiving individual psychotherapy compared with patients in the control condition (9). Some opponents of group support for cancer patients have questioned whether exposure to others who are distressed and physically deteriorating might not be frightening and alienating. In a study on support groups for metastatic breast cancer patients, adverse news about group members was found to influence the content but not the affective tone of group discussions (26). Even during a year when one-quarter of the group died, mood disturbance declined

# 3  Impact of psychosocial interventions on health outcome

## 3.1  PAIN AND TREATMENT SIDE-EFFECTS

Treatment side-effects and pain due to cancer have both physical and psychological repercussions. Certain therapeutic techniques can be useful in helping patients reduce pain and treatment side-effects. Reductions in the physical sensations (such as pain, nausea, and vomiting) can also be expected to reduce psychological distress.

Most notable among these strategies is hypnosis. The efficacy of hypnosis as a component of group therapy for women with metastatic breast cancer has been demonstrated (27). Women who participated in support groups that included self-hypnosis exercises had significantly better ability to control pain sensation compared with women in the group support without hypnosis or women in the control condition. By the end of the intervention year, treated women reported half the pain of those in the control condition. Furthermore, decreased pain sensation was correlated with decreased total mood disturbance.

Cancer patients frequently experience discomfort due to chemotherapy or radiation therapy. Systematic desensitization using progressive muscle relaxation and individual counselling were compared as potential treatments for chemotherapy-induced nausea and vomiting (28). Significantly fewer patients receiving desensitization therapy reported anticipatory nausea and vomiting than those receiving individual counselling or in the control group. There were similar findings in a study examining the efficacy of relaxation and imagery techniques for patients undergoing chemotherapy (29). A relaxation and imagery technique was compared with a 'therapist-present' control and a no-treatment control. The relaxation intervention group demonstrated significantly less nausea than the other two groups, both by their own and others reports. This group also experienced significantly less anxiety and depression, whilst also lowering their pulse rates and systolic blood pressure.

Self-hypnosis and relaxation/imagery techniques involve teaching cancer patients how to control their bodily experience. In addition, they can be used to help patients establish new ways of dealing with their thoughts and feelings about cancer and its side-effects.

3.2 SURVIVAL TIME

As discussed earlier, psychosocial interventions have been shown to enhance the quality of life of cancer patients. However, few studies have examined the effect of psychosocial interventions on survival rates for breast cancer patients. Five studies have addressed this question, three with breast cancer patients (30–32) and two with other types of cancer patients (9, 33). Their findings are inconclusive.

There have been two reports of a retrospective matching, follow-up study assessing the impact of a support programme on survival for women with breast cancer (30, 32). The Exceptional Cancer Patients (ECaP) programme consists of weekly, 90-minute, group meetings of 8–10 patients plus relatives and friends. These meetings are intended to provide peer support, family therapy, individual counselling, and instruction in relaxation, meditation, and positive mental imagery. The follow-up study involved a comparison of a group of breast cancer patients who participated in their ECaP programme with a group of patients who had never participated in that programme. The treatment group consisted of 34 women at all stages of breast cancer who had entered their programme between January 1979 and June 1981. They were matched with three women with breast cancer according to race, age at histological diagnosis, stage of disease (localized, regional involvement, or distant), surgery (positive or negative), sequence of malignancy, and date of diagnosis (within one year). The intervention was described as being unstructured, involving discussions of patients' problems, meditation, and mental imagery.

In the first report (30) both the intervention group and the control group were followed retrospectively from the date of cancer diagnosis (1971–1980) until December 1981. There was no difference in survival time between the two groups when time from initial diagnosis to study entry was controlled. Given that their samples included women in all stages of breast cancer, and that some of their participants had only been in the programme for six months, it is not surprising that there was no survival difference.

More recently, a second publication on this retrospective study extended the follow-up period by 10 years, so that both groups were followed from the date of cancer diagnosis until March 1991 (32). Again, there was no statistically significant difference in survival rates between the treatment and control groups. In addition to the problem of including all stages of breast cancer, the women were not randomly assigned to the treatment group. This introduces the possibility of confounding variables that were not controlled for by matching or analytical techniques.

Spiegel and his colleagues investigated the effects of a psychosocial intervention on survival for women with recurrent breast cancer (31). This was a randomized, prospective outcome study on the effects of a one-year psychosocial intervention. The intervention involved weekly, 90-minute, supportive–

expressive group therapy meetings. Groups consisted of women with meta-static breast cancer and were led by a psychiatrist or social worker along with a therapist who had cancer in remission. The focus of the group was to help patients cope with their cancer. This involved discussions of dying and death, the effect of the illness on the family, treatment concerns, doctor–patient relationships, and how to live life fully in the face of a terminal illness. It is important to note that nothing done in the intervention implied to patients that some change in personal attitude or imaging technique would influence survival time.

Eighty-six women with metastatic breast cancer were recruited into the study. Fifty of these women were randomly assigned to the treatment group. The remaining 36 women were assigned to the control group. The two groups were similar on biomedical prognostic variables at the time of entering the study except for a near significant difference in staging at initial diagnosis, with initial staging favouring the intervention group in that there were fewer Stage IV patients. Although initial staging was found to be unrelated to survival, from the time of randomization in the study until death, staging was used as a control variable during the analysis of survival rates.

During the year of treatment, 15 patients in the treatment group died com-pared with 8 patients in the control group. While there was no difference in median survival, 8 months after the intervention ended survival curves for the two groups began to diverge. By 48 months, all of the control patients had died, while a third of the treatment sample was still alive. The average survival time for the treatment group was 36.6 months from the date of randomization to death, compared with 18.9 months for the control group. This difference was statistically significant.

Although this is a randomized study, a critical question needing to be addressed is the success of the randomization. Since the samples were not stratified, it is reasonable to examine the question of whether or not ran-domization successfully provided comparability on salient psychosocial and biomedical prognostic variables. The sample randomized to intervention was higher on socio-economic status (SES) than the control sample, but less likely to be married (57 per cent vs. 70 per cent) (34). While it is true that SES has been linked with health, so have other sociodemographic variables such as marital status. In fact, marital status is a strong predictor of medical outcome in cancer patients (35). While needing to be demonstrated empirically, it is unlikely that the observed difference in SES accounts for the survival differences.

Extensive analyses of medical prognostic variables and their effect on sur-vival time were conducted. There were no significant differences in disease-free interval (time from initial diagnosis to study entry) or time from first metastasis to study entry. There was an average two-month difference in disease-free interval favouring the control group and a two-and-a-half-month difference in time from first metastasis to study entry favouring the intervention group. The intervention patient group was composed of fewer individuals who were Stage IV at first diagnosis, five years before study entry, but this difference in staging was not associated with survival time and, as mentioned, was controlled for in the statistical analyses. The intervention patients had had fewer days of irradiation as well, but this reduction of treatment likewise did not account for differences in survival time when it was statistically controlled. Thus, on the basis of important prognostic variables, such as time from initial diagnosis to first metastasis, the group randomized to the intervention seemed at least as ill as the control population. For those few variables where there appeared to be a difference favouring the intervention group, this difference could not account statistically for the observed difference in survival time.

This study was originally designed to examine prospectively whether a psychosocial intervention regimen could improve quality of life. The test of the effect of psychosocial interventions on survival, on the other hand, was undertaken after the original intervention trial had been completed. For this reason and given the importance of the question, it is essential that this study be replicated. There are several clinical trials underway in the United States, Canada, and Europe to see if these findings can be replicated. This includes our laboratory which is currently conducting a clinical trial designed to replicate the original findings as well as systematically examine mechanisms that could lead to enhanced survival.

The effect of psychosocial intervention has also been investigated in patients with other types of cancers. In one study (9), 120 men with a variety of end-stage cancers were randomly assigned to a counselling or control condition and were followed-up for 12 months. The length or frequency of the intervention is unspecified. No effect of counselling on survival was found. In another study (33), 100 patients with lymphoma and leukemia were randomly assigned to one of four groups; a control condition or various psychosocial treatment groups, involving home visiting and education. The intervention patients were significantly more likely to adhere to their medical treatment, as measured by utilization of allopurinol. However, there was also significantly longer survival in the intervention samples, even when differences in treatment adherence were controlled. Thus, two of three randomized trials have shown an effect of psychosocial intervention on survival time.

# 4  Psychosocial treatment issues

Psychosocial interventions for cancer patients can take a variety of forms. In this section we review the treatment strategies that have been used with cancer patients and discuss their relative strengths and weaknesses. Timing issues and other mediating factors are also considered.

## 4.1 THERAPEUTIC PARADIGMS: COGNITIVE–BEHAVIOURAL VERSUS SUPPORTIVE–EXPRESSIVE

Many of the studies to be reviewed employ highly structured, educational or skills-focused interventions. We refer to these approaches as 'cognitive–behavioural'. Fewer studies have employed the type of intervention where the main focus is support and the expression of illness-related emotions. We describe this second approach as 'supportive–expressive'. The distinction we make in this section is a general one. We believe it reflects two general treatment strategies that are used with cancer patients. In the literature reviewed, a given intervention may have features of each approach. In categorizing each treatment strategy employed according to this typology, we have tried to reflect the main thrust of each intervention.

### 4.1.1   Cognitive–behavioural

Cognitive–behavioural treatment strategies are designed to provide cancer patients with the cognitive and behavioural skills necessary to manage uncomfortable thoughts and problematic behaviours following a diagnosis of cancer. Cancer patients and their families face multiple challenges during the diagnosis and treatment of cancer. Individuals may feel unable to deal effectively with these exceptionally stressful life events. Coping strategies previously used may now be ineffective. Or, patients and families may feel so overwhelmed that such strategies are felt to be useless. Structured interventions can help patients regain a sense of personal control and self-efficacy in dealing with personal crises. Cognitive–behavioural interventions often provide patients with the opportunity to learn and implement new coping strategies, problem-solving techniques, and communication skills.

Cognitive–behavioural interventions are usually structured, brief, and time-limited, with a predetermined set of issues or themes to be dealt with during the course of the intervention. Groups are often given a topic to be discussed at the beginning of each session. This structure is especially important in a brief, time-limited intervention because it ensures that the most common problems faced by this population are addressed. Together with the introduction of specific topics is a discussion of particular coping strategies to deal with the problems raised. Another component often combined in these interventions is education. Patients clearly state a desire for more knowledge of cancer and its treatment following a diagnosis of cancer (36). When education is the focus, relevant information about the disease is dispersed and a forum is provided where patients are encouraged to ask questions regarding areas of concern or confusion. These groups are not intended, necessarily, to deal with emotions triggered by the educational information.

There are several advantages to this approach. Foremost is that patients are forced to deal with issues that might otherwise be avoided because they are too disturbing. For some group members having the issues raised by the leaders may relieve them of a felt need to 'protect' other group members by not voicing their own concerns and worries. Teaching specific coping skills and educating patients about the disease can help patients to take a more active coping orientation to dealing with their illness. A disadvantage to this type of approach is that specific, personal issues of concern to group members may not be addressed. There may also be less opportunity for group members to provide support to one another.

### 4.1.2 Supportive–expressive

Supportive–expressive treatment strategies (37, 38) are designed to provide a forum for the cancer patient to express all concerns she has regarding her illness, with ventilation of associated strong feelings of fear, sadness, and anger. This is the expressive component of the intervention. The assumption is that the full expression of emotions and thoughts regarding one's illness is therapeutic. Typically, cancer patients lack a place where they can speak openly about their fears and anxieties. Often it is difficult to speak freely with family members because of the mutual concern on both sides about causing more distress for one another. However, because of the perceived need to protect each other, cancer patients are often isolated and alone with their fears. A professionally led group or individual therapy can provide the right environment for the cancer patient to express her feelings and concerns (7, 39, 40).

Another equally important component of supportive–expressive interventions is to provide a place where the cancer patient receives emotional support (39, 40). Group interventions are good for this because they are comprised of individuals who are each going through similar experiences. Hearing about how others have dealt with similar situations, or receiving validation from others about the appropriateness of her emotional reactions and concerns, can be deeply reassuring to the patient.

In addition to providing a place where patients can express their concerns and feelings as well as receive support, supportive–expressive interventions involve helping the patient learn new coping strategies (7, 41). Learning new coping strategies often comes out of watching others cope successfully with their disease. This differs from the cognitive–behavioural interventions where patients are explicitly taught particular coping strategies.

These groups are not traditional psychotherapy groups for longstanding personality and relationship problems. Rather, they act as a forum where wellfunctioning women can address issues associated with their cancers. As such, women who would not otherwise seek or be appropriate for 'psychotherapy' receive needed psychosocial services.

### 4.1.3   Cognitive–behavioural versus supportive–expressive

Two studies have attempted to contrast these methods within the research design. The first was a series of studies (16) exploring the relative benefits of patient education and peer support interventions for people with Hodgkin's disease. Patients were recruited into one of two prospective studies involving either a comparison of education (treatment condition) with evaluation-only (control condition), or a comparison of peer support (treatment condition) with evaluation-only (control condition). Forty-seven subjects participated in the education versus control study and 34 subjects participated in the peer support versus control study. In the education condition, patients received a booklet on Hodgkin's disease which discussed diagnosis, staging, treatment methods, and prognosis. In the peer support condition, patients attended 90-minute-long weekly meetings for 8 weeks. Although an oncologist, psychologist, and social worker attended each meeting, they assumed nondirective roles. Results indicated that those patients receiving education had increased knowledge of the disease compared with the control group. Furthermore, they had significant reductions in anxiety, depression, life disruptions, and treatment problems compared with control group subjects. However, on a variable they called 'social competency' the education group worsened while the control group improved. This difference was statistically significant. For those randomized to the peer support arm of the two studies, members of both the experimental and control groups showed improvements in mood, interpersonal problems, personal habits, and treatment problems. The only variable in which there was a statistically significant difference between the two groups was 'activity'. The peer support group's activity worsened significantly more than did the control group.

The second study (42) involved a direct comparison of cognitive–behavioural and supportive–expressive approaches. Forty-one cancer patients with clear evidence of psychosocial distress were randomly assigned to one of three conditions: (1) group coping skills instruction; (2) support group therapy; or (3) no-treatment. The interventions were time-limited, meeting once a week for six weeks. The coping skills group was structured to cover various topics and specific coping strategies for each topic. Structured homework exercises were given at the end of each session. The support group had little structure, simply providing a place for patients to discuss any concerns they had. It did not focus on dealing with strong emotions related to the disease. Results indicated that members of the coping skills group had a significant reduction in distress and increase in self-efficacy at the end of treatment compared with pretreatment. Members of the support group showed no change on these measures and members of the control group demonstrated deterioration (increased distress and decreased self-efficacy). Furthermore, during structured clinical interviews, independent raters found improvement only in the coping skills group.

These studies would seem to suggest that structured, concrete, skills-focused, or educational interventions are preferable to peer-support interventions. In the first study (16), the lack of guidance from mental health professionals may have left the peer support groups without the ability to deal with difficult and frightening issues in a way that is helpful. They might either avoid these topics or deal with them in a way that is demoralizing. However, Telch and Telch (42) provided a comparison of these therapeutic paradigms and found fewer gains from a supportive–expressive approach. What might account for this difference? In both studies the psychotherapeutic interventions were of a short duration (that is six to eight weeks). It is our experience that support groups gain in effectiveness with time, as group members form lasting relationships that allow for mutual support. It is possible that with a very limited amount of time, greater gains are found from structured programmes. For supportive–expressive interventions it is also important that the leaders be trained to help patients focus on the more difficult and threatening aspects of their illness. Finally, the results of supportive–expressive therapies may not be seen immediately. In many studies, the impact of supportive interventions is not seen until later (eight to twelve month) follow-up assessments are conducted (7).

## 4.2 LENGTH OF INTERVENTION

Research is needed to determine the optimal duration for each type of intervention. We would expect brief interventions (four to eight weeks) to be well-suited to the cognitive–behavioural approach while supportive–expressive interventions should require more time. This has to do with the types of goals unique to each intervention. Although these two approaches share similar goals, such as improved coping skills, there are important differences. The cognitive–behavioural approaches aim to change specific coping behaviors, while supportive–expressive interventions aim to provide a new support system, counter disease-related social isolation, bolster family support, enhance emotional expression about all aspects of the cancer experience, and improve coping strategies. Clearly, in assessing the efficacy of each approach, the outcome measures must also be chosen to reflect these differences.

## 4.3 GROUP VERSUS INDIVIDUAL INTERVENTIONS

Only one study has addressed the structure of the intervention by comparing group therapy with individual therapy (1). Eighty women with cancer were randomly assigned to one of three conditions: (1) group psychosocial intervention; (2) individual psychosocial intervention; and (3) routine oncological care. In both intervention conditions, patients received eight weekly sessions that were structured to systematically cover eight, predetermined topics of common concern to cancer patients, for example, impact of treatment on body image.

At one to two weeks post-treatment, members receiving individual intervention were significantly less anxious than subjects in the group intervention or control conditions. However, by six-month follow-up, participants in both psychosocial interventions were less depressed, less anxious, and better adjusted than members of the control group. This study demonstrates that breast cancer patients can benefit from individual and group therapy. One could argue that, with individual therapy, patients do not risk potential mood disturbance provoked by facing one's own and others' potential for disease progression. However, there are several reasons why we believe group therapy is preferable to individual psychotherapy for cancer patients.

An often noted benefit of support groups is that members can relate to each other in special ways that are different from how they relate to professional group leaders (17, 18). In one study approximately half of the self-help group members felt that only other persons with similar problems could understand and be helpful to them (18). Cancer patients find it helpful when other patients model successful coping (43), thereby providing them with hope. Support in a group setting provides what has been called the 'helper therapy' principle (44); patients gain in self-esteem through their ability to help others. The tragedy of having cancer is converted into an asset, enabling one patient to provide concrete help to another. Being part of a group can afford cancer patients a sense of community necessary for successful coping and provide opportunities to learn from one another.

One final and significant reason to advocate group therapy is that it is more cost-effective than individual therapy. One study examined the effect of psychosocial intervention on newly referred patients within tertiary ambulatory clinics, including an oncology clinic (45). The results of this study suggest that any intervention that increases psychosocial adjustment increases the cost-effectiveness of treatments overall by reducing unnecessary treatment. Thus, group therapy is clearly more cost-effective in that it makes resources available to many more women, including under-served populations. Economically, group therapy may be up to four times more affordable for patients and for institutions (46, 47). The relationship between psychosocial adjustment and cost-effective treatment is of major importance considering the prevalence of (one in eight women will be affected during their lifetimes), and mortality due to, breast cancer (50000 deaths per year in the USA, the second leading cancer killer of women after lung cancer).

## 4.4 TIMING OF INTERVENTION

The timing of the psychosocial intervention may be important for both psychosocial adjustment and, possibly, for survival. One study compared the effects of the same psychosocial intervention at two different windows of time following diagnosis (48). The first intervention occurred approximately 11 weeks, and the other approximately 28 weeks, post-diagnosis. The two groups were evaluated every four months during a one-year period following diagnosis. The timing of the intervention did not appear to make a difference until the eight-month assessment. At this time the late intervention group was significantly less depressed, less anxious, had less intrusive thoughts, and had a greater sense of personal control than those in the early intervention group. By the 12-month assessment, the early intervention group remained more distressed only in terms of intrusive thought. These findings may be confounded, however, since it appears that the early intervention group may have been significantly more distressed at baseline compared with the late intervention group.

This study raises some important questions. For example, what is the natural course of distress in cancer patients following diagnosis? Most patients are likely to react with shock and distress, but how many of these patients will still be experiencing intense distress six months later? Is there an optimal time to provide an intervention? Does it depend on the type of intervention offered or on the patient? Certain factors may mediate distress in breast cancer patients. Younger patients seem to experience more distress at early stages of diagnosis (49), have more fears of recurrence (23), and feel that the cancer is a greater threat to their quality of life than do older patients (50).

Other issues that should be considered in providing psychotherapeutic interventions to cancer patients include the stage of the diagnosed cancer. Primary breast cancer patients deal with different issues than do metastatic cancer patients. While metastatic cancer patients may express a fear of dying and pain involved in this process, primary breast cancer patients are more likely to express fears of recurrence. Similarly, many primary breast cancer patients can realistically expect to be 'cured' and, therefore, may openly resist any exploration of existential issues. Likewise, if the cancer is not found until it has metastasized, these women are likely to experience great distress, feeling relatively unprepared for such a blow. Clearly cancer patients share many of the same feelings and fears regardless of their stage or prognosis. However, it is necessary for psychosocial interventions to be sensitive to the varying needs of cancer patients.

The timing of the evaluation appears to be important when assessing the effects of a psychosocial intervention. Several studies have demonstrated the importance of continued follow-up with patients participating in psychosocial intervention studies as the impact of the intervention may not be immediately observable (7–9). Patients receiving a supportive–expressive group intervention had lower total mood disturbance scores on the Profile of Mood States one year after enrollment in the study than did patients in the control condition (7). These differences were noticeable four and eight months post-enrollment but were not statistically significant at those times. Likewise, in a study with melanoma patients, trends toward less mood disturbance were found among their treatment group at the six-week follow-up, but these differences did not become significant until the six-month follow-up (8). Specifically, melanoma patients receiving group support and education were less confused, depressed, and fatigued, and had less total mood disturbance than members of an evaluation-only control group. On the other hand, another study demonstrated significant differences in depression between treatment and control subjects at the three-month follow-up, but these differences had disappeared by the six-month follow-up (9).

Cancer type may affect the outcome of a treatment. Of the participants in one psychosocial treatment study, breast and lung cancer patients were significantly less depressed and anxious at follow-up than controls (10). However, the melanoma patients participating in the treatment group did not differ significantly on depression or anxiety measures in contrast to the controls. As these studies suggest, improved psychosocial adjustment following a psychosocial intervention may be conditional on multiple factors. Increased psychosocial adjustment is likely for breast cancer patients providing the intervention is of sufficient duration and includes opportunities for both emotional expression, social support and the measurement of the long-term effects of these interventions.

# 5   Possible mediators of disease progression and survival time

## 5.1   DIET, SLEEP, AND EXERCISE

There are a variety of mechanisms through which psychotherapy may mediate disease progression and survival time in breast cancer patients. At a behavioural level, psychosocial interventions may affect diet, sleep, and exercise (51, 52). Interventions may have the effect of instilling hope and active coping styles in breast cancer patients (51).

## 5.2 COMPLIANCE WITH MEDICAL TREATMENT

Compliance with the treatment regimen, defined as the match between the patient's behaviour and health care advice (53), is important because compliance to the treatment regimen may prolong disease-free and overall survival time (33, 54, 55). Compliance issues may be particularly important for cancer treatment regimens due to their complexity, intensity, and side-effects. However, there is little systematic research on compliance with treatment among cancer patients (56). In one survey of 246 randomly selected oncologists (54), the most frequently reported compliance problem was failure to return for the recommended out-patient treatment following initial evaluation. Other major problems included failure to keep subsequent appointments, patient refusal of the recommended in-patient and/or out-patient treatments, and noncompliance with the prescribed home medication regimen (57).

The existing data suggests that noncompliance to treatment regimens is high among cancer patients. In one study, 23 per cent of patients did not keep their appointment for the administration of chemotherapy (57). Withdrawal from the recommended treatment protocol is estimated to range from 16–33 per cent (58–61).

Variables which have been shown to affect compliance include: demographics; patient perceptions of their illness and their role in its treatment; social support; the costs and benefits of compliance from the patient's perspective; and an intention to comply (56). All of the psychosocial factors in this model, except demographics, may be influenced by psychosocial interventions. Psychosocial interventions may increase patients' knowledge, change their attitudes about treatment, and help them to overcome practical obstacles to compliance. Other factors, such as educating patients about the efficacy of treatment, produce better compliance with medication regimens (62–63). To the extent that psychosocial interventions help patients take an active collaborative role in their medical treatment, there is likely to be greater satisfaction and compliance (64, 65). Thus, there is reason to expect that psychosocial interventions can improve compliance by helping patients to: better manage the anxiety that is interwoven with treatment; better comprehend the reasoning behind treatment decisions; feel more in control of the course of their treatment through clearer communication with their physicians; and more effectively mobilize support from family and friends for participating in the treatment.

## 5.3 STRESS AND IMMUNE FUNCTION

The stress of having cancer is quite different from the every-day type of stress. For patients with a diagnosis of malignant disease, stress occurs at many levels. First, there is the physical stress of the disease itself developing within the body. Second, there is the physical effect of treatments: chemotherapy, radiation therapy, surgery, and hormonal treatment, with serious side-effects such as nausea and energy depletion. Third, physical symptoms trigger other psychological stresses. Pain, for example, is compounded by the psychological stress of interpreting the pain as a possible indicator of disease recurrence and progression. Not only are cancer patients dealing with the normal daily hassles of life, now compounded by illness, but they must deal with constant reminders that they have a serious and perhaps terminal disease. Given that stress is ubiquitous in the life of a cancer patient and that the immune system may play a role in inhibiting cancer progression, the possibility of a detrimental effect of stress on immune function is important. A breast cancer patient's immune system is already compromised because of the cancer, but following diagnosis she has the additional emotional and psychological stress of *knowing* that she has a life-threatening disease. Learning how to manage this stress in the context of a solid support system may be one among a number of variables to influence the rate of disease progression.

Over the last 15 years evidence has accumulated addressing the connections between stress and immune function. There are conflicting views, however, on whether this relationship has been unequivocalty demonstrated. Kiecolt-Glaser and Glaser (66) argue that the evidence shows immunosuppression can result from psychological distress. What has not been demonstrated, they suggest, is the *degree* of immunosuppression required for there to be health consequences. They propose that the population most at risk from stress-related immunosuppression will be those individuals already suffering from weakened immune systems. Schulz and Schulz (67) reviewed the literature and found conflicting evidence on the proposed link between psychosocial factors and immune function. Their review demonstrated the importance of addressing four major parameters: psychosocial conditions, immunological factors, mediating variables, and disease outcome.

The existing research on the immunological effects of chronic stressors has focused on such stressors as bereavement, separation and divorce, care givers of patients with Alzheimer's disease, and residents of Three Mile Island. Viewed together, these studies suggest that chronic stress in humans results in immunologic disruption.

In the literature on married and unmarried individuals, marital distruption has been associated with an increased morbidity and mortality (66, 69). Following the death of a spouse, bereaved individuals have been shown to have significant deficits in immune function (70–73). A study (72) comparing-recently bereaved wives, women whose husbands were terminally ill, and women whose husbands were healthy, found that bereaved women had reduced natural killer cell activity (NKCA) and increased plasma cortisol levels compared with controls. Likewise, for women who were anticipating a loss, NK activity was lower than it was for controls; although, no differences were found in plasma cortisol levels. Another study (70) examined the immune function of bereaved subjects at two and six weeks following bereavement, comparing them with controls who were matched for age, sex, and race. They found their T-cell response *in vitro* to phytohemagglutinin at six weeks was significantly lower in the bereaved group than the control group. This effect was not found at two weeks following bereavement, suggesting that the immunological consequences of such a chronic stressor may build up over time.

In a prospective bereavement study of men whose wives had advanced metastatic breast cancer, lymphocyte stimulation responses *in vitro* were measured at six to eight week intervals before the death of their spouses and at similar intervals over the course of a year following the death (73). Compared with prebereavement, subjects showed suppressed lymphocyte stimulation responses to phytohemagglutinin, concanavalin A, and pokeweed mitogen during the first two months following the loss. The lymphocyte stimulation responses to bereavement following the first two months were intermediate between the prebereavement and initial postbereavement responses. This suggests that as the bereaved spouse slowly adjusts to the loss there is a gradual return to prebereavement levels.

Marital disruption has been shown to be a major stressor with both emotional and physical consequences (68). In particular, separation and divorce have been shown to affect immune responses (74). Kiecolt-Glaser and colleagues compared a group of separated/divorced women with a group of married women who were sociodemographically matched. Women who were separated/divorced within a year of being tested showed the greatest immune deficiency, having lower percentages of helper T-lymphocytes and NK cells, along with higher antibody titres to Epstein–Barr virus (EBV) viral capsid antigen. Shorter separation time and continued attachment was also associated with decreased immune response, as was poorer marital quality within the married group.

Two studies examined the relationship between marital quality and immune function (74, 75). Poorer marital quality for women was strongly positively correlated with dysphoria, loneliness, and EBV antibody titres, indicating lower cellular immune control of viral latency (76). Similarly, married men with poorer marital quality had greater distress and lower T-helper/suppressor cell counts and ratio, as well as poorer response to EBV antibodies (75).

Being a caregiver for a family member with Alzheimer's disease is another chronic stressor associated with suppressed immune response (76). Family caregivers of Alzheimer patients were compared with a group of sociodemographically matched controls and, as expected, were found to be more distressed and have poorer immune function. Caregivers had lower percentages of total T-lymphocytes and helper T-lymphocytes, and lower helper–suppressor cell ratios. There was also an increased level of EBV antibodies in the bloodstream.

Residents of the Three Mile Island area were followed-up for six years after the damaged nuclear power plant was in danger of causing a devastating disaster (77). Compared to a control group subjects living in the Three Mile Island area had fewer B-lymphocytes, natural killer (NK) cells, and T-suppressor/cytotoxic lymphocytes. They also occasionally showed higher levels of cortisol.

As this brief review suggests, changes in immune function caused by stress have been documented in the literature. Similarly, the benefits of psychosocial interventions for cancer patients dealing with stress have been shown. However, few studies have documented immune changes in cancer patients as a function of psychosocial interventions. One study delineated such effects following completion of a structured intervention for melanoma patients (78). Patients who participated in a six-week structured group intervention demonstrated significant immune changes compared with a control group at a six-month follow-up assessment. Changes included increased percentages of large granular lymphocytes and NK cells, and increased NK cytotoxicity. Furthermore, there was a reduction in the CD4 helper/inducer T-cells for the treatment group at six months.

### 5.3.1   Social support

Social support has been shown to be an important factor in coping with stress. For instance, married cancer patients survive longer than unmarried patients (35). Indeed, several large epidemiological studies demonstrate a strong relationship between social integration and reduced all-cause mortality (79).

Although interpersonal relationships can be a source of stress and have adverse effects on the immune system (74), they can also play an important mediating role in buffering the effect of stress on immune function (80). Loneliness has been found to be related to lower levels of NK activity, poorer T-lymphocyte response to phytohemagglutinin, and higher levels of urinary cortisol in psychiatric patients (81). Immune function has also been found to be related to loneliness in medical students (82, 83). For instance, lonely medical students had significantly lower levels of NK activity than students who felt less lonely during examination periods (82).

A number of studies have examined the relationship between perceived social support and NK activity in patients with breast cancer (84–86). NK activity at baseline (85) and three months into treatment (84) has been found to be related to fatigue/depression and a lack of social support. These findings are all the more striking given that NK activity at three months did not appear to be affected by chemotherapy and/or radiotherapy, treatments that are immunosuppressive. In another report of this study, high quality emotional support from a spouse or intimate friend, perceived social support from one's physician, and actively seeking social support were found to be related to higher NK activity (86). The salience of NK activity to breast cancer progression is demonstrated by a study from this group which showed a relationship between cancer progression and a decline in NK activity (84). This association does not imply causation: the debilitation caused by advanced disease could retard NK activity, or the reduced activity could hamper effective immune response to disease progression.

Breast cancer is a hormone-sensitive tumour, hence the widespread and effective use of oestrogen receptor-blocking agents such as tamoxifen in the treatment of this illness. These oestrogen and progesterone receptors may be occupied and activated by related steroid hormones such as cortisol, which are secreted in higher amounts in response to stress (87). Other stress hormones, such as prolactin, have been observed to promote breast tumour growth in tissue culture (88, 89). It thus makes sense that an alteration in the internal hormonal environment resulting in a reduction of endogenously secreted stress hormones might reduce the rate of tumour proliferation. One such experimental model was developed by Levine and colleagues (90). Squirrel monkeys exposed to a stressful stimulus show a consistent elevation in plasma cortisol. When exposed to the same aversive stimulus in the company of one friend, the elevation in plasma cortisol is only half as great. When five friends are present in that situation, there is no increase at all in plasma cortisol in response to the stressor. This provides a model for social support being a buffer against the physiological consequences of stress. Psychotherapeutic support may provide a similar buffering in the face of disease-related stress, thereby reducing endogenous stress hormone secretion.

### 5.3.2   Sense of control over the stressor

Breast cancer patients vary widely in how they appraise their situation. Some view it as something over which they have control, others feel helpless. Some blame themselves and their lifestyles; others see it as an unlucky turn of fate. A more favourable medical outcome has been found for cancer patients who initially react to their cancer diagnosis with denial or a fighting spirit compared with those who reacted with stoic acceptance, helplessness, or hopelessness (91), suggesting that appraisal of the situation may influence the course of the disease. The extent to which a particular stressor is experienced as stressful may depend on the individual's appraisal of the situation which, in turn, may affect the immune response (92) and thereby disease outcome. For separated men, a sense of control over the course of the relationship has been shown to make a difference (75). In a study of the relationship between marital status and immune function, separated or divorced men, who were found to be generally more distressed and lonely than married men, showed lower antibody-titres to herpes viruses than their married counterparts. However, those who had separated within the past year and who initiated the separation showed better EBV titres than separated men who reported less control over the separation. Unfortunately, the interpretation of these findings is not clear; it may be that it is not so much an issue of lack of control but rather that it is distressing to be rejected.

The immunosuppressive effects of having no control over a stressor was studied directly in a study on uncontrollable noise (93). Subjects who perceived themselves as having no control over noise showed suppressed NK activity immediately following the noise stressor, as well as 72 hours later. On the other hand, there was no immune suppression among subjects who perceived they had control over the noise, or for subjects in the no-noise condition.

In the light of these findings, psychosocial interventions may promote a sense of control, if not over the disease itself, at least over one's psychological response to it and to some extent its medical management.

### 5.3.3 Mood and emotional expression

There have been many studies examining the link between depression and immune function (see Chapter 1). In a review of the literature, Stein and colleagues (94, 95) have concluded that findings in this area are not consistent or conclusive. Nevertheless, in spite of conceptual and methodological limitations in this research, they suggest that there may be subsets of individuals who have alterations in their immune system due to depression, such as the elderly and severely depressed. As mentioned previously, depression/fatigue, along with social support, has been shown to predict NK cytotoxicity in breast cancer patients (84). This suggests that, along with social support, mood may have clinical relevance.

There have been several large epidemiological studies examining the link between depression and the risk of cancer (96–101). These studies have tended to show weak relationships or none at all. One study focused specifically on the risk of death from breast cancer (99) and found no relationship. However, it is premature to rule out the significance of depression as a mediating variable. As Stein (94) has pointed out, there may be subpopulations of cancer patients whose immune systems would benefit from effective treatment of their depression.

In the study with melanoma patients presented earlier (78), a structured group intervention resulted in significant immune changes compared with the control group at six-month follow-up. Of interest here is that these immune changes were correlated with decreased depression and anxiety and increased anger, but were unrelated to coping strategies. In another study (102) bereaved spouses who could express their feelings more fully had increased T-cell and NK numbers than those who had lower expressiveness scores on the Courtauld Emotional Control Scale. These studies suggest that a possible mediator between psychosocial intervention and immune functioning could be expression of affect. Further investigation is needed to assess this hypothesis.

### 5.3.4 Personality

There has been much research investigating the proposed link between certain personality characteristics and risk of cancer; although the findings have received mixed reviews (92, 103–107). The type 'C' personality, which has been proposed to predispose such individuals to cancer (108), is characterized as stoic, unassertive, compliant, and unexpressive of negative emotions (especially anger) (104). The proposed link between expression of emotion and cancer has been examined in several studies with inconsistent results (109) Nevertheless, lack of emotional expression appears to be related to cancer incidence and progression. Some argue that the evidence is most clear for psychosocial factors, such as personality style, influencing disease progression (110).

## 6 Conclusion

The literature reviewed here makes it clear that psychotherapy has an important place in the management of breast cancer. Numerous interventions have been shown to affect various aspects of quality of life, somatic symptoms, immune function, and even survival time. While at first this may seem startling, it makes sense from a psychophysiological perspective which takes into account the complex inter-relationships between mind and body. Breast cancer, its type, aggressiveness, degree of spread, and sensitivity to hormonal influence are clearly important prognostic parameters. However, the tumour is invading a body designed to resist such attack with hormonal, immune, and other physiological processes, which are susceptible to varying degrees of control by the central nervous system. It makes sense that variables such as social support, affect regulation, self-efficacy, and mood disturbance could impinge on the body's resistance to cancer progression.

Future research could productively address the following questions.

1. What are the most efficacious components of psychotherapy for breast cancer patients (for example, supportive/expressive versus cognitive/behavioural interventions; groups versus individual psychotherapy), and what is the optimal length and timing of such interventions?

2. What are the physiological effects of such psychotherapies? Do they affect the rate of disease progression and survival time? Our laboratory at Stanford is currently investigating these questions with recurrent breast cancer patients. This is a prospective randomized clinical trial designed to test the

psychosocial and medical effects of supportive–expressive group therapy with metastatic breast cancer patients.

3. Which physiological mechanisms might underlie any effects on disease progression: for example health maintenance behaviors, adherence to medical treatment, endocrine and immune function? We are also attempting to address the question of the role of endocrine and immune function in our recurrent breast cancer study by examining measures of immune and endocrine function over time. In addition to periodic measures of immune and endocrine function during the course of the study, we are examining the immunological consequences of experiencing a stressor. The effect of supportive–expressive group therapy on health maintenance behaviors and adherence to medical treatment is also being addressed in the recurrent breast cancer study as well as in a prospective randomized clinical trial with primary breast cancer patients.

4. How can such interventions be integrated into health care service delivery?

5. What are the cost benefits of such interventions? Further exploration is needed to demonstrate the financial benefits of psychosocial interventions to the patient, health care providers, and institutions responsible for paying for health care costs.

Psychotherapeutic intervention has demonstrated its value as a component rather than an adjunct or alternative to standard medical treatment for breast cancer. Few individuals are well prepared by life for the confrontation with disfigurement, pain, and mortality which breast cancer poses. Most would benefit in some way from such psychotherapeutic support.

## 7   References

1.  Cain, E., Kohorn, E., Quinlan, D., Latimer, K., and Schwartz, P. (1986). Psychosocial benefits of a cancer support group. *Cancer*, 57, 183–189.
2.  Worden, J. and Weisman, A. (1984). Preventive psychosocial intervention with newly diagnosed cancer patients. *Gen. Hosp. Psychiatry*, 6, 243–249.
3.  Forester, B., Kornfeld, D., and Fleiss, J. (1985). Psychotherapy during radiotherapy: Effects on emotional and physical distress. *Am. J. Psychiatry*, 142, 22–27.
4.  Christensen, D. (1983). Postmastectomy couple counselling: An outcome study of a structured treatment protocol. *J. Sex Marital Ther.*, 9, 266–275.
5.  Heinrich, R. and Coscarelli-Schag, C. (1985). Stress and activity management: Group treatment for cancer patients and spouses. *J. Consult. Clin. Psychol.*, 53, 439–446.
6.  Capone, M., Good, R., Westie, K., and Jacobson, A. (1980). Psychosocial rehabilitation of gynecologic oncology patients. *Arch. Phys. Med. Rehabil.*, 61, 128–132.

7. Spiegel, D., Bloom, J. R., and Yalom, I. D. (1981). Group support for patients with metastatic cancer: A randomized prospective outcome study. *Arch. Gen. Psychiatry*, **38**, 527–533.
8. Fawzy, F., Cousins, N., Fawzy, N., Kemeny, M., Elashoff, R., and Morton, D. (1990*a*). A structured psychiatric intervention for cancer patients: Changes over time in methods of coping and affective disturbance. *Arch. Gen. Psychiatry*, **47**, 720–728.
9. Linn, M., Linn, B., and Harris, R. (1982). Effects of counseling for late stage cancer patients. *Cancer*, **49**, 1048–1055.
10. Gordon, W. A., Freidenbergs, I., Diller, L. *et al.* (1980). Efficacy of psychosocial intervention with cancer patients. *J. Consult. Clin. Psychol.*, **48**, 743–759.
11. Lazarus, R. and Folkman, S. (1984). *Stress, Appraisal, and Coping*. Springer-Verlag, New York.
12. Dunkel-Schetter, C., Feinstein, L. G., Taylor, S. E., and Falke, R. L. (1992). Patterns of coping with cancer. *Health Psychol,*, **11**, 79–87.
13. Fallowfield, L. J., Hall, A., Maguire, G. P., and Baum, M. (1990). Psychological outcomes of different treatment policies in women with early breast cancer outside a clinical trial. *Br. J. Med.*, **301**, 575–580.
14. Kaplan, H. S. (1992). A neglected issue: The sexual side effects of current treatments for breast cancer. *J. Sex Marital Ther.*, **18**, 3–18.
15. Ferlic, M., Goldman, A., and Kennedy, B. (1979). Group counseling in adult patients with advanced cancer. *Cancer*, **43**, 760–766.
16. Jacobs, C., Ross, R., Walker, I., and Stockdale, F. (1983). Behavior of cancer patients: A randomized study of the effects of education and peer support groups. *Am. J. Clin. Oncol.*, **6**, 347–350.
17. Tracey, G. and Gussow, Z. (1976). Self-help groups: A grass-roots response to a need for services. *J. Appl. Behav. Sci.*, **12**, 381–396.
18. Toseland, R. and Hacker, L. (1982). Self-help groups and professional involvement. *Soc. Work.*, 341–347.
19. Taylor, S. and Lobel, M. (1989). Social comparison activity under threat: Downward evaluation and upward contracts. *Psychol. Rev.*, **96**, 569–575.
20. Bloom, J. R. and Spiegel, D. (1984). The relationship of two dimensions of social support to the psychological well-being and social functioning of women with advanced breast cancer. *Soc. Sci. Med.*, **119**, 831–837.
21. Bloom, J. R., Fobair, P., Spiegel, D., Cox, R. S., Varghese, A., and Hoppe, R. (1991). Social supports and the social well-being of cancer survivors. *Adv. Med. Soc.*, **2**, 95–114.
22. Bloom, J. R. (1982). Social support, accommodation to stress and adjustment to breast cancer. *Soc. Sci. Med.*, **16**, 1329–1338.
23. Spiegel, D., Bloom, J., and Gottheil, E. (1983). Family environment of patients with metastatic carcinoma. *J. Psychosoc. Onc.*, **1**, 33–44.
24. Hinton, J. (1975). The influence of previous personality on reactions to having terminal cancer. *Omega*, **6**, 95–111.
25. Friedman, L. C., Baer, P. E., Nelson, D. V., Lane, M. Smith F. E., and Dworkin, R. J. (1988). Women with breast cancer: Perception of family functioning and adjustment to illness. *Psychosom. Med.*, **50**, 529–540.

26. Spiegel, D. and Glafkides, M. (1983). Effects of group confrontation with death and dying. *Int. J. Group Psychother.*, 33, 433–447.

27. Spiegel, D. and Bloom, J. (1983). Group therapy and hypnosis reduce metastatic breast carcinoma pain. *Psychosom. Med.*, 45, 333–339.

28. Morrow, G. and Morrell, C. (1982). Behavioural treatment for the anticipatory nausea and vomiting induced by cancer chemotherapy. *N. Engl. J. Med.*, 307, 1476–1480.

29. Lyles, J., Burish, T., Krozely, M., and Oldham, R. (1982). Efficacy of relaxation training and guided imagery in reducing the aversiveness of cancer chemotherapy. *J. Consult. Clin. Psychol.*, 50, 509–524.

30. Morgenstern, H., Gelert, G. A., Walter, S. D., Ostfeld, A. M., and Siegel, B. S. (1984). The impact of a pychosocial program on survival with breast cancer: the importance of selection bias in program evaluation. *J. Chronic Dis.*, 37, 273–282.

31. Spiegel, D., Bloom, J., Kraemer, H., and Gottheil, E. (1989). The beneficial effects of psychosocial treatment on survival of metastatic breast cancer patients: A randomized prospective outcome study. *Lancet*, 2, 888–891.

32. Gellert, G. A., Maxwell, R. M., and Siegel, B. S. (1993). Survival of breast cancer patients receiving adjunctive psychosocial support therapy: A 10-year follow-up study, *J. Clin. Oncol.*, 11(1), 66–69.

33. Richardson, J. L., Shelton, D. R., Krailo, M. *et al.* (1990). The effect of compliance with treatment on survival among patients with hematologic malignancies. *J. Clin. Onc.*, 8, 356–364.

34. Spiegel, D., Bloom, J., and Yalom, I. D. (1989). Effect of psychosocial treatment on survival of patients with metastatic breast cancer. *Lancet*, 888–901, October 14.

35. Goodwin, J. S., Hunt, W. C., Key, C. R., and Samet, J. M. (1987). The effect of marital status on stage, treatment and survival of cancer patients. *JAMA*, 258, 3125–3130.

36. Liang, L., Dunn, S., Gorman, A., and Stuart-Harris, R. (1990). Identifying priorities of psychosocial need in cancer patients. *Br, J. Cancer*, 62(6), 1000–1003.

37. Spiegel, D. and Spira, J. (1991). Supportive–expressive group therapy. A treatment manual of psychosocial intervention for women with recurrent breast cancer. Psychosocial Treatment Laboratory, Department of Psychiatry and Behavioural Sciences, Stanford University, California, USA.

38. Classen, C., Diamond, S., Soleman, A., Fobair, P., Spira, J., and Spiegel, D. (1993). Brief supportive–expressive group therapy for women with primary breast cancer: A treatment manual. Stanford, CA: Psychosocial Treatment Laboratory, Department of Psychiatry and Behavioural Sciences.

39. Spiegel, D. (1979). Psychological support for women with metastatic carcinoma. *Psychosomatics*, 20, 780–787.

40. Spiegel, D. and Yalom, I. D. (1978). A support group for dying patients. *Int. J. Group Psychother.*, 28, 233–245.

41. Adams, J. (1979). Mutual-help groups: Enhancing the coping ability of oncology clients. *Cancer Nurs.*, 2, 95–98.

42. Telch, C. and Telch, M. (1986). Group coping skills instruction and supportive

group therapy for cancer patients: A comparison of strategies. *J. Consult. Clin. Psychol.*, **54**, 802–808.

43. Taylor, S. and Dakof, G. (1988). Social support and the cancer patient. In *The Social Psychology of Health: The Claremont Symposium on Applied Social Psychology*, (ed. S. Spacapan and S. Oskamp), pp. 95–116. Sage, Newbury Park, CA.

44. Reissman, F. (1965). The 'helper therapy' principle. *Soc. Work*, **10**, 27–32.

45. Browne, G., Arpin, K., Corey, P., Fitch, M., and Gafni, A. (1990). Individual correlates of health service utilization and the cost of poor adjustment to chronic illness. *Med. Care*, **28**, 43–58.

46. Hellman, C., Budd, M., Borysenko, J., McClelland, D., and Benson, H. (1990). A study of the effectiveness of two group behavioural medicine interventions for patients with psychosomatic complaints. *Behav. Med.*, **16**, 165–173.

47. Yalom, V. and Yalom, I. (1990). Brief interactive group psychotherapy. *Psychiatric Annals*, **20**, 362–367.

48. Edgar, L., Rosberger, Z., and Nowlis, D. (1992). Coping with cancer during the first year after diagnosis: Assessment and intervention. *Cancer*, **69**, 817–828.

49. Northhouse, L. L. and Swain, M. A. (1987). Adjustment of patients and husbands to the initial impact of breast cancer. *Nurs. Res.*, **36**, 221–225.

50. Vinokur, A. D., Threatt, B. A., Vinokur-Kaplan, D., and Satariano, W. A. (1990). The process of recovery from breast cancer for younger and older patients: Change during the first year. *Cancer*, **65**, 1242–1254.

51. Stones, M. J., Dornan, B., and Kozma, A. (1989). The prediction of mortality in elderly institution residents. *J. Geront.*, **44**, 72–79.

52. Berkman, L. F. and Syme, S. L. (1979). Social networks, host resistance, and mortality: a nine-year follow-up study of Alameda County residents. *Am. J. Epidemiol.*, **109**, 186–204.

53. Haynes, B. R., Taylor, D. W., and Sackett, D. L. (eds) (1979). *Compliance in Health Care*. Johns Hopkins University Press, Baltimore, Maryland.

54. Hoagland, A. C., Bennett, J. M., Morrow, G. R., and Carnile, C. L. M. (1983). Oncologists' views of cancer patient noncompliance. *Aim. J. Clin. Oncol. (CCT)*, **6**, 239–244.

55. Steckel, S. B. (1982). Predicting, measuring, implementing and following up on patient compliance. *Nurs. Clin. North Amer.*, **17**, (3), 491–498.

56. Given, B. A. and Given, C. W. (1989). Compliance among patients with cancer. *Oncol. Nurs. Forum*, **16**, 1, 97–103.

57. Itano, J., Tanabe, P., and Lum, J. (eds) (1983). Compliance and noncompliance in cancer patients, In *Advances in cancer control*, pp. 483–495. Allen Liss, New York.

58. Glass, A., Wieand, H. S., Fisher, B., Bedmond, C., Erner, H., Wolter, J. *et al.* (1981). Acute toxicity during chemotherapy for breast cancer. *Cancer Treat. Res.*, **65**, 5, 363–376.

59. Laszlo, J., Lucas, V. S., and Huang, R. (1981). Emesis as a critical problem in chemotherapy. *N. Engl. J. Med.*, **305**, 16, 948–949.

60. Lee, Y-TN. (1983). Adjuvant chemotherapy (CMF) for breast cancer carcinoma: Patient compliance and total dose received. *Am. J. Clin. Oncol. (CCT)*, **6**, 1, 25–30.

# 160      *C. Classen et al.*

61. Wilcox, P. M., Fetting, J. S., Nettesheim, K. M., and Abelof, M. D. (1982). Anticipatory vomiting in women receiving cyclophosphamide, methotrexate, and 5-FU (CMF) adjuvant chemotherapy for breast carcinoma. *Cancer Treat. Res.*, **66**, 8, 1–4.

62. Ferguson, K. and Bole, G. G. (1979). Family support, health beliefs, and therapeutic compliance in patients with rheumatoid arthritis. *Patient Couns. Health Educ.*, **1**, 101–105.

63. Beck, N. C., Parker, J. C., Frank, R. G. *et al.* (1988). Patients with rheumatoid arthritis at high risk for noncompliance with salicylate treatment regimens. *J. Rheumatol.*, **15**, 1081–1084.

64. Eisenthal, S., Emery, R., Lazare, A., and Udin, H. (1979). 'Adherence' and the negotiated approach to patienthood. *Arch. Gen. Psychiatry*, **36**, 393–398.

65. Wyszynski, A. A. (1990). Managing noncompliance in the 'difficult' medical patient: The contributions of insight. *Psychother. Psychosom.*, **54**, 181–186.

66. Kiecolt-Glaser, J. K. and Glaser, R. (1991). Stress and immune function in humans. In *Psychoneuroimmunology*, (2nd edn), (ed. R. Ader, D. L. Felten, and N. Cohen). Academic Press, New York.

67. Schulz, K. H. and Schulz, H. (1992). Overview of psychoneuroimmunological stress and intervention studies in humans with emphasis on the uses of immunological parameters. *Psycho-oncology*, **1**, 51–70.

68. Bloom, B. L., Asher, S. J., and White, S. W. (1978) Marital disruption as a stressor: A review and analysis. *Psychol. Bull.*, **85**, 867–894.

69. Verbrugge, L. M. (1979). Marital status and health. *J. Marriage Fam.*, **41**, 267–285.

70. Bartrop, R. W., Luckhurst, E., Lazarus, L., Kiloh, L. G., and Penny, R. (1977). Depressed lymphocyte function after bereavement. *Lancet*, i, 834–836.

71. Irwin, M., Daniels, M., Smith, T. L., Bloom, E., and Weiner, H. (1987). Impaired natural killer cell activity during bereavement. *Brain Behav. Immun.*, **1**, 98–104.

72. Irwin, M., Daniels, M., Risch, S. C., Bloom, E., and Weiner, H. (1988). Plasma cortisol and natural killer cell activity during bereavement. *Biol. Psychiatry*, **24**, 173–178.

73. Schleifer, S. J., Keller, S. E., Camerino, M., Thornton, J. C. and Stein, M. (1983). Suppression of lymphocyte stimulation following bereavement. *JAMA*, **250**, 374–377.

74. Kiecolt-Glaser, J. K., Fisher, L., Ogrocki, P., Stout, J. C., Speecher, C. E., and Glaser, R. (1987). Marital quality, marital disruption, and immune function. *Psychosom. Med.*, **49**, 13–34.

75. Kiecolt-Glaser, J. K., Kennedy, S., Malkoff, S., Fisher, L., Speecher, C. E., and Glaser, R. (1988). Marital discord and immunity in males. *J. Behav. Med.*, **50**, 213–229.

76. Kiecolt-Glaser, J. K., Glaser, R., Shuttleworth, E. C., Dyer, C., Ogrocki, P., and Speecher, C. E. (1987). Chronic stress and immune function in family caregivers of Alzheimer's disease victims. *Psychosom. Med.*, **49**, 523–535.

77. McKinnon, W., Weisse, C. S., Reynolds, C. P., Bowles, C. A., and Baum, A. (1989). Chronic stress, leukocyte subpopulations, and humoral response to latent viruses. *Health Psychol.*, **8**, 389–402.

78. Fawzy, F., Kemeny, M., Fawzy, N., Elashoff, R., Morton, D., Cousins, N. *et al.* (1990b). A structured psychiatric intervention for cancer patients: Changes over time in immunological measures. *Arch. Gen. Psychiatry*, **47**, 729–735.

79. House, J. S., Landis, K. R., and Umberson, D. (1988). Social relationships and health. *Science*, **241**, 540–545.

80. Kennedy, S., Kiecolt-Glaser, J. K., and Glaser, R. (1988). Immunological consequences of acute and chronic stressors: Mediating role of interpersonal relationships. *Br. J. Med. Psychol.*, **61**, 77–85.

81. Kiecolt-Glaser, J. K., Ricker, D., George, J., Messick, G., Speecher, C. E., Garner, W. *et al.* (1984). Urinary cortisol levels, cellular immunocompetency, and loneliness in psychiatric impatients. *Psychosom. Med.*, **46**, 15–23.

82. Kiecolt-Glaser, J. K., Garner, W., Speecher, C. E., Penn, G. M., Holliday, J.E., and Glaser, R. (1984). Psychosocial modifiers of immunocompetence in medical students. *Psychosom. Med.*, **46**, 7–14.

83. Glaser, R., Kiecolt-Glaser, J. K. Speecher, C. E., and Holliday, J. E. (1985). Stress-related impairments in cellular immunity. *Psychiat. Res.*, **16**, 233–239.

84. Levy, S., Herberman, R., Lippman, M., and d'Angelo, T. (1987). Correlation of stress factors with sustained depression of natural killer cell activity and predicted prognosis in patients with breast cancer. *J. Clin. Oncol.*, **5**, 348–353.

85. Levy, S., Herberman, R., Maluish, A., Schlien, B., and Lippman, M. (1985). Prognostic risk assessment in primary breast cancer by behavioural and immunological parameters. *Health Psychol.*, **4**, 99–113.

86. Levy, S. M., Herberman, R. B., Whiteside, T., Sanzo, K., Lee, J., and Kirkwood, J. (1990). Perceived social support and tumor estrogen/progesterone receptor status as predictors of natural killer cell activity in breast cancer patients. *Psychosom. Med.*, **52**, 73–85.

87. Rose, R. M. (1984). Overview of endocrinology of stress. In *Neuroendocrinology and Psychiatric Disorder*, (eds G. M. Brown, S. H. Koslow, and S. Reichlin), pp. 95–122. Raven Press, New York.

88. Israel, L. (1989). Psychological supports for cancer patients. *Lancet*, ii, 1209.

89. Malarkey, W. B., Kennedy, M., Allred, L. E., and Milo, G. (1983). Physiological concentration of prolactin can promote the growth of human breast tumor cells in culture. *J. Clin. Endocrinol. Metast.*, **56**, 673–77.

90. Levine, S., Coe, C., and Wiener, S. (1989). Psychoneuroendocrinology of stress: A psychobiological perspective. In *Psychoendocrinology*, pp. 341–377. Academic Press, New York.

91. Greer, S., Morris, T., and Pettingale, K. W. (1979). Psychological response to breast cancer: Effect on outcome. *Lancet*, **2**, 785–787.

92. Eysenck, H. J. (1987). Anxiety, learned helplessness, and cancer: A causal theory. *J. Anxiety Disorders*, **1**, 87–104.

93. Sieber, W. J., Rodin, J., Larson, L., Ortega, S., Cummings, N., Levy, S. *et al.* (1994). Modulation of human natural killer cell activity by exposure to uncontrollable stress. In preparation.

94. Stein, M. (1989). Stress, despression, and the immune system. *J. Clin. Psychiatry*, **50**, (suppl. 5), 35–40.

95. Stein, M., Miller, A. H., and Trestman, R. L. (1991). Depression, and immune system, and health and illness. *Arch. Gen. Psychiatry*, **48**, 171–177.

96.  Shekelle, R. B., Raynor, W. J., Ostfeld, A. M., Garron, D. C., Bieliauskas, L. A. , Lui, S. C. *et al.* (1981). Psychological depression and 17-year risk of death from cancer. *Psychosom. Med.*, **43**, 117–125.

97.  Persky, V. W., Kempthorne-Rawson, J., and Shekelle, R. B. (1987). Personality and risk of cancer: 20 year follow-up of the Western Electrick study. *Psychosom. Med.*, **49**, 435–449.

98.  Kaplan, G. A. and Reynolds, P. (1988). Depression and cancer mortality and morbidity: Prospective evidence from the Alameda County study. *J. Behav. Med.*, **11**, 1–13.

99.  Hahn, R. C. and Petitti, D. B. (1988). Minnesota Multiphasic Personality Inventory—rated depression and the incidence of breast cancer. *Cancer*, **61**, 845–848.

100. Linkins, R. W. and Comstock, G. W. (1988). Depressed mood and development of cancer. *Am. J. Epidemiol.*, **262**, 1191–1195.

101. Zonderman, A. B., Costa, P. T., and McCrae, R. R. (1989). Depression as a risk for cancer morbidity and mortality in a nationally representative sample. *JAMA*, **262**, 1191–1195.

102. Pettingale, K. W., Watson, M., Tee, D. E., Inayat, Q. *et al.* (1989). Pathological grief, psychiatric symptoms, and immune status following conjugal bereavement. *Stress Med.*, **5**(2), 77–78.

103. Greer, S. and Morris, T. (1975). Psychological attributes of women who develop breast cancer: A controlled study. *J. Psychosom. Res.*, **19**, 147–153.

104. Temoshok, L. (1987). Personality, coping style, emotion and cancer: Towards an integrative model. *Cancer Surveys*, **6**, 545–567.

105. Fow, B. H. (1983). Current theory of psychogenic effects on cancer incidence and prognosis. *J. Psychosoc. Oncol.*, **1**, 17–31.

106. Angell, M. (1985). Disease as a reflection of the psyche. *N. Engl. J. Med.*, **312**, 1570–1572.

107. Cassileth, B. R., Lusk, E. J., Miller, D. S., Brown, L. L., and Miller, C. (1985). Psychosocial correlates of survival in advanced malignant disease? *N. Engl. J. Med.*, **312**, 1551–1555.

108. Morris, T. and Greer, S. (1980). A 'Type C' for cancer? Low trait anxiety in the pathogenesis of breast cancer. *Cancer Det. Prev.*, **3**(l), Abstract 102.

109. Gross, J. (1989). Emotional expression in cancer onset and progression. *Soc. Sci. Med.*, **28**, 1239–1248.

110. Levenson, J. and Bemis, C. (1991). The role of psychological factors in cancer onset and progression. *Psychosomatics*, **32**, 124–132.

# 5

# Synergistic interaction between psychosocial and physical factors in the causation of lung cancer

H. J. EYSENCK

## 1 Introduction

There is no doubt that there are numerous risk factors for cancer. Smoking, genetics, exposure to radon gas or asbestos, drinking, eating patterns, sexual excesses, and many other factors have been isolated. This fact alone makes *univariate* analyses unacceptable; such analyses cannot tell us anything about the precise contribution of one factor, when the possible involvement of other factors is disregarded. The Surgeon-General, the Royal College of Physicians, and other medical bodies have published statements about the number of deaths caused by smoking. Thus the Health Education Council, jointly with the British Medical Association (1), stated that smoking kills 77 774 people annually (55 107 men and 22 667 women) in England and Wales, and because of their smoking, some 108 218 people are hospitalized each year because of smoking-related diseases. Such figures are based on extrapolations of data listing differences in mortality between smokers and non-smokers, but disregard all other risk factors. Given that such risk factors usually appear jointly, rather than singly, such a *univariate* treatment of the figure is clearly inappropriate. A person might be certified as having died of lung cancer who, during his life, smoked heavily, worked in an asbestos factory, lived in a house with radon gas present, was exposed to X-rays while in hospital, drank heavily and unwisely, and had three first-degree relatives who died of lung cancer. Here we have seven risk factors, interacting in a complex manner, all or any of which might have been the 'cause' of death, yet in the statistics of the Surgeon-General and the Royal College of Physicians *smoking* would have been the only factor noted. This problem invalidates much of the evidence implicating any single cause, like smoking, particularly when added to the poor methodology and the inappropriate statistics so characteristic of this whole field (2–6).

Given the multiplicity of risk factors, clearly their *mode of interaction* is of crucial interest. It is possible that the interaction is additive, that is the effects of Factor A are simply added to those of Factor B if both are present. Alternatively, effects may multiply to produce a synergistic effect. If multiple risk factors act synergistically, the usual method of determining mortality as due to one factor only becomes even more unscientific and misleading, and the need for multivariate methods of analysis becomes even more essential.

## 2   Models of interaction

There is a good deal of evidence to show that *physical* risk factors in major decisions act synergistically rather than additively (7–17). There is now accumulating evidence that *psychosocial* factors also interact synergistically with physical factors (3, 18–22). If this hypothesis of synergistic interaction between psychosocial and physical risk factors is correct, it has tremendous implications for the analysis and interpretation of epidemiological data, as pointed out above.

The hypothesis to be tested is that *single* risk factors, (for example smoking, drinking, stress, genetic predisposition, etc.) have relatively little influence on mortality from cancer, but that their effects may be synergistic, in the sense that these universal effects do not *add* (the additive hypothesis) but *multiply*. This problem has been attacked along several different lines, using different samples and different methods (3). Some of these studies have been referred to above. There are many different ways of looking at this problem, and different statistical tests; this variety raises problems some of which are discussed in this chapter.

The term 'synergism' may at first appear to be perfectly clear in its meaning;

it is usually defined as the combined effect of drugs, behaviours, genetic factors, etc. that exceeds the sum of their individual effects. However, the precise operational definition of the term has given rise to many difficulties (23), and apparently contradictory results have been obtained by workers using different models for identical data. We may use an *additive* model looking simply at *differences between proportions*, or a *multiplicative* one which works with *ratios of proportions*, or relative risks. As Everitt and Smith (23) point out, 'it is quite possible for the two models to lead to seemingly conflicting results when applied to the same set of data' (p. 582). They also point out, in answer to the question of which model is the correct one, that 'unfortunately there is no absolute answer, and in practice the choice between them may depend on rather complex reasoning' (3, p. 582).

Cornfield (24) is credited with first introducing the multiple logistic function, in his analysis of the factors related to the occurrence of coronary heart disease (CHD). Then in 1968, Selikoff, Hammond and Chang (25) showed that the combined exposure to tobacco smoking and to asbestos was associated with a lung cancer risk far exceeding that expected from the separate exposure to each of these agents, indicating the occurrence of an interaction between the two agents. Saracci (15) has published a survey of interactions of tobacco smoking and other agents in cancer a etiology, concluding that 'a multiplicative relation of the relative risks for tobacco smoking and for another agent can at present be regarded either as an approximately satisfactory representation of the data, or, at the worst, as an upper limit of the strength of the interaction' (p. 190).

How is synergism measured? According to Saracci, we observe relative risks among subjects exposed to smoking alone $(R_s)$, to the other agent alone $(R_o)$, or to both agents $(R_{so})$, all relative risks here being calculated taking the subjects not exposed to either agent as reference. A *zero* difference between the observed value of $R_s$ and the value of $R_s + R_o - 1$ defines zero interaction, that is a simple additive relation or model. A value greater than zero defines a positive interaction (synergism) (12, 14).

Perkins (9) uses a similar model. He follows Kleinbaum, Kupper, and Morganstern (10) in not using 'synergism' as a synonym for 'interaction'. As he points out, non-linear, multiplicative models, such as logistic regression, widely used in recent years, '. . . allow for simultaneous control of the effects of converging risk factors of interest, but they may also hide the existence of risk factor interactions as defined above, by deviations from additivity [(11, 12, 17)]. Therefore, a primary reason that these interactions have gone unrecognized may be that most epidemiologic studies of CHD have used predictive models which are generally incompatible with the detection of such interactions.' (9).

In other words, when synergism so defined is present, even on simple inspection of the four-fold table, this additive model is not the only one available

(26–30). There is also a *multiplicative*, logistic model (31) and the two models may give apparently different answers, as Everitt and Smith (23) point out in discussing alternative interpretations of identical data by Brown and Harris (31) and Tennant and Bebbington (32).

I have used both types of approach, wherever applicable, to a variety of data, some previously published, others not; the tables will be able to give evidence concerning synergism, as defined by Saracci and Perkins, but are also adequately described by logistic models in which effects act independently. A more technical discussion of the issues involved is given in Section 6.


## 3   Smoking and stress in lung cancer

Let us consider a particular example before turning to a more sophisticated look at the statistical problems involved. Table 1 gives data on lung cancer mortality from a study carried out on 2374 healthy probands who were followed-up for 10 years and finally rated on the basis of death certificates as having died of lung cancer, or not having died of lung cancer, that is either still being alive, or having died of some other cause. They were subdivided into smoking or not smoking groups, and again into suffering or not suffering from stress. Stress was defined in terms of a pattern of questionnaire answers suggesting the presence of a stress, and inability to cope with the stress experienced. Details concerning all these points can be found elsewhere (3).

The background factor is a mortality of .35 per cent in the non-smoking, non-stress group. For the non-smoking cancer-prone group it is 2.89 per cent, giving an excess of 2.54 per cent (2.89 per cent–.35 per cent). For smoking in non-cancer-prone probands, the effect is .45 per cent (.80 per cent–.35 per cent), that is about a fifth of that of personality. The *combined* effect of

**Table 1**   Lung cancer mortality of 2374 probands followed-up over a ten-year period (33). Lung cancer as a function of smoking and stress

|                | No stress | Stress | Stress effect |
|----------------|-----------|--------|---------------|
| No smoking     | 0.35%     | 2.89%  | $(2.89\% - 0.35\%) = 2.54\%$ |
| Smoking        | 0.80%     | 15.56% |               |
| Smoking effect |           | $(0.80\% - 0.35\%) = 0.45\%$ | |
| $N = 2374$     | Real combined effect  $(15.56\% - 0.35\%) = 15.21\%$ | | |
|                | Additive effect        $( 0.45\% + 2.54\%) = 2.99\%$ | | |
|                | Difference (Synergistic effect)        12.22% | | |

smoking and personality is 15.21 per cent (15.56 per cent–.35 per cent), which is five times the effect expected from a simple addition of the smoking and personality effects (.45 + 2.54 per cent = 2.99 per cent). This calculation takes into account 2374 people, giving 77 cases of lung cancer mortality. The results are suggestive, but the number of deaths is not large enough to take the results as anything but a very rough-and-ready guideline. Also the bringing together of two different populations (Yugoslav and German), differing in age and stress, might be criticized, although the results when analysed separately for the two groups are not dissimilar.

Consider now a *standard logistic model* applied to the data. Table 2 shows the model.

For the *Stress and Smoking* model the estimated parameters are as follows.

$$\begin{aligned} \text{Grand Mean} &= -6.277 \ (0.4191) \\ \text{Stress} &= \phantom{-}2.872 \ (0.3557) \\ \text{Smoking} &= \phantom{-}1.689 \ (0.3078) \end{aligned}$$

(Standard errors are given in parentheses.)

A comparison of observed, fitted, and standardized residual values for this model indicates that the fit is extremely good.

Being in the stress group rather than the non-stress group increases the odds (in favour of dying from cancer) by 2.872 with an approximately 95 per cent confidence interval (2.161, 3.585). Converting this to the 'odds' scale gives a confidence interval (8.68, 35.98).

Being a smoker rather than a non-smoker increases the odds (in favour of dying from cancer) by 1.689 with an approximately 95 per cent confidence

**Table 2** Standard logistic model of data in Table 1

| Model | Chi-Square | d.f. | P |
|---|---|---|---|
| Grand mean | 167.85 | 3 | 0.000 |
| Stress | 42.20 | 2 | 0.000 |
| Smoking | 117.22 | 2 | 0.000 |
| Stress and smoking | 1.49 | 1 | 0.222 |

**Table 3** Fit of model in Table 2

| | Observed | Fitted | Residual |
|---|---|---|---|
| No smoking/No stress | 3 | 1.50 | 1.11 |
| No smoking/Stress | 10 | 11.41 | −0.42 |
| Smoking/No stress | 6 | 7.41 | −0.52 |
| Smoking/Stress | 86 | 66.59 | 0.10 |

interval $(1.073, 2.305)$. Converting this to the 'odds' scale gives a confidence interval $(2.924, 10.242)$.

Lastly, and perhaps most importantly the model implies that smoking and stress act *independently*; so on this particular scale there is little need to postulate interactions between conditions.

What is happening? How can identical data give rise to apparently contradictory conclusions? The answer lies in the use of *logarithms* in the standard logistic model. As will be well known, to *multiply* numbers we *add* logarithms; in other words, the multiplication of effects in the raw data becomes an additive effect in the logarithmized data. The appendix to this chapter will serve to clarify the argument for readers interested in the statistical issues involved. What has to be remembered is simply that the results are not contradictory, but distribute the synergistic effects differently — one over the interaction between raw data, the other over the addition of logarithms. We are safe in inferring synergistic interaction in the data even though the interaction term in the logistic model is insignificant.

Are the data replicable? We (33) have reported a study similar to the one given in Table 1, but carried out on a different population of 1914 probands (Table 4). We again found an additive effect (0.95 per cent) which is clearly lower than the true combined effect of stress and smoking (9.90 per cent), giving a synergistic effect of 8.95 per cent. The outcome is rather similar to that reported in Table 1. In the causation of lung cancer, smoking and stress clearly act in a synergistic fashion.

# 4   Interaction of several risk factors

How about the interaction of more than two factors? Consider the following analysis.

Table 4   Replication of study in Table 1 (33). Lung cancer as a function of smoking and stress

|  | No stress | Stress | Stress effect |
|---|---|---|---|
| No smoking | 0.69% | 2.09% | $(2.09\% - 0.69\%) = 1.40\%$ |
| Smoking | 0.24% | 10.59% |  |
| Smoking effect |  | $(0.24\% - 0.69\% = 0.45\%)$ | |
| | Real combined effect | $(10.59\% - 0.69\%) = 9.90\%$ | |
| $N = 1914$ | Additive effect | $(1.40\% - 0.45\%) = 0.95\%$ | |
| | Difference (Synergistic effect) | 8.95% | |

This study began in 1972, when some 16 000 males, aged between 32 and 66 years, constituting a random sample of the male population between these age limits, were interviewed and asked if they had any relatives or friends characterized by the following risk factors for lung cancer. This group consisted of people who were heavy smokers, and/or had one or more close relatives who had died, or were suffering from lung cancer, or from severe bronchitis for more than 5 years. Persons suffering from only one of these risk factors for lung cancer could also be nominated. After consultation with the person so nominated, 798 were nominated, but 54 refused to participate, leaving 744 in all. This is our sample, the members of which are clearly far from random, but who are well suited to investigate the effects of single risk factors as compared with different combinations of two, three, or four such risk factors.

Members of the group filled in a questionnaire as follows:

1. Of your parents or grandparents, are any ill with lung cancer, or have any died of lung cancer? If yes, how many? In which clinic was the diagnosis made? What treatment was administered? How long did your relatives live after diagnosis?

2. Do you smoke? If yes, for how long have you smoked, and how many cigarettes did you smoke a day during the past five years?

3. Have you been suffering from bronchitis, as diagnosed by a physician, for more than five years?

4. Are you suffering from high blood pressure? What is the reading?

5. Are you suffering from high cholesterol levels? What is the reading?

6. Are you suffering from diabetes mellitus? If yes, for how long?

In addition, participants were given a personality questionnaire which is reproduced in full elsewhere (34); this questionnaire is the same as that used in the study reported in Table 4. This gives scores to each person on six type-factors, of which three (factors 1, 2, and 5) are prognostic of stress-induced disease, particularly cancer and CHD, while the other three (factors 3, 4, and 6) are prognostic of absence of disease. We used the formula: $(1 + 2 + 5) - (3 + 4 + 6) > 0$ as our measure of (psychological) stress. We thus have four two-value (YES or NO) risk factors: H (hereditary predisposition), C (cigarette smoking), B (bronchitis), and S (stress), as defined by answers to the interviewer-administered questionnaires. Mortality was ascertained in 1986, that is after 13 years; cause of death was taken from the death certificates.

Results are shown in Table 5, giving mortality figures for cancer of the lung, and for all other causes, as well as the mean ages of the groups concerned. We compared mortality rates for groups having only one risk factor, two risk factors, three risk factors, or all four risk factors. It was not possible to find sufficient persons to fill all possible 'cells'; thus there are no persons in the table *only* suffering from bronchitis. However, for all combinations of two, three, or four risk factors, we were able to find sufficient subjects to make up groups of reasonable size, the smallest consisting of 26 members.

What does Table 5 tell us? Looking at lung cancer first of all, we see that the risk factors taken singly do not lead to mortality in these groups. Bronchitis, as already mentioned, is missing, but it is not associated with mortality even when associated with other risk factors, so that we may perhaps be justified in assuming that it is innocent when present alone. Thus our four risk factors, taken one at a time, produce 0 deaths in 209 subjects. For combination of two risk factors, there are 3 deaths in 356 subjects, that is a rate of 1 per cent. For three risk factors, we have 17 deaths, in a population of 127 subjects, giving a rate of 13 per cent. For the 26 subjects showing all four risk factors, there are 8 deaths, amounting to 31 per cent. Thus there is a steep rise in mortality as we go from one to two, three and four risk factors: 0 per cent, 1 per cent, 13 per cent, 31 per cent. This is far removed from an additive model, and indicative of synergistic actions.

We now turn to 'other causes of death'. Here for single risk factors we have 33 deaths for H, C, or S alone, for 209 subjects, or 16 per cent. If we add half of the deaths from H + B, C + B, and B + S, to take the place of B alone, we have 13 additional deaths for 209 subjects, that is 16 per cent overall. For combinations of two risk factors, we have 61 deaths for 356 subjects, equal to 17 per cent. For three risk factor combinations, there are 29 deaths for 127 subjects, or 23 per cent. Finally, for all four risk factors in combination, there

**Table 5** Lung cancer and other causes of death as a function of Bronchitis (B), Cigarette-smoking (C), Stress (S), and Heredity (H) (33)

| Combination of risks | N | Lung cancer | Percentage | Other causes of death | Percentage | Average age |
|---|---|---|---|---|---|---|
| Only H | 50 | 0 | 0 | 5 | 10 | 51 |
| Only C | 100 | 0 | 0 | 12 | 12 | 52 |
| Only S | 59 | 0 | 0 | 16 | 27 | 52 |
| H + C | 50 | 1 | 2 | 4 | 8 | 53 |
| H + B | 52 | 0 | 0 | 8 | 15 | 51 |
| C + B | 55 | 0 | 0 | 11 | 20 | 52 |
| C + S | 100 | 2 | 2 | 21 | 21 | 53 |
| H + S | 49 | 0 | 0 | 9 | 18 | 54 |
| B + S | 50 | 0 | 0 | 8 | 16 | 53 |
| C + H + B | 26 | 2 | 8 | 5 | 19 | 51 |
| C + H + S | 50 | 10 | 20 | 14 | 28 | 51 |
| C + B + S | 51 | 5 | 10 | 10 | 20 | 51 |
| H + C + B + S | 26 | 8 | 31 | 8 | 31 | 52 |

are 8 deaths for 26 subjects, that is 31 per cent. Thus for 'other causes of death' the progression is 16 per cent, 17 per cent, 23 per cent, and 31 per cent. This is very different from the progression in the case of deaths from lung cancer, suggesting quite a different pattern of interaction.

Applying statistical procedures to the data, we find the following, treating the number of risk factors (NRF) as forming a kind of dose–response curve. The results of fitting a series of logistic models for the cancer deaths are shown in Table 6.

The quadratic term significantly improves the fit and so is retained in the final model which is therefore:

$$\ln \frac{P}{1-p} = -16.22 + 7.588 \text{ NRF} - 0.934 \text{ NRF} \times \text{NRF}$$

This model is essentially a simple 'dose–response' curve which one would not normally think of in terms of synergistic effects, although it is clear that the odds of dying from cancer increases considerably as the number of risk factors increases. Again, the synergistic effect is somewhat hidden by the use of logarithms.

# 5  Extension of the model to other carcinomas

Another study (34) shows the synergistic effects of stress, smoking, and alcohol on cancer of the mouth and pharynx. The number and proportion of probands either with ($n = 34$) or without ($n = 1706$) zero, one, two, or all three risk factors was ascertained, and the results are shown in Table 7. It is clear that none of the cancer cases had experienced none or only one of these risk factors, while 30 per cent of healthy people had. Any combination of two risk factors occurred in 21 per cent of the cancer cases, but in 44 per cent of health probands. It is when all three occur that the two groups are differentiated—79 per cent of cancer patients, but only 26 per cent of healthy people are so characterized.

Two further studies may be of interest in demonstrating that synergistic interaction is equally observable in the case of other types of cancer, and is not restricted to lung cancer. Both come from a large-scale prospective study

**Table 6**  Analysis of Table 5 data for lung cancer

| Model | Chi-square | d.f. | P |
|---|---|---|---|
| Grand mean | 69.85 | 3 | 0.001 |
| N.R.F (Lin) | 5.51 | 2 | 0.064 |
| N.R.F (Quad) | 0.03 | 1 | 0.862 |

**Table 7** Cancer patients and healthy probands showing different combinations of three risk factors for cancer (34)

| Risk factors | Cancer | | Population | |
|---|---|---|---|---|
| | *n* | Percentage | *n* | Percentage |
| None | 0 | 0 | 137 | 8 |
| Smoking | 0 | 0 | 64 | 4 |
| Personality only | 0 | 0 | 151 | 9 |
| Drinking only | 0 | 0 | 158 | 9 |
| Smoking + Stress | 3 | 9 | 52 | 3 |
| Drinking + Stress | 3 | 9 | 447 | 26 |
| Smoking + Drinking | 1 | 3 | 256 | 15 |
| Smoking + Drinking + Stress | 27 | 79 | 441 | 26 |
| | 34 | 100 | 1706 | 100 |

carried out by Dr R. Grossarth-Maticek with the assistance of the Psychological Department of the Heidelberg University Clinic (to be published shortly). In the first study, four groups of 179 women were chosen from a total of 6051 healthy women originally studied in 1973, and followed-up until 1988; choice was based on high or low psychosocial stress, and high or low physical stress factors. The dependent variables were (1) breast carcinoma, and (2) carcinoma of other types. Table 8 shows the results. There is a clear synergistic effect for breast cancer but not for other cancers (significance estimated after Vetter (35).

From the same sample, Table 9 gives results for Stress/No stress groups having respectively zero, one, two, or three first-degree relatives who died of breast cancer. The results again show synergistic interaction between stress and heredity, using the Vetter (1988) test.

# 6  Additive vs. multiplicative models

Let us return to Table 1. There are three approaches to analysing such 2 × 2 data tables.

## 6.1  AN ADDITIVE EFFECT MODEL

A model that calculates the expected proportion in cell P4 based upon taking the difference between cells P2 and P1, and cells P3 and P1. The logic behind such an operation is that the combined effect of stress and smoking is predicted from a simple additive function of the two factors. Given the background mortality rate (cell P1) of no smoking and no stress, the effects of each factor are separately computed, then added to the background rate to

**Table 8** Breast carcinoma and other carcinomas as a function of psychosocial and physical risk factors (36)

|  | N: No psychosocial | Psychosocial |
|---|---|---|
| No physical | 1 (0.5%) | 3 ( 1.6%) |
|  | 7 (3.9%) | 35 (19.5%) |
| Physical | 2 (1.1%) | 25 (13.9%) |
|  | 8 (4.4%) | 36 (20.1%) |

Breast carcinoma on top; other carcinomas below. (N = 179 in each cell)

**Table 9** Breast carcinoma as a function of psychosocial and genetic risk factors (36)

|  | No stress | | Stress | |
|---|---|---|---|---|
|  | n: | Breast cancer | n: | Breast cancer |
|  |  | Percentage |  | Percentage |
| No genetic predisposition | 306 | 1 ( 0.3) | 238 | 1 ( 0.4) |
| One relative | 208 | 3 ( 1.4) | 141 | 6 ( 4.1) |
| Two relatives | 70 | 3 ( 4.2) | 68 | 6 ( 8.8) |
| Three relatives | 28 | 3 (10.7) | 29 | 11 (37.9) |

produce the proportion expected to be observed in cell P4 (the joint effect). Specifically:

Stress effect = P2 − P1 = 0.0289 − 0.0035 = 0.0254
Smoking effect = P3 − P1 = 0.0080 − 0.0035 = 0.0045
Stress and Smoking = 0.0254 + 0.0045 = 0.0299
Expected proportion for cell P4 = 0.0299 + 0.0035 = 0.0334

As can be seen, the expected proportion is computed in a purely additive, linear, fashion. In this form of analysis, the hypothesis is specific and targeted on one cell only. That is, do the joint effects of factors 1 and 2 (in the case above, stress and smoking) act in an additive fashion when they occur jointly? The alternative hypotheses are that the factors act in a simple multiplicative or a synergistic fashion. The simple multiplicative model is described below in detail but is characterized by a simple multiplier function of the P1, background mortality, cell. The synergistic model is one that proposed that the factors act in a complex multiplicative fashion, generally taken to be some form of exponential increase in proportionate mortality when the two factors occur together. The probability of observing a proportion in cell P4, given the expected 'calculated' proportion can be assessed using the binomial distribution. Approximating the binomial distribution by the normal distribution, we can compute a standardized normal deviate by examining the difference between the observed and expected frequencies, given the observed and expected proportions. The probability of observing such a deviate is a direct measure of the goodness of fit of the additive model. Note that in this model, the table of expected frequency marginals does not fit the observed marginals, neither is the odds ratio equal to 1. Both conditions are required for a typical contingency table chi-square analysis.

## 6.2 A SIMPLE MULTIPLICATIVE MODEL

This model calculates the expected proportion in cell P4 based upon the ratio (or odds) between cells P2 and P1, and cells P3 alnd P1. The logic behind such an operation is that the combined effect of stress and smoking is predicted from a simple multiplicative function of the two odds ratios. Given the background mortality rate (cell P) of no smoking and no stress, the effect of each factor is separately computed, then multiplied with the background rate to produce the proportion expected to be observed in cell P4 (the joint effect). Specifically:

Stress effect = P2/P1 = 0.0289/0.0035 = 8.2571
Smoking effect = P3/P1 = 0.0080/0.0035 = 2.2857
Stress and Smoking = 8.2571 × 2.2857 = 18.8735
Expected proportion for cell P4 = 18.8735 × 0.0035 = 0.0661

As with the additive model above the probability of observing the number of deaths, given the expected number computed from the calculated proportion, is provided by the normal approximation to the binomial test. Note that in this particular model, the odds ratio is always 1.0, although the marginals remain unequal due to there being no constraint in the model fitting process. Thus, a contingency table chi-square test would also seem to be inappropriate here. Note that in both this model and the one above, cells P1, P2, and P3 are fixed. Only cell P4 can be estimated.

## 6.3 COMPLEX MULTIPLICATIVE MODELS

These models are tested using the techniques of log-linear analysis and logit analysis (logistic regression). Essentially, these models always produce expected marginal frequencies that fit the observed marginal frequencies and odds ratios equal to 1.0 (under the hypothesis of independent effects). In order to focus on one particular model, it can be noted that the logit is 0.5 × log (odds). Within a log-linear 2 × 2 analysis, three 'effect' parameters can be estimated that will explain the observed frequencies exactly. In our example above, one is stress, the other smoking, and the third a stress × smoking interaction parameter. Now, the form of this saturated log-linear model (expressed in its direct exponential form rather than its logarithmically transformed form) is

$$F_{ij} = \eta \tau_i^{St} \tau_j^{Sm} \tau_{ij}^{StSm}$$

where $F_{ij}$ = the expected frequency in cell position $i = 1, 2$ rows and $j = 1, 2$ cols; $\eta$ = the geometric mean of the number of cases in each cell of the table; $\tau_i^{St}$ = the tau effect that Stress has on the frequencies in cells $i$; $\tau_j^{Sm}$ = the tau effect that Smoking has on the frequencies in cells $j$; $\tau_{ij}^{StSm}$ = the tau effect that Stress and Smoking have on the frequencies in cells, $ij$.
For example,

$$\tau^{St} = \left( F_{11} F_{12} / F_{21} F_{22} \right)^{1/4}$$

and, more specifically, for cell $i$

$$\tau_i^{St} = \frac{(F_{i1} F_{i2})^{1/2}}{(F_{11} F_{12} F_{21} F_{22})^{1/4}} \, .$$

Also, given that the tau coefficients can be seen to represent the ratio of the number of expected frequencies in one category to the geometric average of the expected frequencies in all categories, it becomes readily apparent that the model being fitted is a complex multiplicative function of the marginal odds and odds ratios within the table of data. Although an interaction term can be examined as part of the model fitting procedure, it is clear that this interaction is accounting for cell frequency disparities based upon multiplicative, independent, functions of both row and column factors (stress and smoking). Essentially, the interaction term in a 2 × 2 table is examined indirectly via the null hypothesis that the row and/or column frequencies, *acting independently*, can sufficiently account for the observed frequencies. In this model, the expected frequencies are those as given by the more familiar chi-square contingency table analysis. That is, the expected proportions for each row or colum factor are set equal to the observed marginal proportion, then multiplied by the observed marginal number of observations for the corresponding row or column. The null hypothesis is essentially one of equal proportions within each factor. Note that the additive and simple multiplicative models above take the observed proportions as fixed, and compute the joint effect frequency/proportion based upon these fixed values.

Everitt and Smith's (23) observation that additive vs. multiplicative models can lead to conflicting results is obviously correct. However, in understanding the computational background of the hypothesized interaction between two variables, it becomes apparent that the fault lies not with the statistical methods but with the *choice* of method given the null hypothesis proposed. It is quite inappropriate to use a multiplicative model if the null hypothesis is one concerning additive, conjoint, effects. Testing a hypothesis that attempts to specify the independence of two effect variables, using a multiplicative effects model, is of no value to a research question that specifies a synergistic effect. Independence does not mean additivity, neither does it equate to a lack of synergy. The factor effects within such models are computed as multi-plicative (synergistic) functions from the outset. The multiplicative relation-ship *between* the variables (the interaction) may be of interest with regard to the size of a synergistic function but is actually irrelevant to demonstrating the presence of such a function.

# 7  Summary and conclusions

The data reviewed here suggest quite strongly that cancer of the lung, and probably other cancers also, are the result of synergistic interaction between several risk factors. In particular, smoking and stress have been studied as examples of *physical* and *psychosocial* risk factors. There are certain problems with the statistical methods used to establish such interactions, but they arise from a failure to recognize the different meanings of the term 'interaction' when raw data and log data are being used.

The results suggest that the use of the epidemiological practice of carrying out *univariate* analyses is mistaken, and may give untrustworthy results. Where it is known that there is more than one risk factor, and where in fact there are numerous such factors, often occurring together (as in lung cancer), only *multivariate* methods of analysis are admissible. This would necessitate a switch from univariate to multivariate methodology and analysis even if risk factors acted independently; the fact that they seem to interact syner-gistically makes such a switch-over even more necessary. Obviously much more work needs to be carried out in this field, using different types of cancer as a target, and different risk factors as the independent variable, but the need for such research is urgent if we wish to understand the complex web of *causation* that the usual epidemiological studies leave unexplored.

# 8  References

1.  Roberts, J. L. and Graveling, P. A. (1986). *The Big Kill*. Health Education Coun-cil and the British Medical Association for N. W. Regional Health Authority.
2.  Eysenck, H. J. (1980). *The Causes and Effects of Smoking*. Sage, Los Angeles.
3.  Eysenck, H. J. (1991). *Smoking, Personality and Stress: Psychosocial Factors in the Prevention of Cancer and Coronary Heart Disease*. Springer Verlag, New York.
4.  Burch, P. A. J. (1976). *The Biology of Cancer: A New Approach*. Medical Technology Publishing, Lancaster.
5.  Burch, P. A. J. (1978). Smoking and lung cancer: The problem of inferring cause. *J. Roy. Stats Soc.*, **141**, 437–477.

6. Burch, P. A. J. (1983). The Surgeon-General's 'epidemiologic criteria for causality': A critique. *J. Chron. Dis.*, **36**, 821–836.

7. Perkins, K. A. (1985). The synergistic effect of smoking and serum cholesterol on coronary heart disease. *Hlth. Psychol.*, **4**, 337–360.

8. Perkins, K. A. (1987). Use of terms to describe results: 'additive', 'synergistic'. *Psychophysiol.*, **24**, 719–730.

9. Perkins, K. A. (1989). Ineractions among coronary heart disease risk factors. *Annals of Behav. Med.*, **11**, 3–11.

10. Kleinbaum, D. G., Kupper, L. L., and Morganstern, H. (1982). *Epidemiological Research: Principles and Quantitative Methods*, pp. 403–418. Lifetime Learning Publications, Belmont, CA.

11. Rothman, K. J. (1974). Synergy and antagonism in cause–effect relationships. *Amer. J. Epidemiol.*, **99**, 385–388.

12. Rothman, K. J. (1976). The estimation of synergy or antagonism. *Amer. J. Epidemiol.*, **112**, 465–466.

13. Kannel, W. B., Neaton, J. D., Wentworth, D. *et al.* (1986). Overall and coronary heart disease mortality rates in relation to major risk factors in 325,348 men screened for the MRFIT. *Amer. Heart J.*, **112**, 825–836.

14. Saracci, R. (1980). Interaction and synergism. *Amer. J. Epidemiol.*, **112**, 465–466.

15. Saracci, R. (1987). The interactions of tobacco smoking and other agents in cancer etiology. *Epidemiol. Rev.*, **9**, 175–193.

16. Walker, A. M. (1981). Proportion of disease attributable to the combined effect of two factors. *Inter. J. Epidem.*, **10**, 81–85.

17. Koopman, J. S. (1981). Interaction between discrete causes. *Amer. J. Epidemiol.*, **113**, 716–724.

18. Grossarth-Maticek, R. (1980). Synergistic effects of cigarette smoking, systolic blood pressure and psychosocial risk factors for lung cancer, cardiac infarction and Apoplexy cerebri. *Psychother, Psychosom.*, **34**, 267–272.

19. Grossarth-Maticek, R. (1989). Disposition, exposition, Vernajtensmuster, Organverschadigung und stimulierung des zenhalen Nerresytems in der Aetiologie des Bronchial-, Magen- und Leber karzinoms. *Deutsche Zeitschrift. fuer Onkologie*, **21**, 62–78.

20. Grossarth-Maticek, R. and Eysenck, H. J. (1990*b*). Personality, smoking, and alcohol as synergistic risk factors for cancer of the mouth and pharynx. *Psychol. Reps.*, **67**, 1024–1026.

21. Grossarth-Maticek, R., Eysenck, H. J., and Vetter, H. (1988). Personality type, smoking habit and their interaction as predictors of cancer and coronary heart disease. *Person. individ. Diff.*, **9**, 479–495.

22. Grossarth-Maticek, R., Vetter, H., Frentzel-Beyme, R., and Heller, W. D. (1988). Precursor lesions of the Gl tract and psychosocial risk factors for prediction and prevention of gastric cancer. *Cancer Detect. Prov.*, **13**, 23–29.

23. Everitt, B. S. and Smith, A. M. R. (1979). Interactions in contingency tables; a brick discussion of alternative definitions. *Psychol. Med.*, **9**, 581–583.

24. Cornfield, J. (1962). Joint dependence of risk of coronory heart disease on serum cholesterol and systolic blood pressure: A discriminant function analysis. In *Fed. Proc.*, **21** (Suppl. 11), 98–116.

25. Selikoff, I. J., Hammond, E. C., and Charg, J. (1968). Asbestos exposure, smoking and neoplasms. *JAMA*, **204**, 104–110.
26. Cox, D. R. (1970). *Analysis of Binary Data*. Chapman and Hall, London.
27. Darrock, J. V. (1974). Multiplicative and additive interaction in contingency tables. *Biometrics*, **61**, 207–214.
28. Galtung, J. (1967). *Theory and Methods of Social Research*. Allen and Unwin, London.
29. Grizzle, J. E., Starmer, C. E., and Koch, G. G. (1969). Analysis of categorical data by linear models. *Biometrics*, **25**, 489–504.
30. Plackett, R. L. (1974). *The Analysis of Categorical Data*. Griffin, London.
31. Brown, G. W. and Harris, T. (1978). Social origins of depression: a reply. *Psychol. Med.*, **8**, 577–588.
32. Tennant, C. and Bebbington, P. (1978). The social causation of depression: a critique of the work of Brown and his colleagues. *Psychol. Med.*, **8**, 565–575.
33. Eysenck, H. J., Grossarth-Maticek, R., and Everitt, B. (1991). Personality, stress, smoking, and genetic predisposition as synergistic risk factors for cancer and coronary heart disease. *Integrat. Physiolog. and Behav. Sci.*, **26**, 309–322.
34. Grossarth-Maticek, R. and Eysenck, H. J. (1990). Personality, smoking and alcohol as synergistic risk factors for cancer of the mouth and pharynx. *Psychol. Reps.*, **67**, 1024–1026.
35. Vetter, H. (1988). Probleme bei der Analyse von Kategorialen abhaugigen Variablen, insbesonden mit SAS-CATMOD. In *Fortschrift der Statistik-software 1*, (eds F. von Faulbaum and H.-M. Vehlinger), pp. 46–53. Fischer Verlag, Stuttgart.
36. Grossarth-Maticek, R. (1992). Die Bedentung den Interaktion Zwischen psycho-sozialen und organischen Risikofaktoren fur die primäre Praevention des Mammakarzinoms. Lecture presented 4.11.92. at the Frauenklinik of the University cf Heidelberg.

# 6

# Unconventional therapies in cancer care

T. A. B. SHEARD

# 1  Introduction

The subject of this chapter is a number of therapeutic approaches which currently lie outside the boundaries of conventional medicine. The lack of a widely accepted word to use as an umbrella term is symptomatic of the fragmentation and controversy surrounding this field and the difficulty, perhaps impossibility, of uniting widely divergent or even incommensurable viewpoints and definitions. I have chosen the term 'unconventional' rather than 'alternative', 'complementary', 'unorthodox', 'unproven', 'fraudulent', 'quack', 'natural', or 'holistic' as a reflection of my viewpoint that the main factor linking them all together is their separation from conventional medicine. In the United Kingdom there is a drift in word usage towards describing those therapies which are used alongside conventional medicine as 'complementary' and those outside this definition as 'alternative'. As will be demonstrated below, some of these approaches are becoming both very popular and increasingly accepted by the medical establishment, and it may be simply a matter of time before they too become incorporated into the term 'conventional'.

## 1.1  A BRIEF OVERVIEW OF UNCONVENTIONAL MEDICINE

The diversity and in some cases simplistic nature of unconventional medicine may have deterred attempts to validate and determine the possible physiological basis for their beneficial effects. Therapies range from traditional Chinese medicine (a complete medical system refined over centuries which includes acupuncture and herbalism), to the apparently ubiquitous spiritual healing, from complex western, professionally organized systems such as osteopathy and chiropractice, to self-help and psychosocial therapies, and finally special diets and latter day medicinal nostrums such as laetrile. These therapies are not united or explicable in terms of a common thread of theory or even ideology. They are united solely by the negative sociocultural factor of their separation from mainstream western medicine.

This divide has unfortunate consequences both clinically and scientifically. It has resulted in a fragmentation of health care services into fiefdoms which rarely communicate, and which may result in divided care and allegiances for distressed individuals. A particularly unfortunate consequence is the potentially vicious circle of exclusion of unconventional therapies from mainstream medicine. They are rejected on the grounds of not having been scientifically evaluated and in turn are not scientifically evaluated because they are outside the scope of a biologically based body of scientific knowledge. This latter is the result of an understandable, but unscientific attitude, frequently seen when doctors encounter a foreign, non-biological medical system or theory, that is the mistaken equation of a specific theoretical framework, in this case biological medicine with 'science' itself (for an example see a 1993 editorial in *The New England Journal of Medicine*) (1). This attitude has impeded evaluation of unconventional medicine and is equivalent to the Guinness advertisement: 'I've never tried it because I don't like it'. Science is not a theory, it is a method used for obtaining reliable, repeatable, shared knowledge, a process which can be applied, in appropriate form, to test any type of medical theoretical system (2, 3). A final consequence of the divide separating the two systems has been the prevention of the transfer of conventional medicine's hard-won professional standards of training, accreditation, registration, supervision, and quality control to the almost wholly deregulated sphere of unconventional medicine.

Table 1 gives an approximate and oversimplified map of the different, partly overlapping, groups of therapies or medical systems, divided up by focus and theoretical base. They highlight both the perplexing diversity and potential richness of health care available in, and generated by, the modern world. The first two categories to a large extent share conventional medicine's mechanistic theoretical base which follows the Cartesian split between mind and body, though, unlike Descartes himself they all appear to actually eliminate the spirit. Their basic orientation, as in conventional medicine, is instrumental, that is towards treatment of symptoms or cure. The medical systems in category three derive from both Asian and Western traditions, they share a tendency to conceptualize mind and body as an indivisible, unified process, often including a spiritual aspect. They frequently place their emphasis on health, well-being, and the 'holistic' unity of the person rather than on pathology. They are sociologically similar to conventional medicine in that they involve a passive patient being treated by an expert with special knowledge, however this is often balanced by an emphasis on psychosocial/lifestyle

**Table 1** Approximate map of types of unconventional therapy

| Category | Type of therapy | Specific therapies | Treatment objectives |
|---|---|---|---|
| 1 | Mechanistic pseudomedical, with limited theoretical base | Megavitamins, laetrile, 'immune' therapies, Gerson, metabolic, and related dietary therapies | Cancer treatment/cure and symptom relief |
| 2 | Mechanistic with systematic theoretical base | Osteopathy, chiropractic, and massage (Swedish) | In the UK the focus is on musculoskeletal problems |
| 3 | Medical systems using theoretical bases fundamentally different from conventional biomedicine | Traditional Chinese medicine (including acupuncture and Chinese herbs), Ayurvedic medicine (Indian tradition), homoeopathy, herbalism, aromatherapy, massage (e.g. 'holistic' massage), anthroposophy, and certain traditions of spiritual healing | Used for specific diseases, symptom control, and promotion of health and well being. Probably rarely used as a treatment for cancer, more for symptoms/well being? |
| 4 | Spiritual/existential: psychological/ theological/philosophical/mystical theoretical base | Spiritual healing or 'laying on of hands', psychotherapies with a prominent existential emphasis (Jungian and transpersonal), and meditation | Aim may be either physical or psychospiritual improvement or both |
| 5 | Integrative: 'holistic' theoretical base | Clinical teams of practitioners using a combination of therapies | Usually aiming for both physical and psychospiritual improvement |
| 6 | Psychosocial: theoretical base psychology, sociology, and politics | Counselling/psychotherapy, relaxation, meditation, imagery, self-help/support groups | Certainly psychosocial benefit, also sometimes physical |

advice. The fourth category, spiritual help, appears to be as old and diverse as humankind. Spiritual healing, as with prayer, is often used in an instrumental way for the relief of symptoms, or, alternatively, in search of peace, spiritual solace, improvement, or development. It usually involves an unusual relationship between client and healer in that 'therapy' is normally given free of charge and is performed in service to a higher power beyond ego volition, or control. The potential importance and indeed dangers of this approach to individuals facing their own mortality are obvious. Psychotherapies, such as Jungian and transpersonal, which emphasize the importance of meaning also contribute to this category. Priests, rabbis, and other institutional mediators of religious experience are probably best regarded as being outside the domain of unconventional medicine; they are generally part of the 'establishment' and work in parallel with conventional medicine. The fifth category, integrated therapies (4), represents an aggregate of various unconventional therapies offered in a clinic or by a single practitioner, such an approach is often described as 'holistic'.

Unconventional therapies are frequently loosely lumped under the umbrella terms 'holistic' or 'whole person' medicine; this degrades the term as they are frequently no more, or less 'holistic' than penicillin. A simple working definition might be 'an approach which seeks to address individuals, or larger units such as families, in terms of their different, but interrelated functioning dimensions, that is physical, psychosocial, and spiritual'. These are understood to interact in a process of growth and development towards wholeness, the whole being greater than the sum of the parts. Using this definition it is unlikely that any of the approaches in Table 1, used either alone, or in isolation from conventional medicine, could be considered holistic. It could be argued that holism is an approach which cannot be achieved in a climate of division: it is an integrative and, as such, a necessarily multidisciplinary model. The sixth category, 'psychosocial' includes some approaches which are fairly routine in psychiatry/psychology and which are increasingly offered in oncology departments. In the context of consumer-driven unconventional therapies it can be understood to be a facet of, or driven by, a specific late-twentieth-century Western cultural movement which emphasizes autonomy, self-help, responsibility, informed choice, and the construction of personal meaning in many spheres of life, particularly health care. It can readily be understood how therapies and models from categories 1, 2, 3, 4, and 5 of Table 1 can all act as vehicles for this way of interacting with, and constructing health care. Viewing unconventional therapies from this sociological perspective forces an understanding of their recent enormous growth as being much more complex and important than a mere explosion of quackery (5). The evidence for this assertion is examined in Section 3.

1.2  SURVEYS OF THE USE OF UNCONVENTIONAL MEDICINE

A search of Medline and Psyclit databases and article bibliographies revealed few published surveys of the use of unconventional therapies in either general or cancer populations. They are consistent in showing a relatively high level of use, particularly in the better educated and more affluent sections of society. Surveys of the general population are considered first. Maddocks (6) cites the Australian Health Survey findings of 1977–1978. Over a four-week period, 2 per cent of Australians consulted a chiropractor, osteopath, or naturopath, accounting for approximately 386 000 consultations. This compares with 17 per cent visiting a doctor in a two-week (*sic*) period, approximately 3 555 200 consultations. Donnelly (7) reported in 1985 a survey of 285 families attending hospital in Australia for treatment of a child with either asthma or a minor surgical condition. Forty-six per cent of families had used unconventional therapies on at least one occasion, chiropractic, osteopathy, naturopathy, and acupuncture forming the bulk of these therapies. No significant demographic pattern of use emerged.

Eisenberg *et al.* (8) reported a national (USA) telephone survey in 1993. They obtained a response rate of 67 per cent, completing interviews with 1539 adult subjects who were demographically representative of the total population but who had a lower rate of 'poor health' than the national (3 per cent against 7 per cent). The operational definition of unconventional was 16 commonly used therapies which were neither commonly taught in US medical schools nor routinely available in hospitals. Thirty-four per cent of respondents had used an unconventional therapy in the previous twelve months, the proportion being approximately 25 per cent for those with serious health problems. Seven out of ten consultations took place unknown to the subjects' doctors. Extrapolating to the whole of the USA these findings imply that approximately 61 million Americans used at least one unconventional therapy in 1990 at an estimated total cost of $13.7 billion. Much of the use of therapies was without professional supervision or advice. Forty-seven per cent had consulted neither a doctor nor unconventional practitioner for the complaint for which they were using the therapy. Of the 83 per cent of respondents who reported a medical condition, 58 per cent saw a doctor but not an unconventional practitioner, only 3 per cent the reverse, and 7 per cent consulted both. Unconventional medicines were found to be used as a supplement to, rather than replacement of, conventional medicine. A clear demographic pattern of use emerged. Users were significantly more likely to be non-black, age 25–49, living in the west, college educated, and earning > $35 000. However, use was not confined to this subpopulation, it ranged from 23–53 per cent over all sociodemographic groups.

Surveys of doctors' attitudes have shown a perhaps surprisingly high degree of acceptance. Reilly (9) surveyed 100 general practice trainees in the UK in 1983. He found that 86 had a positive attitude, 18 were using at least one therapy themselves, 70 wanted some training, and 31 had made referrals for unconventional treatment. Wharton and Lewith (10) surveyed 200 general practitioners in South-West England in 1986. One hundred and forty five responded, 38 per cent had received some training in unconventional therapies, 59 per cent thought them useful, 76 per cent had referred to medically qualified unconventional practitioners, and 72 per cent to non-medically qualified ones. Anderson and Anderson (11) in 1987 sent out questionnaires to 274 general practitioners and received 222 replies. Thirty-one per cent claimed a working knowledge of one or more therapies, 16 per cent practised one or more, 41 per cent had attended courses or classes on unconventional medicine, and 59 per cent had made referrals for unconventional therapy. Knipschild *et al.* (12), in a survey of 400 randomly selected Dutch general practitioners had a 74 per cent response rate: 80 per cent considered 'manual therapies' effective. Furthermore, 50 per cent, 45 per cent, and 17 per cent considered acupuncture, homoeopathy, and healing respectively to be effective in certain conditions.

A greater number of studies have been reported on cancer populations, these are summarized in Table 2. Markle *et al.* in 1978 (13) and Wagenfeld *et al.* in 1979 (14) reported on questionnaires answered by 252 out of approximately 450 attendees at a conference in Michigan, USA sponsored by the Cancer Control Society (linked with laetrile). Sixty-one per cent had received college or higher education although they tended to be of lower occupational prestige. Forty-three per cent claimed to be using laetrile or apricot kernels as part of a cancer prevention approach. The sampling procedure renders the generalisability of these findings difficult to assess. Arkko (15) surveyed 151 out-patient clinic attendees in Finland; 55.6 per cent of women and 29.5 per cent of men had used one or more therapies. The therapies used were largely local folk cancer remedies, the most popular being extract of birch bark ash. There were no significant demographic factors distinguishing users from non-users other than gender. However, confidence in the effectiveness of remedies was 57.5 per cent in those who had received higher education and only 31.6 per cent in those who had not.

Cassileth *et al.* (16) reported, in 1984, a survey of 304 cancer in-patients in Philadelphia (8 per cent refusal rate); of these, 13 per cent had used, or were using unconventional therapies. They also attempted to contact subjects under the care of unconventional practitioners but encountered methodological problems salutary to those seeking to research in this field. Of the 157 unconventional clinics or practitioners contacted only 45 eventually collaborated by supplying names and addresses of individuals with cancer under their care. Of 515 subjects contacted, only 380 were finally interviewed (attrition was due to refusals, death, being too ill, and failure to meet entry criteria). Fifty-three subjects (14 per cent) had rejected conventional care after diagnosis, while 40 per cent of those using both approaches abandoned conventional care after a mean of eight months. Information was not given as

**Table 2**  Surveys of the use of unconventional therapies by subjects with cancer

| Author | Year | Context | Country and place | Medical status | n | % using/used unconventional therapies | Associated demographic factors | Most popular therapies |
|---|---|---|---|---|---|---|---|---|
| Arkko *et al.* (15) | 1980 | Out-patient clinic | Finland | Mixed | 151 | 66% women 30% men | Gender, confidence in effectiveness greater in those with higher education | Extract of birch bark |
| Cassileth *et al.* (16) | 1984 | In-patients and subjects under care of unconventional practitioners | USA Philadelphia and national | Mixed | 684 | 13% in hospital population | Well educated Race: white | Metabolic therapy, diets, imagery, megavitamins, spiritual healing, and immune therapies |
| Eidinger and Schapira (18) | 1984 | Under care of hospital cancer centre | Canada, Saskatchewan | Metastatic | 190 | 7%, but 70% said they would use them if available | Higher level of education correlated with disbelief in effectiveness | Not surveyed |
| Clinical Oncology Group (9) | 1987 | Five cancer treatment centres | New Zealand, five cities | Mixed, one month post diagnosis | 463 | 22.5% intended to use therapies | Not surveyed | Diet most popular preference |
| Zouwe *et al.* (20) | 1988 | Out-patients of general and academic hospitals | Holland | Mixed | 1000 | 10% current, 6% previously | Higher education and income | Moerman diet, iscador, and psychologically oriented techniques |

| Study | Year | Sample | Country | Type | n | Findings | Demographics | Therapies |
|---|---|---|---|---|---|---|---|---|
| Cosh and Sikora (39) | 1989 | Consecutive attenders at oncology department | United Kingdom, London | Mixed | 100 | 10% for cancer, 33% previously, 66% said they would accept unconventional therapies given in the hospital | Not surveyed | Meditation, visualization, and relaxation |
| Downer | Undated | Attenders at oncology department | United Kingdom, London | Mixed | 202 | 16% (psychological excluded) | Not surveyed | Spiritual healing and visualization |
| Sutherland and Goldstein (24) | 1992 | Attenders at initial drop-in orientation meeting at an unconventional centre | USA, California | Mixed | 62 | 60% of attenders continued to attend | High users: women, older, more highly educated, relatively affluent and with no religious affiliation. Non-users lower incomes and greater proportion in work | Main reason for attendance was social support |

to whether these refusers had been offered active, palliative, or no treat-ment. Sixty-four per cent only started unconventional treatment some time after diagnosis (mean, 24 months), often on the detection of secondaries. Use of unconventional therapies was significantly associated with being well educated and white; this association was confirmed in an update on a sample of 1000 subjects (17). The most commonly used therapies were metabolic therapy (diets, enemas, and vitamins), diets, imagery, megavitamins, spiritual healing, and immune therapy. In contrast to Eisenberg et al., 75 per cent had told their physicians, 39 per cent of whom were disapproving and 4 per cent of whom refused to see the person again. It is striking that 60 per cent of the unconventional practitioners were MDs, however this may be in part the result of a consent bias.

Eidinger and Schapira (18) also in 1984 reported a survey of 190 Canadian subjects with metastatic cancer. Only 7 per cent were using, or had used, unconventional therapies but 70 per cent stated they would use them if avail-able locally (that is, in Saskatchewan). Twenty-five per cent believed that laetrile, diets, and vitamins were 'effective in curing cancer' and 40 per cent were doubtful; in this sample higher levels of education correlated with disbelief in effectiveness. The Clinical Oncology Group of New Zealand reported in 1987 a survey in which 463 individuals were interviewed by doctors and nurses one month after their first attendance at one of five cancer centres (19). Thirty-two per cent had been advised, by someone, about unconventional therapies: of these, 68 per cent intended to adopt uncon-ventional therapies. Diet was the most popular preference (77 per cent). One individual, with potentially curable disease refused conventional treatment in favour of unconventional and re-presented five months later with incurable disease. Zouwe et al. (20) surveyed approximately 1000 subjects in Holland: 9.8 per cent were currently using unconventional therapies for cancer and 6.4 per cent had done so before. The most commonly used therapies were the Moerman diet (60 per cent) (21), Iscador (12 per cent) (see below Section 4), and psychological approaches (9 per cent). Use was significantly associated with palliative treatment and again with higher income and education. Sikora (personal communication) in a survey of 100 consecutive attendees at a London cancer centre found that 10 per cent of subjects were using uncon-ventional therapies; 33 per cent had used them previously and 66 per cent would accept them if provided in the department. The therapies most often used were meditation, visualization, and relaxation. Downer et al. (22) at a different London Hospital administered a self-report questionnaire to 202 subjects. Sixteen per cent had used unconventional therapies during their cancer illness, the most commonly used therapies were spiritual healing and visualization (relaxation, counselling, and psychotherapy were not included). McGinnis (23), in her 1990 overview of alternative therapies, quoted a 15 per cent usage by 207 cancer patients surveyed on behalf of the US Department of Health and Human Services' in 1986, and a 9 per cent rate of use in 5047 subjects interviewed in the American Cancer Society's 1988 telephone survey. However, as she points out 10 per cent of individuals living with cancer is equivalent to 600 000 people in the USA alone.

Sutherland and Goldstein (24) reported in 1982 a study of 62 subjects who attended an initial, drop-in orientation meeting at The Wellness Community, a self-help centre in California which now has offshoots scattered around the USA. The Wellness Community's stated aim is to enhance quality of life which in turn 'may enhance the possibility of recovery'. It seeks to work alongside conventional medical and spiritual 'experts'. After baseline interview the subjects were followed-up and classed as high (24), low (13), and non-users (28) of the Wellness Community. High users tended to be women, older, more highly educated, relatively affluent, and with no religious affiliation. Low participants were more likely to be men and less educated, while non-participants had the lowest incomes and the greatest proportion in work. Stage of disease was similar across groups. All subjects had a high level of previous use of unconventional therapies: 54, 31, and 39 per cent respectively. These figures include psychotherapy which was the most commonly used therapy of all.

Even taking the most conservative estimates of use of unconventional therapies by individuals with cancer it is clear that their use constitutes a very significant health care, social, and economic phenomenon. Secondly, perhaps contrary to expectation, this trend is led by the more educated and affluent classes, and for this reason may be expected to both endure and increase. Unfortunately comparatively few studies have been reported. Aggregating the findings into a mean percentage of use is not possible because of: (a) the surveys being widely scattered around the globe; (b) the samples being of people at different stages of disease, at different points in the course of the disease; (c) the use of varying definitions of unconventional therapies; and (d) research interviewers having varying degrees of therapeutic neutrality. Hospital-based surveys present few methodological problems, but accessing users of unconventional therapies at the point of delivery can present, as the study of Cassileth *et al.* (16) showed, considerable problems of accrual and a probable consent bias towards only those clinics and practitioners more favourably disposed towards conventional medicine.

## 2 Beliefs and motivation

A number of papers, editorials, and book chapters have both described and commented on unconventional therapies (23, 25–41). They present a variety of theories as to why people use unconventional therapies: ranging from an ignorant aberration, to an ungrateful response to the triumphs of modern medicine; from a desperate act resulting from being abandoned by doctors, to a more general 'failure' by conventional medicine to address people's needs and suffering; from a result of the appeal of 'common-sense' models of health and illness to a distrust of science; from a form of self-help or way of becoming actively involved, to a form of support; from being a vehicle for exploration of personal and spiritual meaning when confronted with mortality to a search for a mystical side to healing; and finally as a facet of a wider cultural trend towards increasing self-responsibility. Surveys of psychological distress in cancer populations have consistently shown a very high level. It is highly plausible that a significant proportion of the users of unconventional therapies are drawn from this vulnerable subgroup. Unfortunately, there has been little systematic investigation of these hypotheses.

Cassileth *et al.* in the study cited above (16) examined attitudes in three groups: users of conventional medicine alone, of both approaches, or unconventional alone. They found a stepwise progression in attitudes across the groups in terms of: (a) increasing distrust in the effectiveness of conventional medicine; (b) increasing faith in unconventional therapies; (c) decrease in 'good relationships' with physicians; (d) increasing faith in cancer being 'preventable'; and (e) increasing belief in the existence of a national conspiracy to deny the public the use of unconventional therapies, the effectiveness of which was known but deliberately being kept secret. Fifty-nine per cent of those using unconventional therapies believed they could at best cure, or at least halt the growth of their cancers.

Pruyn *et al.* (42) reported in 1985 a survey of individuals with either breast cancer or Hodgkins disease attending for treatment at 15 hospitals in Holland; 25 per cent refused to participate out of 663 contacted. The subjects use of the Moerman diet (21) was examined in relation to psychological factors. They hypothesized that use of the diet would be associated with: (a) a subjective impression of insufficiency and lack of clarity of medical information provided; (b) that this correlation would hold specifically for subjects with high trait anxiety, low self esteem, angry/aggressive coping style, and poor impulse control. The first hypothesis was confirmed and the secondary ones held up well in the Hodgkins but less well in the breast cancer group.

The New Zealand Clinical Oncology Group (19) asked what subjects hoped to gain from the use of unconventional therapies; they could select any or all of only three answers: 'Increase your chance of a cure' (42 per cent), 'Make you feel better' (33 per cent), and 'Anything is worth a try' (50 per cent). Zouwe *et al.* (20) found that the most frequently stated motives were: the benign nature of the unconventional therapies; belief in a possible contribution to cure; and their value in giving increased resistance to disease and treatment side-effects.

Sutherland and Goldstein (24) in their study of The Wellness Community found that satisfaction with medical care was high but participants reported seeking more control in the medical relationship. Non-participants reported greater overall life satisfaction but this difference only achieved statistical significance for work satisfaction. Availability of social support was similar in all groups but the non-participants reported greater satisfaction with their support. Consistent with the findings of Cassileth *et al.* (16), participants were more likely to attribute the cause of cancer to lifestyle or behavioural factors. They felt that a 'positive attitude' was most important in recovery. When asked why they had joined, the great majority indicated 'social support', 25 per cent sought information, and a minority physical improvement. In order to contextualize their findings the authors also used the social research technique of participant observation.

Very few studies have been conducted surveying subjects' motives for using unconventional therapies and the questions asked have tended to focus on the instrumental dimension of possible physical effects on cancer. Pruyn *et al.* generated and tested hypotheses and their findings lent support to the idea that some of the individuals who use unconventional therapies find the doctor–patient relationship inadequate and are a psychologically vulnerable subgroup. The sample of Cassileth *et al.* (16) corresponded to Category 1 of Table 1 (mechanistic pseudomedical therapies used to treat illness) both in terms of type of therapy used and hoped-for therapeutic effect. Conversely, Sutherland and Goldstein's sample corresponded more with Categories 5 and 6 (integrative and psychosocial therapies used to promote quality of life and perhaps improve physical health). Similarly, the sample of Cassileth *et al.* (16) manifested a degree of alienation from conventional care while Sutherland and Golstein's sample only sought greater control in their relationships with their physicians. This suggests the hypothesis that unconventional therapies of different types are being used by subgroups with differing psychosocial profiles and with differing needs and objectives. Further studies are required to test this hypothesis. The available data are scanty but do support the notion of two main groups of subjects, one using pseudomedical therapies with the main intent of treating the disease (and perhaps alienated from conventional medicine) and a second group using predominantly psychosocial–spiritual approaches in a way that is complementary to mainstream medicine. The distinction is unlikely to be sharp as many may be using the Category 1 therapies mainly as a form of self-help and expression of autonomy rather than as a pure treatment of cancer. Reliable research data are required to elucidate the psychosocial characteristics of what is clearly a significant health care phenomenon and, when available, they could inform the provision of mainstream psychosocial cancer care.

## 3   Review of studies assessing the biological effects of unconventional therapies in cancer care

Potential anti-cancer drugs have to successfully pass a rigorous series of tests: *in vitro*, animal tests, phase I (toxicity), phase II (anti-tumour effect), and phase III (survival) clinical trials. A new product can only be released after many years of testing; the vast majority of drugs, some with initial great promise, fail to make it. Unconventional cancer treatments (that is Category 1) have completely bypassed this system and are in general use with little or no knowledge of either their toxicity or therapeutic efficacy. However, a number of studies have been performed, and a full review can be found in the only major resource publication in this field: the 1990 report by the Office of Technology Assessment, US Congress on 'Unconventional Cancer Treatments' (43). A brief review of the major studies is presented below.

### 3.1   LAETRILE

Laetrile (or amygdalin), a cyanide-containing drug extracted from apricot kernels and speciously described as a 'vitamin' by one of its principal promoters, is often regarded as the emblematic health fraud of the twentieth century (37, 43). Unfortunately, it has rivals for this status. Cassileth (17), in a historical review, demonstrated a cycle of new wonder cures being promoted, enjoying similar popularity to laetrile, and then fading away. It is estimated that in its heyday, laetrile was used by tens of thousands of American cancer sufferers (37, 43) and was legalized in 27 states. It was promoted as a cancer treatment and became big business.

Scientific investigation proceeded from negative *in vitro* studies (43) to a nationwide request from the National Cancer Institute of the USA (via nearly half a million letters, press coverage, and direct contact with laetrile groups) for any cases who had appeared to respond (44). The NCI hoped for a large series of 'best cases' but finally accrued only 93 cases out of an estimated 70 000 laetrile users. Sixty-eight were evaluable and their records mixed with the case histories of 68 conventionally treated and 24 untreated subjects. The 160 records were assessed by a panel of 12 oncologists blind to treatment modality. Six laetrile treated subjects were judged to have responded: four complete and two partial, an inconclusive finding from such a potentially large sample. Phase I and II trials followed (45, 46). An uncontrolled group of 178 subjects were given laetrile in standard doses along with metabolic therapy (an unspecified diet, enzymes, and vitamins). The anti-tumour effects and symptom relief were then assessed. Only one out of 178 subjects had a transient partial response, there was no significant improvement in symptoms and survival times were comparable to national norms. Significant cyanide blood levels and toxicity were observed, with a very narrow therapeutic index when apricot kernels were eaten in addition to oral laetrile. These results are quite conclusive; laetrile is dangerous and can be assumed with confidence to be ineffective as a treatment of cancer.

3.2 VITAMIN C

The use of high doses of ascorbic acid in the treatment of cancer was initiated by Ewan Cameron, a surgeon practising in Scotland. Cameron and Linus Pauling (a biochemistry Nobel Laureate) hypothesized that vitamin C increased host resistance to cancer spread, as opposed to having a direct anti-tumour effect. In 1974 Cameron and Campbell (47) reported an uncontrolled series of fifty subjects with advanced cancer treated with high dose ascorbate. They documented five cases of partial or complete response (histological diagnosis absent on either one or two) and other examples of improvement in symptoms and performance status. This was followed by two reports (48, 49) comparing ascorbate-treated subjects with advanced cancer with similar controls pulled from the hospital files. The second study used better matched controls (sex, age, histological type, primary site, time from diagnosis of primary, secondary, or local invasion), but used the same experimental group bar ten subjects who were substituted because of their rare tumour type. Survival was measured from the time diagnosed as 'untreatable'. The first study showed a survival advantage for the ascorbate-treated group of a factor of 4.2; the second study an even better one with mean survival advantage of 300 + days. These results provoked considerable interest and controversy. A phase III, double-blind randomized trial was conducted on 150 subjects with advanced cancer at the Mayo clinic in the USA (50). There was no significant difference in either survival or symptoms between the two groups, although both experimental and placebo-control groups did show an improvement in symptoms. Pauling and Camerons' main criticism of this study was that a substantial proportion of subjects had already received chemotherapy, potentially compromising their immune function. A second randomized double-blind study (51) was then performed on a sample of chemotherapy-naive subjects with advanced bowel cancer (untreatable with chemotherapy at that time). The ascorbate-treated group did not show any tumour regression, nor any difference in interval to progression or significant advantage in either symptom control or survival. Indeed, there were substantially more long-term survivors in the placebo group. Pauling criticized these results on the basis that Vitamin C treatment was stopped when marked progression was evident, rather than continued until death as in the original studies (52). It is difficult to see how this could have significantly altered the outcome. These two phase III trials of vitamin C represent the most rigorous and scientifically satisfactory therapeutic evaluations of any unconventional therapy. They would appear to have closed the case on vitamin C. However the debate continues, Campbell (53) of the original 1974 paper reported in 1992 the 17-year follow-up of a man with reticulum cell sarcoma who has had two separate well documented complete responses to Vitamin C in the absence of any other treatment.

## 3.3 ISCADOR

Widely used in North-Western Europe, and available on the National Health Service in the UK, iscador, which is derived from mistletoe, is available in an injectable or oral preparation. It was developed within Rudolf Steiner's Anthroposophical system of medicine and is understood to act by strengthening the 'higher organizational forces' of the organism which are thought to be weakened in cancer. However it has been extensively evaluated within a biomedical model, a search in 'medline' 1966–1992 for iscador, mistletoe, and viscum album produced over 100 citations in English and German. The Office of Technology Assessment review (43) reported conflicting *in vitro* and animal studies, a demonstration of immune cell stimulating properties and seriously flawed clinical studies from which conclusions could not be drawn.

## 3.4 DIETS

Special cancer diets, as demonstrated above, are frequently used and are probably now the most controversial area of unconventional cancer therapy. Reasonably detailed descriptions are available in a number of reviews (55–59). For mainstream practitioners, the long list of potentially serious side-effects (increased risk of malnutrition in a disease which commonly causes it anyway, disruption of family life, diminished quality of life through unpalatable food and the hard work of preparing the diet, promotion of guilt, and amplification of obsessionality based on fear) coupled with the absence of any evidence of therapeutic effect, is a potent, provocative, and dangerous mixture. For persons with advanced cancer, a diet may represent the last psychological defence against the crushing realization of their impending death or, conversely, a reasoned attempt at using a self-help activity which can constructively involve all family members. Despite the heated debate there has been little attempt to assess dietary therapies. Gerson presented a series of best cases (60) claiming numerous successes with his very arduous regime of vegetable juices, coffee enemas, liver extract, potassium supplementation, and enzymes. Reviewers have found that Gerson's cases lack sufficient documentation to form a secure basis for claims of objective regression (43, 61). Reed *et al.* visited the Gerson clinic in Mexico and assessed a new series of best cases, finding no evidence of exceptional outcome (62). However, they noted a high level of perceived support among the subjects and adequate analgesia in the absence of opiates, which they found surprising considering the advanced stage of disease. Metabolic therapy is largely derived from Gerson's diet, subjects given laetrile in Moertel's phase II study described above (46) were also offered metabolic therapy. Subjects' compliance with this regime was not reported and, therefore, its contribution is not assessable (63).

## 3.5 LIVINGSTONE-WHEELER REGIME

Virginia Livingstone-Wheeler was a doctor and former Associate Professor of Microbiology at the University of San Diego who believed that all cancers were the result of an infection by a microorganism which she claimed to have isolated and called *progenitor cryptocides* (43). Treatment consists of a special vaccine, immune-stimulating drugs including BCG, blood transfusions, a 75 per cent raw vegetarian diet, vitamins, and enemas. Cassileth *et al.* reported a controlled study in 1991 (64). Seventy-eight subjects attending the Livingstone-Wheeler Clinic in California, of mixed diagnostic types and advanced disease, were matched with controls from Philadelphia (matched for sex, race, age < or > 59 years, diagnosis, and date of metastatic or recurrent disease). Follow-up was for a maximum of three years by which time only four subjects were still alive. There was no significant difference in survival or performance status between the two groups, the survival curves were remarkably close. The only significant predictor of longer survival was gender. Quality of life was assessed using the Functional Living Index-Cancer, a self-report instrument validated on cancer subjects. The Livingstone-Wheeler sample had a significantly poorer quality of life at recruitment and this was maintained at follow-up interviews every two months: the quality of life plots for the two samples were parallel. Chemotherapy was examined as a confounding factor but had no detectable effect on quality of life. Symptoms of loss of appetite, pain, nausea, and breathing difficulties were assessed: more adverse effects were reported in the Livingstone-Wheeler group, suggesting a possible causal connection. The clear strengths of this study are the rigorous attempt at matching the samples and the assessment of quality of life as an outcome in addition to physical indices. The obvious methodological weakness, discussed by the authors, is the self-selection of the experimental group. The potential for significant selection bias precludes any firm conclusions. Other weaknesses are the lack of blindness of the assessors (due to geography), inclusion being based merely on compliance with injections of the special vaccine twice a week for one month (that is a fraction of the complete programme), the lack of more extensive assessment of psychological status, the apparent lack of matching for time between diagnosis of primary and progression to advanced disease, and finally the experimental group commencing with a significantly lower quality of life, a possible independent predictor of length of survival (65). The researchers encountered a logistical difficulty:

matching the subjects so closely led to enrolment of the control group taking three and a half years.

### 3.6 INTENSIVE MEDITATION

Ainslie Meares, an Australian psychiatrist developed a meditation procedure for individuals with cancer involving profound relaxation which he likened to a form of prayer in which individuals 'experience God' or 'that aspect of God which is within themselves' (66). Subjects were required to attend a daily meditation group and also to meditate for three hours a day. He reported a few cases of apparent regression of cancer (66–70) which have not been independently assessed. Unfortunately, following his death, there have been no reports of continuing research.

### 3.7 THE SIMONTONS' APPROACH

The work of Carl Simonton (a radiation oncologist) and Stephanie Matthews-Simonton was popularized in their book 'Getting Well Again' (71). They used relaxation, group and individual psychotherapy, and the technique for which they became well known: visualization. This involved individuals finding an image for their cancer and then imagining it being destroyed by overwhelming forces. These forces were symbolic of either the immune system, conventional cancer treatment, or both. Findings of a 'pilot' study were published in 1980 (72), the median survival of 225 subjects of mixed diagnoses was found to be 'as much as twice as long' compared with national averages. Entry criteria were having advanced cancer and being willing to do the therapy. No data were presented on refusal rate, the duration of survival of those who refused to participate, or on staging/prognostic factors. A separate paper, a transcript of a lecture (73), reported that usually more than 50 per cent of subjects turned down the therapy. A second paper was published in 1981 (74), apparently an update on the 1980 paper, as 20 subjects had been added with essentially the same results. The profound methodological flaws, that is the non-representative nature of the sample and lack of crucial medical data dictate that these studies can tell us nothing about any possible effect of the therapy. Data on tumour regression would have been informative as would data on the findings of the standardized psychological tests which were administered.

### 3.8 THE 'EXCEPTIONAL CANCER PATIENT' (ECaP) PROGRAMME: THE WORK OF DR BERNARD SIEGEL

Siegel, a surgeon, popularized his approach with the book 'Love, Medicine and Miracles' (75). The group psychosocial support programme uses group psychotherapy, meditation, and visualization. Morgenstern *et al.* (76), in their survival study summarized the programme aims as: 'to get patients to accept their disease, to get them to take charge of their lives, and to give them hope' in order to improve both their quality of life and length of survival. The survival study was retrospective, comparing 34 women with breast cancer who had gone through the programme with 102 controls selected from files. Three controls were matched with each experimental subject for a number of medical and demographic variables. Follow-up was for between 6 and 34 months depending on date of entry into the programme. Complex statistical analysis revealed two factors significantly associated with survival: chemotherapy (negative, presumably as it was given to women with more advanced disease) and the ECaP programme (positive: $p = 0.066$, marginal significance). This lent support to the hypothesis that the programme would lengthen survival, however a selection bias was then detected. Women entering the programme did so a mean of 18 months after diagnosis, up to a maximum of 10 years, but over the equivalent period a number of the controls had died, while the ECaP subjects, by definition, could not have done so. *Post hoc* adjustment for this bias was attempted by two methods both of which removed the apparent survival advantage of the ECaP group. This study was an important object lesson in the profound methodological difficulties inherent in trying to adequately match self-selected subjects with non-randomized controls.

### 3.9 THE WORK OF THE BRISTOL CANCER HELP CENTRE IN THE UK

Opened in 1980, the Bristol Cancer Help Centre initially promoted a regime in which a variant of metaboric therapy was prominent (77). In particular it became known for advocating a restricted form of vegan diet (78). The regime became less extreme over time (79) and moved towards a position where psychosocial–spiritual aspects and quality of life were the principal focus. About the mid-point of this transition a prospective survival study, conducted by an independent research team from the Institute of Cancer Research was initiated and reported by Bagenal *et al.* in 1990 (80). The research team's request to conduct a randomized study was refused by the Cancer Help Centre. Three hundred and thirty four women with breast cancer who had attended the Cancer Help Centre on at least one occasion were compared with 461 controls attending two hospitals in and around London and followed-up for at most two years. Controls were matched initially only on diagnosis, age (<50, 50 and over) and year of diagnosis (1979–1983, 1983 onwards). Medical data (including T and N status) were recorded for each group and entered into a Cox regression analysis, psychological indices were not assessed. The selection bias problem identified in the ECaP study was taken into account. The Bristol group were significantly younger/premenopausal

$(p < 0.001,\ p = 0.001)$, and had more extensive surgery $(p = 0.07)$. For those metastasis-free at entry, metastasis-free survival was significantly poorer (hazard ratio: 2.85) and for relapsed subjects survival was significantly shorter (hazard ratio: 1.81). Revised statistics were published later as local recurrence had been identified as a confounding factor: the hazard ratio for metastasis-free survival was reduced from 2.85 to 1.79 and rose above the 5 per cent significance threshold $(p = 0.07)$ (81). The results, given the relatively benign nature of the Bristol regime, were 'intrinsically implausible' (82). Published correspondence on the substance of these findings (83–89) focused on three themes: the comparability of the experimental and control group for prognostic/psychological factors, statistical procedures, and 'compliance' (that is the lack of any documentation as to whether the experimental group adopted any of the Bristol regime or as to what proportion of the controls were themselves using unconventional therapies). Even with the revised statistics the difference in overall survival remained significant and for metastasis-free survival became borderline significant. It is of particular note that the (negative) effect size was considerably greater than the (positive) effect sizes of either tamoxifen or adjuvant chemotherapy. This study illustrated the perils even of carefully conducted non-randomized survival studies and the peculiar problems faced in the evaluation of unconventional therapies (see Section 6).

### 3.10 THERAPIES OUTSIDE THE SCOPE OF THIS REVIEW

Psychotherapy and counselling are reviewed in subsequent chapters of this book, they span the ill-defined border between conventional and unconventional medicine. For these reasons they will not be considered further in this chapter. The use of unconventional therapies in symptom control is also not reviewed, examples are the use of relaxation, visualization, and acupuncture in the treatment of chemotherapy-associated nausea and emesis (90, 91), and acupuncture and hypnosis in pain control (92–94). Again little research has been carried out in this area but it is clearly an important focus for further study.

### 3.11 SUMMARY

There have been few attempts to objectively evaluate the biological impact of unconventional therapies in cancer. Series of 'best cases' presented as showing tumour regression have been inconclusive. Indeed, phase I and II trials of laetrile showed it to be ineffective and dangerous. The unreliability of the non-randomized survival study is well demonstrated by this field. All of the non-randomized studies bar one, (the Livingstone-Wheeler study) produced results which were initially statistically significant. Corrections for selection bias in the ECaP and Bristol studies eliminated initially significant overall survival advantage in the former, and negative metastasis-free survival in the latter. The statistically significant negative association between the Bristol therapies and overall survival still stands, but therapeutic causality is rendered highly implausible through the magnitude of the effect. The apparent beneficial effects of Vitamin C, which included cases of tumour regression, were shown to be dubious by two rigorous double-blind placebo control trials. Quality of life was assessed in only one study (64), none of the remaining studies reported documented any psychosocial indices.

There has, therefore, been no positive effect demonstrated for unconventional therapies in cancer either in terms of tumour response or increased duration of survival. The odd result of the Bristol study can be assumed to be due to hidden selection bias. Psychosocial factors, either as independent or dependent variables, have not been evaluated.

## 4 Toxicity/side-effects of unconventional therapies

### 4.1 PHYSICAL

Few studies or case histories have been reported. A number are briefly reviewed but it is of note that the negative effects are largely the result of failure to exercise professional standards rather than being dangers intrinsic to the actual therapies. Significant cyanide toxicity, with a narrow therapeutic index for those supplementing oral laetrile with apricot kernels, has been demonstrated (45, 46). Analysis of pooled human blood products used in immuno-augmentative therapy suggested contamination with HIV and hepatitis B (95). Very severe amoebiasis following colonic irrigation at a Chiropractic clinic in the USA occurred in 36 people, leading to 10 colectomies and 6 deaths (96). Two case histories of deaths associated with the use of coffee enemas were reported in 1980 (97); cause of death was thought to be severe electrolyte imbalance resulting from the enemas. Three similar but less detailed cases, in addition to a woman with gastric carcinoma who had bilateral chemical phlebitis following intravenous injection of ozone, were reported in 1985 (98).

Excessive pyridoxine use has been associated with a sensory neuropathy (99) but fears that megadoses of vitamin C might cause renal calculi have not been confirmed (50, 51). There have been unpublished clinical anecdotes of hypervitaminosis A perhaps contributing to hepatic dysfunction and of orange-coloured individuals taking large doses of beta carotene. Finally there have been many anecdotes of individuals suffering from malnutrition when using special diets, however this has yet to documented in case reports or to be systematically investigated.

## 4.2 EDUCATIONAL

Coward, in her book 'The Whole Truth: The Myth of Alternative Health' (100) and Sontag in 'Illness as Metaphor' (101) explore in depth some of the ideas and in some cases misconceptions underlying unconventional medicine. The appeal of the 'common sense' theories of some unconventional therapies has been described by Gillick (25), such theories match persons' experiences of themselves a way that biomedicine cannot hope to emulate. It is difficult to make the complex mechanistic theories of cancer biology both under-standable and meaningful, their meaning can only be mechanistic and, there-fore, nihilistic. This coupled with a perhaps exaggerated public perception of treatment toxicity and the absence, in many cases of an explanation for the cause of cancer leaves oncology with an uphill public relations task. Sophisticated holistic health approaches which include both conventional medicine and a perspective more sensitive to subjective experience and which recognizes a person's need for meaning and active participation in their health may well become the established practice in the future. In contrast, the more simplistic models, though superficially attractive, contain considerable dangers of misinformation. Causes of cancer, for example dietary, are con-fused with treatments. This is equivalent to suggesting that smokers with lung cancer can cure their condition if they stop smoking. Self-help, psychosocial approaches enhancing individual effectiveness and 'control', the healing of emotional wounds, and the adoption of a fighting spirit can readily be con-fused with actual control over the cancer itself (see Section 4.4). There is a developing viewpoint that illness is entirely avoidable if one eats the right food, takes enough vitamins, exercises regularly, relaxes, meditates, thinks positive, and undergoes some kind of regular psychic spring cleaning. A kind of alternative medicine superman has been created (the down side of this is examined in Section 4.4). If only life were that simple. This attitude can become more extreme in 'holistic fundamentalism'. I use this term to describe that attitude in which oncology is rejected out of hand as 'cutting, burning and poisoning' while unconventional medicine is embraced as 'natural' and an *a priori* good.

## 4.3 REFUSAL OF CONVENTIONAL TREATMENT

This is a major concern but again has been little documented and studies are required which give a reliable indication of the prevalence of refusal of conventional treatment. The data in the survey of Cassileth *et al.* (16) are cause for concern and give some credence to the often expressed fear that the main danger in unconventional therapies lies in seducing people away from potentially curative treatment. However, the nature of the conventional treatment rejected, whether potentially curative, palliative, or simply a watching brief was not specified. Conversely, the New Zealand survey (19) identified one out of 463 subjects who refused potentially curative treatment and died. Eisenberg *et al.* in the US national telephone survey found that all respondents with serious illness (including cancer) were still seeing their doctors (8), similarly the sample from the Wellness Community were still having conventional treatment (24). More precise documentation of the scale of this problem could be obtained by surveying non-attendees for treatment/ follow-up following the initial diagnosis of cancer. The conflicting evidence cited above may support the hypothesis that there is a small, 'hard-core' group of users of Category 1 therapies (see Table 1) who actually reject conventional therapies, but that the (probably great) majority use them as a complement to conventional treatment.

### 4.4 PSYCHOSOCIAL SIDE-EFFECTS

These are potentially severe; the notion that individuals can control the progression of cancer either through a specific therapy like a diet, or through psychological means such as visualization shifts some of the burden of responsibility for treatment away from the health care professionals and onto the sick person. This can result in a positive sense of involvement and control but also guilt at progression which can be construed as a personal failure. This is often compounded by the stress models of carcinogenesis, a person may feel that not only have they brought their cancer on themselves but that it has progressed because they did not fight it hard enough. This burden may also be reinforced, or indeed be imposed by relatives or friends who may be only trying to help, be unable to face the loss, or are perhaps angry at the person for dying. Gray and Doan have written an illuminating discussion of this problem (102). A further problem, particularly for the Category 1 therapies, or of misguided therapists, is their potential to be the anchor of a dysfunctional extension of denial, of fear expressed through obsessionally pursuing a therapy right up to death, inhibiting the individual's and the family's process of adjustment.

# 5 Specific methodological considerations

### 5.1 CONVENTIONAL RESEARCH PROCEDURES

The double-blind, randomized placebo-controlled trial has been established over the last few decades as the gold standard for clinical trials. This model provides the best possible conditions for minimizing the intrusion of bias derived from the experimenters' expectations, the experimental subjects' expectations (placebo effect), or from the selection of the two or more groups to be compared. Using this procedure permits a good degree of confidence in attributing any observed differences in outcome to the treatment being assessed. Applying this model to the evaluation of Category 1, pseudomedical therapies such as laetrile or vitamin C (Table 1) is both desirable and entirely satisfactory as their hypothesized mode of action is purely biological. The model needs to be extended to include psychosocial indices when evaluating more sophisticated therapies in which effects may be mediated physically, psychologically, or both. The effects, if any, even of apparently physical therapies, such as diets may be mediated psychologically through the diet acting as a behavioural focus and reinforcement for a particular coping style. This would seem more plausible than a direct (that is physically mediated) effect on tumours. The tools and methods appropriate to investigating such a putative neuro-immune/endocrine pathway are described elsewhere (Section III) in this book. The randomized control trial has been used successfully in the evaluation of unconventional therapies used for conditions other than cancer (103–109). However, the model is corroded by the individual volition and choice which is so central to the use of many unconventional therapies; this is explored in Sections 5.2 to 5.6 of this chapter.

## 5.2 MOTIVATION VERSUS RANDOMIZATION

Certain diets are very arduous, unpleasant, and require a considerable change in lifestyle; undertaking them demands considerable motivation. Attempting randomization in a clinical trial of such a diet would be likely to result in a high rate of refusal to consent followed by a high drop-out rate/poor 'compliance' in the experimental group. There are no known examples of this having been attempted with cancer patients. However Kjeldsen-Kragh *et al.* have reported a successful randomization of subjects with rheumatoid arthritis to a partial fast followed by lacto-vegetarian diet on a health farm (103). For therapies where randomization is not possible the best mode of evaluation would be assessment of anti-tumour effects rather than risking the vagaries of the non-randomized control trial.

## 5.3 CHOICE VERSUS COMPLIANCE

For therapies requiring less extreme motivation, subject choice can still conflict with 'compliance'. This is a term belonging to a medical culture where the only active role required of the 'patient' is to be compliant in taking the treatment prescribed. This supine posture is not consistent with much of the culture of unconventional medicine. Subject choice or preference for unconventional therapies may not fit the trial protocol, in particular subjects who actively want a therapy may find themselves randomly allocated to the control condition. In contrast to conventional drug trials they have the means readily to defy their control status and use the therapy in another context. Brewin and Bradley (110) have proposed an interesting model (tested in the evaluation of self-care in diabetes), to address this problem. They propose identifying the motivation of the subjects before randomization, highly motivated subjects are then allocated to the experimental condition, low motivation ones to the control, and the 'don't minds' are randomized. The utility of this model could be compared with a simple assessment of motivation/preference as a significant variable in a normally structured randomized trial. The possible effect of subject's 'intentionality' on studies has been examined by Heron (111) and Anthony (112) and has expanded the theme that only particular subgroups within a population may show a positive, or conversely a negative, therapeutic effect.

## 5.4 MONITORING ADHERENCE TO PROTOCOLS

A corollary of subjects' exercise of choice and their ready access to unconventional therapies is the need for unusual rigour in documenting not only the actual use of the therapy being evaluated by the experimental group, but also inquiring as to whether the control group has also used it or a similar therapy. This would be superfluous in a normal medical trial but its absence in a study of unconventional therapies is a serious weakness. This is negatively illustrated by both the Livingstone-Wheeler (64) and Bristol Cancer Help Centre (80) studies where it was respectively vestigial and omitted; and positively in the vitamin C studies (50, 51) in which subjects in each condition had random urine tests for vitamin C metabolites.

## 5.5 UNDERLYING MOTIVES IN USING UNCONVENTIONAL THERAPIES VERSUS CONSENT TO RESEARCH

The surveys reviewed in Section 3.2 confirmed that one common motive for using unconventional therapy is the hope of a cure or longer survival. It can be hypothesized that some of this hope is a genuine rational expectation and some is a hope borne of the need for illusion/denial (113, 114). Clinical work with people dying of cancer very quickly illustrates how completely contradictory thoughts and expectations can coexist. One day an individual might talk of the inevitability of imminent death, the next of plans for a holiday the following year. Maintaining the coexistence of such mutually exclusive constructs may be facilitated by the contradiction having an external anchor, such as the divide between conventional and unconventional medicine. In this case conventional medicine and doctors, as the messengers of bad news, would represent the rational and bleak expectation of death, while in contrast unconventional therapies would represent the warm glow of hope (see

Gray and Doan regarding therapy 'gurus' (102)). Subjects struggling to maintain their psychological defences in this way may well refuse consent for inclusion in clinical research, a study monitoring tumour status could be too threatening.

## 5.6 RANDOMIZATION VERSUS THERAPEUTIC CULTURE

Just as relative patient passivity is an essential feature of conventional medical culture so too the self-selected nature of unconventional medicine consumers both reflects and constructs the nature of the therapies. Randomizing subjects to unconventional therapies who would otherwise not have used them would change both the way they could be practised and the clinical milieu. The experimenter inevitably interferes with the system being assessed. This problem could become serious in the evaluation of clinics in which shared belief systems, often focused on a charismatic leader, are central to the therapeutic milieu. Randomization of subjects to such a context could undermine or even destroy the hope-maintaining culture and thus the main therapeutic process. This problem could be tackled in two stages. First an evaluation of the existing programme, (involving the usual self-selected subjects), in terms of tumour response, perhaps indices of immune function, sociodemographic data, psychosocial indices, and statements of subjectively perceived motivation in attending, benefits, and adverse effects. This could be supplemented by participant observation, as in the study of the Wellness Community (24), or cooperative inquiry (Section 5.8). The second phase, if appropriate, would be a randomized study using subjects attending nearby oncology centres. The subjects in the experimental group would be offered a modified version of the clinic's programme tailored to their different needs. Alternatively, therapists from the clinic could deliver an adjusted programme in the hospital.

## 5.7 INVOLVING OTHER DISCIPLINES

A more comprehensive study of the phenomenon of unconventional medicine can only be achieved by using the research approaches of sociology, anthropology, and theological/spiritual studies in addition to medicine and psychology. The paucity and narrow scope of research reported to date is out of all proportion to the importance of unconventional therapies as a health care, social, economic, and political issue.

## 5.8 NEW RESEARCH MODELS

Heron (111) and Reason (115, 116) have described and used new research models such as cooperative inquiry which involve subjects as co-researchers rather than as 'objects of research'. This is done (in sharp contrast to the randomized trial) in an attempt to reduce or eliminate the distortions introduced by attempts to achieve objective generalizations which, by their very nature, necessitate a reductive and depersonalizing approach to human experience. An illustration: this approach could be used in investigations of a patient's spiritual response to cancer or the subjective experiences of those receiving spiritual healing.

## 5.9 SUMMARY

Randomized clinical trials are the research procedure of choice in evaluating unconventional therapies. Randomization can probably be successfully used for most therapies but subject preference and motivation for the therapy must be assessed pre-randomization. There are circumstances, such as extreme diets, where randomization is not feasible because of the degree of subject motivation required to endure and carry out the therapy. Survival studies using non-randomized controls are very unreliable and probably obsolescent. This point is well illustrated by the results of the non-randomized studies of Vitamin C (48, 49), the Simontons approach (72, 74), the ECaP program (76), the Bristol Cancer Help Centre (80, 81), and finally the Livingstone-Wheeler regime (64) which was the only study producing a first time null result. If a non-randomized study is precluded then a study of tumour response, rather than survival is most probably the best approach. Studies of side-effects, both physical and psychological are also required. Assessment of psychosocial indices must also be routinely included in all studies in order to investigate potential psychological confounding or mediating factors.

To date, the research agenda has been largely biomedical in focus, the questions asked have largely been limited to the frame of investigating unconventional therapies as a *treatment of cancer as a disease* rather than as part of an individual's multifaceted *response to the experience of having cancer*. The experience of having cancer has social, psychological, medical/physical, and spiritual dimensions. Sociological and psychological studies are required to investigate the prevalence of use of therapies, motivation in using them, subjectively perceived benefits, and adverse effects, and also users' psychological adjustment, vulnerability, and morbidity compared with non-users. Anthropological studies would place their use in the wider context of cross-cultural medical systems and a different perspective on intracultural use of different practices and belief systems. This could be integrated with a theological perspective on therapies addressing spiritual and existential issues (see Csordas' study of faith healing in Roman Catholic Evangelicals (117)). Procedures such as cooperative inquiry can contribute to an understanding of subjective experiences.

# 6  Summary and conclusions

The small number of reported studies surveying the use of unconventional therapies in cancer care are consistent in demonstrating that they are widely used. A conservative estimate would be 10 per cent, the proportion may be growing and appears to be led by the educated middle classes. Very few studies have examined the motives for using unconventional therapies; however the limited evidence available supports the hypothesis that there are two main, overlapping subgroups: those who are somewhat alienated from conventional medicine and predominantly use pseudomedical therapies to treat the disease and a second group which uses therapies in a complementary fashion and with more of an emphasis on psychosocial–spiritual benefit. Well designed studies of the impact of unconventional therapies on tumours and survival have shown no positive effect. Non-randomized survival studies involving self-selected subjects have proved unreliable. With one exception, (64), these studies did not include psychological indices which may be confounding or mediating factors. There have not been any studies evaluating psychosocial and spiritual effects (bar quality of life in one, (64)) of the use of unconventional therapies, despite this being the more plausible area of benefit.

Research methodology problems posed by this field have been described. Unconventional therapies present a challenge to expand the conventional research model into a bio–psychosocial–spiritual framework. To achieve this would require the collaboration of researchers from diverse academic disciplines. Similarly unconventional therapies provide impetus to the further development of a multidisciplinary, 'whole person' model of clinical care capable of addressing the multidimensional problems presented by cancer.

6.1 ACKNOWLEDGEMENTS

I would like to thank Bridget Prescott Thomas, James Brennan, and Michael Parle for their helpful *comments on drafts of this* chapter and the Cancer Research Campaign for funding my *clinical research training* fellowship. However any errors or misrepresentations within the text are wholly my responsibility.

# 7  References

1.  Campion, E. W. (1993). Why unconventional medicine? *N. Engl. J. Med.*, **328**(4), 282–283.

2. Lakatos, I. and Musgrave, A. (eds) (1970). *Criticism and the Growth of Knowledge*. Cambridge University Press.

3. Kuhn, T. S. (1962). *The Structure of Scientific Revolutions*. Chicago University Press.

4. Lerner, M. and Remin, N. (1985). A variety of integral cancer therapies. *Advances: J. Inst. Advancement of Health.*, **2**(3), 14–33.

5. Cassileth, B. R. (1989). The social implications of questionable cancer therapies. *Cancer*, **63**, 1247–1250.

6. Maddocks, I. (1985). Alternative medicine. *Med. J. Aust.*, **142**, 547–550.

7. Donnelly, W. J., Spykerboer, J. E., and Thong, Y. H. (1985). Are patients who use alternative medicine dissatisfied with orthodox medicine? *Med. J. Aust.*, **142**(10), 539–541.

8. Eisenberg, D. M., Kessler, R. C., Foster, C., Norlock, F. E., Calkins, D. R., and Delbanco, T. L. (1993). Unconventional medicine in the United States: prevalence, costs, and patterns of use. *N. Engl. J. Med.*, **328**(4), 246–252.

9. Reilly, D. T. (1983). Young doctors' views on alternative medicine. *Br. Med. J.*, **287**, 337–341.

10. Wharton, R. and Lewith, G. (1980). Complementary medicine and the general practitioner. *Br. Med. J.*, **292**, 1498–1500.

11. Anderson, E. and Anderson, P. (1987). General Practitioners and alternative medicine. *J. R. Coll. Gen. Pract.*, **37**, 52–55.

12. Knipschild, P., Kleijnen, J., and Ter Riet, G. (1990). Belief in the efficacy of alternative medicine among general practioners in the Netherlands. *Soc. Sci. Med.*, **31**(5), 625–626.

13. Markle, G. E., Petersen, J. C., and Wagenfeld, M. O. (1978). Notes from the cancer underground: participation in the laetrile movement. *Soc. Sci. Med.*, **12**, 31–37.

14. Wagenfeld, M. O., Vissing, Y. M., Markle, G. E., and Petersen, J. C. (1979). Notes from the cancer underground: health attitudes and practices of participants in the laetrile movement. *Soc. Sci. Med.*, **13A**, 483–485.

15. Arkko, P. J., Arkko, B. L., Kari-Koskinen, O., and Taskinen, P. J. (1980). A survey of unproven cancer remedies and their users in an out-patient clinic for cancer therapy in Finland. *Soc. Sci. Med.*, **14A**, 511–514.

16. Cassileth, B. R., Lusk, E. J., Strouse, B., and Bodenheimer, B. J. (1984). Contemporary unorthodox treatments in cancer medicine: a study of patients, treatments and practitioners. *Ann. Int. Med.*, **101**, 105–112.

17. Cassileth, B. R. (1986). Unorthodox cancer medicine. *Cancer Invest*, **4**(6), 591–598.

18. Eidinger, R. N. and Schapira, D. V. (1984). Cancer patients insight into their treatment, prognosis and unconventional therapies. *Cancer*, **53**, 2376–2740.

19. Clinical Oncology Group (1987). New Zealand cancer patients and alternative medicine. *N.Z. Med. J.*, **100**, 100–113.

20. Zouwe, N. v. d., Renrink, I., Dam, F. S. A. M. v., Aaronson, N., Hanewald, G. J. P. F., and Rumke, P. (1988). Concurrent use of unorthodox and conventional cancer therapies in *Current Concepts in Psycho-Oncology and AIDS* (eds J. C. Holland, J. Massie, and L. Lesko), p. 331. Memorial Sloane Kettering, New York.

21. Deplazes, G. and Hauser, S. (1982–1992). *Cancer cure by the Moerman diet*. File number 24E for the study group on 'Unproven Methods in Oncology'. Swiss Society for Oncology, Swiss Cancer League. Available in German, French and English from The Swiss Cancer League, P.O. Box 2284, CH-3001, Bern, Switzerland.

22. Downer, S., Cody, M., and Slevin, M. (1989). The practice and popularity of complementary/alternative therapies in a group of National Health Service cancer patients receiving conventional treatment: Unpublished abstract. St. Bartholomew's Hospital, London.

23. McGinnis, L. S. (1991). Alternative therapies 1990: an overview. *Cancer*, **67**, 1788–1792.

24. Sutherland, C. E. and Goldstein, M. S. (1992). Joining a healing community for cancer: who and why? *Soc. Sci. Med.*, **35**(3), 323–333.

25. Gillick, M. R. (1985). Common-sense models of health and disease. *N. Engl. J. Med.*, **313**(11), 700–703.

26. Ingelfinger, F. J. (1976). Quenchless quest for questionable cure. *N. Engl. J. Med.*, **295**(15), 838–839.

27. Relman, A. S. (1979). Holistic Medicine. *N. Engl. J. Med.*, **300**(6), 312–313.

28. Janssen, W. F. (1979). Cancer quackery: The past in the present. *Sem. Oncol.*, **6**(4), 526–536.

29. Editorial (1980). The flight from science. *Br. Med. J.*, **280**, 1–2.

30. Henney, J. E. (1982). Unproven methods of cancer treatment in *Principles and Practice of Oncology*, (eds DeVita, V. T., Hellman, S., and Rosenberg, S. A.), pp. 1878–1887. Lippincott, Philadelphia.

31. Holland, J. C. (1982). Why patients seek unproven cancer remedies: a psychological perspective. *CA*, **32**, 10–14.

32. Smith, A. (1983). Alternative medicine. *Br. Med. J.*, **287**, 307–308.

33. Editorial (1983). Alternative medicine no alternative. *Lancet*, Oct. 1, 773–774.

34. Baum, M. (1983). Quack cancer cures or scientific remedies? *Clin. Oncol.*, **9**, 275–280.

35. Howard-Ruben, J. and Miller, N. J. (1983). Unproven methods of cancer management part I: Background and historical perspectives. **10**(4), 46–52.

36. Sub-committee on unorthodox therapies, American Society of Clinical Oncology (1983). Ineffective cancer therapies: A guide for the layperson. *J. Clin. Oncol.*, **1**(2), 154–163.

37. Lerner, I. J. (1984). The why's of cancer quackery. *Cancer*, **53**, 815–819.

38. Holohan, T. V. (1987). Referral by default: the medical community and unorthodox therapy. *JAMA*, **257**(12), 1641–1642.

39. Cosh, J. and Sikora, K. (1989). Conventional and complementary treatment for cancer: time to join forces. *Br. Med. J.*, **298**, 1200–1201.

40. Holland, J. C., Geary, N., and Furman, A. (1990). Alternative cancer therapies in *Handbook of Psycho-Oncology*, (eds J. C. Holland, and J. H. Rowland), pp. 508–515. Oxford.

41. Murray, R. H. and Rubel, A. J. (1992). Physicians and healers, unwitting partners in health care. *N. Engl. J. Med.*, **326**, 61–64.

42. Pruyn, J. F. A., Rijckman, R. M., Brunschot, C. J. M. v., and Borne, H. W. v. d. (1985). Cancer patients personality characteristics, physician-

patient communication and adoption of the Moerman diet. *Soc. Sci. Med.*, 20(8), 841–847.

43. Office of Technology Assessment, Congress of the United States (1990). *Unconventional Cancer Treatments*. US Government Printing Office, Washington DC 20402 9395.

44. Ellison, N. M., Byar, D. P., and Newell, G. R. (1978). Special report on laetrile: The NCI laetrile review. *N. Engl. J. Med.*, 299, 549–542.

45. Moertel, C. G., Ames, M. M., Kovach, J. S., Moyer, T. P., Rubin, J. R., and Tinker, J. H. (1981). A pharmacologic and toxicological study of amygdalin. *JAMA*, 245(6), 591–595.

46. Moertel, C. G., Fleming, T. R., Rubin, J., Kvols, L. K., Sarna, G., Koch, R. *et al.* (1982). A clinical trial of amygdalin (laetrile) in the treatment of human cancer. *N. Engl. J. Med.*, 306(4), 201–206.

47. Cameron, E. and Campbell, A. (1974). The orthomolecular treatment of cancer II. Clinical trial of high-dose ascorbic acid supplements in advanced human cancer. *Chem. Biol. Interacts.*, 9, 285–315.

48. Cameron, E. and Pauling, L. (1976). Supplemental ascorbate in the supportive treatment of cancer. Prolongation of survival times in terminal human cancer. *Proc. Natl. Acad. Sci. USA*, 73(10), 3685–3689.

49. Cameron, E. and Pauling, L. (1978). Supplemental ascorbate in the supportive treatment of cancer: reevaluation of prolongation of survival times in terminal human cancer. *Proc. Natl. Acad. Sci. USA*, 75(9), 4538–4542.

50. Creagan, E. T., Moertel, C. G., O'Fallon, J. R., Schutt, A. J., O'Connell, M. J., Rubin, J. *et al.* (1979). Failure of high-dose vitamin C (ascorbic acid) therapy to benefit patients with advanced cancer a controlled trial. *N. Engl. J. Med.*, 301(13), 687–690.

51. Moertel, C. G., Fleming, T. R., Creagan, E. T., Rubin, J., O'Connel, M. J., and Ames, M. M. (1985). High-dose vitamin C versus placebo in the treatment of patients with advanced cancer who have had no prior chemotherapy: a randomised double-blind comparison. *N. Engl. J. Med.*, 312(3), 137–141.

52. Pauling, L. (1986). A proposition: Megadoses of vitamin C are valuable in the treatment of cancer. *Nutrition Reviews*, 44(1), 28–29.

53. Campbell, A., Jack, T., and Cameron, E. (1991). Reticulum cell sarcoma: Two complete 'spontaneous' remissionsin response to high dose ascorbic acid therapy: a report on subsequent progress. *Oncology*, 48, 495–497.

54. Office of Technology Assessment, Congress of the United States (1990). *Unconventional Cancer Treatments*, pp. 81–86. US Government Printing Office, Washington DC 20402 9395.

55. Schils, M. E. and Hermann, M. G. (1982). Unproven dietary claims in the treatment of patients with cancer. *Bull. N. Y. Acad. Med.*, 58(3), 323–340.

56. Bowman, B. B., Kushner, R. F., Dawson, S. C., and Levin, B. (1984). Macrobiotic diets for Cancer Treatment and prevention. *J. Clin. Oncol.*, 2(6), 702–711.

57. Herbert, V. (1986). Unproven (questionable) dietary and nutritional methods in cancer prevention and treatment. *Cancer*, 58, 1930–1941.

58. Hunter, M. (1988). Unproven dietary methods of treatment of oncology patients. *Rec. Res. Cancer Res.*, 108, 235–238.

59. Office of Technology Assessment, Congress of the United States (1990). *Unconventional Cancer Treatments*, pp. 41–64. US Government Printing Office, Washington DC 20402 9395.

60. Gerson, M. (1958). *A Cancer Therapy: Results of Fifty Cases*. Totality Books, Del Mar, California.

61. Office of Technology Assessment, Congress of the United States (1990). *Unconventional Cancer Treatments*, pp. 55–58. US Government Printing Office, Washington DC 20402 9395.

62. Reed, A., James, N., and Sikora, K. (1990). Mexico: juices, coffee enemas, and cancer. *Lancet*, **336**, 677–678.

63. Office of Technology Assessment, Congress of the United States (1990). *Unconventional Cancer Treatments*, pp. 107–111. US Government Printing Office, Washington DC 20402 9395.

64. Cassileth, B. R., Lusk, E. J., Guerry, Du-P., Blake, A. D., Walsh, W. P., Kascius, L. *et al.* (1991). Survival and quality of life among patients receiving unproven as compared with conventional cancer therapy. *N. Engl. J. Med.*, **324**(17), 1180–1185.

65. Coates, A. (1993). Prognostic implications of quality of life. *Cancer Treat. Reviews*, **19**, 53–57.

66. Meares, A. (1977). Atavistic regression as a factor in the remission of cancer. *Med. J. Aust.*, **2**, (July 23), 132–133.

67. Meares, A. (1976). Regression of cancer after intensive meditation. *Med. J. Aust.*, **2**(5), (July 31), 184.

68. Meares, A. (1978). Regression of osteogenic sarcoma metastases associated with intensive meditation. *Med. J. Aust.*, **2**(9), Oct 21, 433.

69. Meares, A. (1979). Regression of cancer of the rectum after intensive meditation. *Med. J. Aust.*, **2**(10), (Nov 17), 539–540.

70. Meares, A. (1982–83). A form of intensive meditation associated with regression of cancer. *Am. J. Clin. Hypn.*, **25**(2–3), 114–121.

71. Simonton, O. C., Matthews-Simonton, S., and Creighton, J. L. (1978). *Getting Well Again*. Bantam Books, Toronto.

72. Simonton, O. C. and Matthews-Simonton, S. (1975). Belief systems and the management of the emotional aspects of malignancy. *J. Transpersonal Psychol.*, **7**, 29–47.

73. Simonton, O. C., Matthews-Simonton. S., and Sparks, T. F. (1980). Psychological intervention in the treatment of cancer. *Psychosomatics*, **21**(3), 226–233.

74. Simonton, O. C. and Matthews-Simonton, S. (1981). Cancer and stress, counseling the cancer patient. *Med. J. Aust.* June 27, 679–683.

75. Siegel, B. S. (1986). *Love, Medicine and Miracles*. Harper and Row, New York.

76. Morgenstern, H., Gellert, G. A., Walter, S. D., Ostfeld, A. M., and Siegel, B. S. (1984). The impact of a psychosocial support program on survival with breast cancer: the importance of selection bias in program evaluation. *J. Chron. Dis.*, **37**(4), 273–282.

77. Kidman, B. (1983). *A Gentle Way with Cancer*. Century, London.

78. Forbes, A. (1984). *The Bristol Diet*. Century, London.

79. Brohn, P. (1986). *The Bristol Programme*. Century, London.

80. Bagenal, F. S., Easton, D. F., Harris, E., Chilvers, C. E. D., and McElwain, T. J. (1990). Survival of patients with breast cancer attending Bristol Cancer Help Centre. *Lancet*. **336**, 606–610.

81. Chilvers, C. E. D., Easton, D. F., Bagenal, F. S., Harris, E. and McElwain, T. J. (1990). Bristol Cancer Help Centre. *Lancet*, **336**, 1186–1188.

82. James, N. and Reed, A. (1990). Bristol Cancer Help Centre *Lancet*, **336**, 744.

83. Sheard, T. A. B. (1990). Bristol Cancer Help Centre. *Lancet*, **336**, 683.

84. Heyse-Moore, L. (1990). Bristol Cancer Help Centre. *Lancet*, **336**, 743.

85. Wright, S. (1990). Bristol Cancer Help Centre. *Lancet*, **336**, 743.

86. Boulter, P. S. (1990). Bristol Cancer Help Centre. *Lancet*, **336**, 744.

87. Hayes, R. J., Smith, P. G., and Carpenter, L. (1990). Bristol Cancer Help Centre. *Lancet*, **336**, 1185.

88. Sheard, T. A. B. (1990). Bristol Cancer Help Centre. *Lancet*, **336**, 1185–1186.

89. Bodmer, W. (1990). Bristol Cancer Help Centre. *Lancet*, **336**, 1188.

90. Carey, M. and Burish, T. G. (1988). Etiology and treatment of the psychological side effects associated with cancer chemotherapy: A critical review and discussion. *Psychol. Bull.*, **104**(3), 307–325.

91. Dundee, J. W., Ghaly, R. G., Fitzpatrick, K. T., Abram, W. P., and Lynch, G. A. (1989). Acupuncture prophylaxis of cancer chemotherapy-induced sickness. *J. R. Soc. Med.*, **82**(5), 268–71.

92. Spiegel, D. and Bloom, J. R. (1993). Group therapy and hypnosis reduce metastatic breast carcinoma pain. *Psychosom. Med*, **45**(4), 333–339.

93. Filshie, J. and Redman, D. (1985). Acupuncture and malignant pain problems. *Eur. J. Surg. Oncol.*, **11**, 389–394.

94. Filshie, J. and Morrison, P. J. (1988). Acupuncture for chronic pain: a review. *Pall. Med.*, **2**, 1–14.

95. Curt, G. A., Katterhagen, G., and Mahaney, F. X. (1986). Immunoaugmentive therapy: a primer on the perils of unproved treatments. *JAMA*, **255**(4), 505–507.

96. Istre, G. R., Kreiss, K., Hopkins, R. S., Healy, G. R., Benziger, M., Canfield, T. M. *et al.* (1982). An outbreak of amoebiasis spread by colonic irrigation at a chiropractic clinic. *N. Engl. J. Med.*, **307**(6), 339–342.

97. Eisele, J. W. and Reay, D. T. (1980). Deaths related to coffee enemas. *JAMA*, **244**(14), 1608–1609.

98. Markman, M. (1985). Medical complications of 'alternative cancer therapy'. *N. Engl. J. Med.*, **312**, 1640.

99. Schaumburg, H., Kaplan, J., Windebank, A., Vick, N., Rasmus, S., Pleasure, D. *et al.* (1983). Sensory neuropathy from pyridoxine abuse: a new megavitamin syndrome. *N. Engl. J. Med.*, **309**(8), 445–448.

100. Coward, R. (1989). *The Whole Truth: the Myth of Alternative Health*. Faber and Faber, London.

101. Sontag, S. (1977). *Illness as Metaphor*. Penguin Books, Harmondsworth, UK.

102. Gray, R. E. and Doan, B. D. (1990). Heroic self-healing and cancer: clinical issues for the health professions. *J. Pall. Care*, **6**(1), 32–41.

103. Kjeldsen-Kragh, J., Haugen, M., Borchgrevink, C. F., Laerum, E., Eek, M., Mowinkel, P. *et al.* (1991). Controlled trial of fasting and one year vegetarian diet in rheumatoid arthritis. *Lancet*, **338**, 899–902.

104. Simon, A., Worthen, D. M., and Mitas, J. A. (1979). An evaluation of iridology. *JAMA*, **242**(13), 1385–1389.
105. Shipley, M., Berry, H., Broster, G., Jenkins, M., Clover, A., and Williams, I. (1983). Controlled trial of homoeopathic treatment of osteoarthritis. *Lancet*, Jan 15, 97–98.
106. Gibson, R. G., Gibson, S. L. M., MacNeill, A. D., and Watson, W. (1980). Homoeopathic therapy in rheumatoid arthritis: evaluation by double-blind clinical therapeutic trial. *Br. J. Clin. Pharmac.*, **9**, 453–459.
107. Meade, T. W., Dyer, S., Browne, W., Townsend, J., and Frank, A. O. (1990). Low back pain of mechanical origin: randomised comparison of chiropractic and hospital outpatient treatment. *Br. Med. J.*, **300**, 1431–1437.
108. Sheehan, M. P., Rustin, M. H. A., Atherton, D. J., Buckley, C., Harris, D. J., Brostoff, J. *et al.* (1992). Efficacy of traditional Chinese herbal therapy in adult atopic dermatitis. *Lancet*, **340**, 13–17.
109. Benor, D. J. (1990). Survey of spiritual healing research. *Complementary Med. Res.*, **4**(3), 9–33.
110. Brewin, C. R. and Bradley, C. (1989). Patient preferences and randomised clinical trials. *Br. Med. J.*, **299**, 313–315.
111. Heron, J. (1986). Critique of conventional research methodology. *Complementary Med. Res.*, **1**(1), 12–22.
112. Anthony, H. (1986). Post-script: a further critique of conventional trials methodology: implications for research into orthodox and complementary therapies. *Complementary Med. Res.*, **1**(1), 48–54.
113. Taylor, S. E. (1983). Adjustment to threatening events, a theory of cognitive adaptation. *Am. Psychol.*, **38**, 1161–1173.
114. Taylor, S. E. (1988). Illusion and well-being: A social psychological perspective on mental health. *Psych. Bull.*, **103**(2), 193–210.
115. Reason, P. (1986). Innovative research techniques. *Complementary Med. Res.*, **1**(1), 23–39.
116. Reason, P. (ed.) (1988). *Human Inquiry in Action*. Sage, London.
117. Csordas, T. J. (1983). The rhetoric of transformation in ritual healing. *Cult. Med. Psych.*, **7**, 333–375.

# 7

# Life events and the outcome of breast cancer

## J. BARRACLOUGH

The belief that psychological stress may contribute to onset or progression of cancer is ingrained in popular culture, providing a continual impetus for research. 'Life events' such as bereavement or divorce are one common source of stress, and this chapter is concerned with clinical and epidemiological studies of their possible relationship with breast cancer.

## 1 Life events and illness: researching the links

That adverse life events cause adverse effects on health may seem self-evident. Research on the measurement of life events and their relationship with illness has flourished in the past few decades, with earlier studies focused on psychiatric illnesses such as depression. By the late 1970s, life event stress could be considered an established risk factor for such conditions (1). Later studies have found evidence for a causal relationship between adverse life events and some types of physical illness. Before describing the work about breast cancer, some general issues regarding the methodology of life event research (2) will be discussed.

Dating must be established accurately, both for life events and illness onset. In interview studies, dating of life events largely depends upon the memory of the respondents, which is likely to be less accurate for events far back in time. For illnesses of acute onset, timing can be checked from medical records, but this is less satisfactory for chronic conditions which develop gradually.

Independence of life events from the subject's behaviour is important because some events might be a consequence, rather than a cause, of the illness. Only a few events, natural disasters for example, can be considered completely independent. Many others, such as the death of a relative, are usually independent but not always so. A further group of life events, such as divorce or the loss of a job, are clearly not independent and might have been at least partly brought about by the subject's own unrecognized failing health.

Biased reporting of events is a risk in retrospective studies in which subjects are interviewed after the illness in question has already developed. Sick people seeking an explanation for their plight unwittingly tend to exaggerate the significance of trivial incidents ('effort after meaning'). Deliberate falsification is probably rare, but some subjects may omit or distort life events if they feel ashamed of them.

Circumstances surrounding the event may be important. The adverse impact of life events can be partially 'buffered' by a strong family and social network providing emotional and practical support. The subjective impact of an event may not correspond with its objective features, because emotional significance for the individual is coloured by personality and past experience. However, some major events such as the death of a close relative are virtually always distressing and it is probably legitimate to rate their severity on standard measures.

Life event stress must clearly be considered in the context of all the other factors which influence vulnerability to disease. Not all subjects fall ill after life event stress, and not all of those who do, develop the same sort of illness. Besides the psychological and social variables mentioned above, biological factors such as genetic constitution, infection, diet, smoking, and exposure to toxic chemicals contribute in varying degree to the aetiology of many disease conditions.

Any relationship between life event stress and decreased resistance to disease is unlikely to follow a simple linear model. If adverse life events lower the immune defences, maybe pleasant life events promote immunity. Maybe too little life event stress is just as bad for health as too much, with a moderate quantity providing just enough stimulation for optimum mental and physical functioning. Animal experiments (3) suggest that events beyond the subject's control may be more detrimental to health than those which offer scope for mastery and challenge.

Finding a robust association between life events and illness does not necessarily imply a direct causative process, mediated through the immunological and/or hormonal pathways described elsewhere in this book. Any link might be brought about by behavioural means, for example change in diet, smoking, or drinking habits, or compliance with health care.

As this brief consideration of methodological issues shows, it is no simple task to investigate even some of the links in the postulated chain of external stressor, emotional and physiological reaction, and altered susceptibility to cancer. Life event research is fraught with pitfalls. Overcoming these suffi- ciently to yield credible results poses a formidable challenge.

The choice of an instrument to measure life events is clearly of crucial importance. Some studies have employed a checklist such as the 'Schedule of Recent Experiences' or SRE (4). Subjects are presented with a list of pre- determined items and asked to endorse those which have happened to them over a given period, say in the year before interview. Each item on the list is assigned a standard score, the maximum being 100 (for 'death of a spouse'). The checklist approach has the merit of economy and simplicity, but several limitations. Items are vaguely defined, for example 'illness in the family' could range from the trivial to the catastrophic. Circumstances surrounding the event are ignored. There is no attempt to date events in relation to disease onset, or establish the direction of causality.

Various other instruments for measuring life event stress have been published and the Life Events and Difficulties Schedule (LEDS) is the most detailed and sophisticated of these. Developed at Bedford College in London, the LEDS is a semi-structured interview designed to cover all aspects of the subject's recent life experience using a narrative style. Discrete, datable life events (for example deaths) are distinguished from long-term social difficulties (for example poor housing). The interviewer is obliged to ask certain core questions but has freedom to probe for more detail in relevant areas. Timing is determined by careful questioning, relating each event to other significant dates or anniversaries, and checking with documentary evidence such as diaries. An early application of the LEDS was in a community survey regarding depression among women; the book '*Social Origins of Depression*' (5) gives a full description of this work, and contains the actual interview schedule.

A key concept in the LEDS is that of 'contextual' threat; rating the severity of each event or difficulty according to the impact it would be expected to have upon the average person, given similar circumstances. The individual background history of the person concerned is taken into account when making contextual ratings, but the person's actual emotional response is not, subjective response being rated separately as the 'reported' threat. The reasons for distinguishing contextual from reported threat are to avoid bias arising from 'effort after meaning' and from the tendency of sick people, especially those who are depressed, to emphasize the negative aspects of any given event.

Rules exist as to the inclusion, or otherwise, of certain events. For example, deaths or illnesses of other people are only included if they affect a first-degree relative or a close confidant of the subject, or if the subject was directly involved, for example being in a car crash in which the other driver was killed. No predetermined list of events is given, as no list could adequately cover the enormous range of potential experiences. However, events can be grouped into certain predetermined categories, and classified on many different parameters. Use of the LEDS requires a fortnight's training course, and regular consultation with a large manual of examples. Interviews are tape-recorded and relevant sections transcribed. The factual details of each event are discussed with one or more other trained people, who are kept in ignorance of the subject's reported reaction to the event and of any putative consequences for the subject's health, in order to agree upon consensus ratings.

The LEDS represents a more satisfactory approach to the measurement of life event stress than any checklist, and its correct use should minimize the problems discussed above. The LEDS has now been applied in many research studies to investigate relationships between life event stress and various medical conditions, both physical and psychiatric, with the majority yielding positive associations. Such studies are drawn together in the book '*Life Events and Illness*' (6). This book does not contain a chapter about cancer, and the majority of pubished studies on life events and cancer have not employed the LEDS.

## 2   Studies on life events and breast cancer

Breast cancer has attracted more life event research than any other type of cancer. The hormone sensitivity of many breast cancers provides a rational basis for this choice, whereas the high incidence of this disease among relatively young and articulate women, who are willing to cooperate in psychosocial research, provides a pragmatic justification.

The majority of clinical studies have been designed to explore the idea that life event stress contributes to the primary onset of breast cancer, as opposed to the prognosis of the disease once diagnosed. Their interpretation is hampered by the question of timing. While it is recognized that a latent period of several years may elapse between initiation of a malignant breast tumour and its clinical presentation, there is no valid method of dating this interval and therefore no way of knowing whether a given life event occurred before or after onset of the disease. This is obviously a crucial problem if life event stress is postulated to be an initiating factor, triggering the beginning of the cancer process, but less important if stress were to act as a promoting factor, speeding up the growth of an existing tumour.

Many clinical studies (6–14) have taken patients with benign breast disease as a comparison group. Women presenting for investigation of breast lumps are interviewed about their life event experience, before the final diagnosis is known. Results for those whose lumps later turn out to be malignant are compared with those whose final diagnosis is benign breast disease. This research design, though convenient, is flawed in its implicit assumption that patients referred to hospital for investigation of breast lumps which prove to be benign are representative of women in the general population. Like other groups of hospital attenders, these women probably have high rates of recent mood disorder and life event stress (15). In several of the quoted studies the benign breast patients were younger than the cancer ones, and life event experience is known to alter with age. Benign breast disease is itself one of the risk factors for breast cancer in later life, so that some overlap between the two groups is likely. Lastly, even if the life event interviews are carried out before biopsy results are known, a high proportion of patients have correctly guessed their diagnosis by that time (16). This group of studies has yielded inconsistent findings. The advent of breast screening programmes, involving mammography on large populations of asymptomatic women, has permitted improvements in research design. A study of 1052 women undergoing breast screening (17) found few relationships between psychological variables, including life events, and breast cancer.

Epidemiological methods offer a different approach. A ten-year follow-up of widowed subjects, identified through the 1971 census for England and Wales, revealed only a small excess of new cancer registrations (18). A study from Denmark (19) reported a similar lifetime frequency of both widowhood and divorce for 1792 women registered with breast cancer and for 1739 general population controls. While epidemiological methods are limited in that they can given no information about other psychological or social factors, they have the considerable merit of being based on large populations, and accurately dated events of an indisputably stressful kind.

Whether life event stress affects the outcome of breast cancer, after diagnosis and treatment, is a somewhat different question and this can be investigated by prospective follow-up of a cohort of recently diagnosed patients. A similar research design has previously been used to assess the prognostic influence of attitude to disease (20), and of mood (21). No published studies, other than the one to be described in this chapter, have used this design in relation to life events, but several other pieces of work are relevant. The epidemiological study already quoted (18), linking national cancer registration data to census data on marital status, found that for married women already diagnosed with breast cancer, widowhood was followed by a long-term increase in breast cancer mortality but the effect size was small. Subjective life event stress and lack of social support during the five years preceding breast cancer diagnosis was found in one interview study (22) to predict a decreased twenty-year survival, though not for women between 40 and 60 years old. This design did not take account of life events occurring during the postoperative disease-free interval. Another interview study (23) assessed 204 patients with advanced cancer and 155 with operable cancer, including breast cancer, on the following variables: social ties and marital history, job satisfaction, use of psychotropic drugs, general life evaluation/satisfaction, subjective view of adult health, hopelessness/helplessness, and amount of adjustment required to cope with diagnosis. None of these proved to be related to survival time in the first group, nor the length of disease-free interval in the second. In a retrospective study carried out at Guy's Hospital in London (24), the LEDS was administered to 50 recently relapsed breast cancer patients, and to 50 control patients matched on physical characteristics and date of original presentation but still in remission. Relapsed patients reported significantly more severe life events and difficulties since surgery than controls. A subsequent analysis of this data suggested that the link between stress and relapse was confined to women with hormone receptor-positive tumours (25).

A recent review (26) covers the wider field of psychosocial factors in the outcome of breast cancer.


## 3 The present study

The present study was designed to test the hypothesis that experience of adverse life events shortens the disease-free interval following primary treatment for operable breast cancer. This was a purely clinical project, not including measurements of immunological or hormonal parameters. A descriptive account of the work is given here, a more detailed version including data tabulations having been published elsewhere (27, 28).

The aim was to recruit a series of women recently treated for operable breast cancer, without clinical evidence of metastatic disease at entry to the study, and to carry out serial interview follow-up of this cohort, documenting and dating both experience of life events and social difficulties, and onset of symptoms of breast cancer relapse. Consecutive new breast cancer patients who had presented to the breast clinics at the Royal South Hants Hospital in Southampton or Queen Alexandra Hospital in Portsmouth, between February 1986 and August 1987, were identified through surgical records. Exclusion criteria were: age over 70, clinical evidence of tumour spread beyond the ipsilateral axilla, and/or a past history of breast cancer.

Providing the family doctor agreed, potential subjects were approached by a letter explaining the project in general terms as being concerned with the links between stress and physical illness. Three home interviews, timed at four, 24, and 42 months postoperatively, were planned for each participant. Each interview inquired about the experiences of the previous 18 months, yielding data about the period from one year before breast cancer surgery until three-and-a-half years afterwards.

The LEDS, which has been described above (5), was the chief instrument used at interview. After some questions about the subject's family composition and social circumstances, including availability of confiding relationships, this schedule inquires about experience of life events (for example bereavements) and social difficulties (for example unemployment). The section about the subject's own health was left to the end, to minimize any bias which might arise from the interviewer's knowledge about the dating of relapse. Symptoms of major depression were elicited using DSM-III criteria (29). Each interview, lasting between one and three hours, was tape recorded and transcribed, and the abstracted material discussed at a weekly meeting between the investigators. Events and difficulties were rated according to the following parameters: classification by domain of life involved (for example own health, others' health, bereavement, marital); severity, according to short- and long-term threat, both 'contextual' (objective) and 'reported' (subjective); independence from the patient's own behaviour or state of health; and timing, determined at interview with reference to written evidence such as diaries and medical records when available.

Fixed variables, including sociodemographic characteristics of the patient and details of the breast cancer and its treatment, were recorded on entry to the study. Time-dependent variables, including experience of psychosocial stressors and physical symptoms, were recorded on a monthly basis. The end-point of the study for patients who relapsed was taken as either local recurrence or distant metastasis, with histological and/or radiological confirmation, and timed from the month when clinical symptoms or signs began.

Of 246 consecutive patients who fulfilled the selection criteria, 204 (83 per cent) accepted the first home interview. Non-participants tended to be younger and to have less favourable physical prognostic features than those interviewed. No systematic information about the psychosocial characteristics of the non-participants was available; while it seems likely that some of the women in this group had particularly severe emotional problems, others may have made a good psychological adjustment and wanted to resume a normal life. Of the 204 patients taking part in the first interview, two declined the second and one declined the third. Eleven of the follow-up interviews were conducted with a close relative because the patients themselves were terminally ill or had died; in ten of these cases, this relative had previously been nominated by the patient herself as a full confidant. For two other deceased patients, the next-of-kin refused an interview.

Some characteristics of the 204 participants at entry to the study are as follows. Age ranged from 20 to 70, with a mean of 54 years. The majority, 77 per cent, were living with a husband or partner; 13 per cent lived alone. As a crude indicator of socioeconomic status, 78 per cent lived in owner-occupied housing. Mastectomy was performed in 60 per cent of patients, followed by radiotherapy in a few cases, and 40 per cent had local excisions with postoperative radiotherapy. Axillary lymph node involvement was histologically demonstrated in 39 per cent of the surgical specimens. Cytotoxic chemotherapy was not given, but 26 per cent of patients received the anti-oestrogen drug tamoxifen.

Life events and difficulties were common, the total being 1995 events (range 0–45 per patient), and 924 difficulties (range 0–12 patient). Events and difficulties were often linked; to take a simple example, a husband's heart attack (other's health event) followed by his being unwell for several months (other's health difficulty), then his death (bereavement event), and its aftermath (bereavement difficulty). Such a sequence might well be more complicated, for example if the patient gave up her job to nurse her husband or if a family dispute over his will led to interpersonal or financial problems. Of particular interest were 'severe' events, those which carried a high long-term contextual threat. During the year before breast cancer surgery, 54 patients (27 per cent) reported one or more severe experiences, not counting those involving their own health, and 103 patients (51 per cent) did so during the follow-up period. Death of a husband, child, or grandchild constituted the most severe events reported. Death of a parent or sibling, and marital separation or divorce, was rated severe in almost all cases. Other examples of severe events include the house burning down, a son sent to prison, or a major family rift. For difficulties, common examples are the chronic illness of close relatives, bereavements, and marital discord.

Overall, 30 per cent of events and 40 per cent of difficulties were rated independent of the patient. Independence was related to domain of life involved; whereas illnesses and deaths of other people were usually independent, items concerned with interpersonal relationships were not. Only 4 per cent of events and 1 per cent of difficulties appeared to be an obvious direct result of the patient's breast cancer, for example giving up a heavy manual job, the onset of sexual or marital difficulties, and being rehoused on medical grounds. Causative links of a more subtle kind could have existed in other cases; breast cancer could be a contributory factor towards moving house, a daughter's marriage, or a husband's dismissal from work, though such a link would be impossible to prove or quantify.

Major depression lasting three months or more affected 45 patients (23 per cent) during the follow-up period; the more severe and prolonged depressions often pre-dated the breast cancer diagnosis and could not necessarily be attributed to it. The majority (83 per cent) of patients reported one or more full confidants at the outset of the study, and availability of confidants remained fairly constant during follow-up.

Relapse of breast cancer was confirmed in 47 (23 per cent) of the 204 patients, and 28 of these (14 per cent of the 204) had died by the end of the follow-up period, that is 42 months after primary surgery. One other patient died from a stroke, classed as not related to cancer. Review of the case-notes of the non-participants showed them to have a somewhat less favourable prognosis, with relapse confirmed in 17 (40 per cent) of the 42 patients and 10 of these (24 per cent of the 42) being dead by the end of the 42-month follow-up period. One possible explanation is that some of these patients refused to take part because, when approached about the study, they already felt unwell.

As the fieldwork progressed, any expectations of finding a positive relationship between life event stress and relapse receded. Most strikingly, all thirteen patients who experienced the most stressful life events of all (death of a husband, child, or grandchild) remained in remission during the follow-up period. Conversely, many relapses seemed to develop in the context of quiet, contented lives. Clinical impressions, however, can be misleading and a formal statistical analysis is necessary to take account of the fixed biological variables which are known to influence prognosis, and of the different time periods for which different patients were exposed to the postulated psychosocial risk factors. Analysis was carried out using the Cox proportional hazards model with allowance for time-dependent variables (30). The fixed co-variates were examined first to find those most strongly related to outcome, in order to allow for these when modelling the time-dependent ones. This procedure showed axillary lymph node involvement, large tumour diameter, and younger age to be associated with increased risk of relapse, in keeping with other published studies (31). Axillary lymph node involvement was the single most important factor, being associated with a hazard ratio of 4.50 (95 per cent confidence interval 2.41 to 8.42, significance level <0.001).

Turning to the relationship between life events and other psychosocial variables, and the subsequent risk of relapse, a large number of preliminary analyses revealed no striking relationships. The final model used in the analysis of the time-dependent psychosocial risk factors included adjustment for age group and lymph node involvement. Tumour size was not included in the model because it added no contribution after the first two factors had been entered. The following measures of psychosocial stress were chosen: severe events and/or difficulties, divided into own-health and other categories, major depression over three months' duration, and lack of a full confidant. The hazard ratio associated with severe life events and/or social difficulties (excluding own-health ones) during the year before breast cancer surgery was 0.43 (95 per cent confidence interval 0.20 to 0.93); for those during the follow-up period it was 0.88 (0.48 to 1.64). For prolonged major depression before surgery and during the follow-up period, hazard ratios were 1.26 (0.49 to 3.26) and 0.85 (0.41 to 1.79) respectively. For absence of a full confidant the figures were 0.93 (0.42 to 2.09) and 0.86 (0.38 to 1.93). None of these reach the conventional 0.05 level of statistical significance.

An unexpected finding to emerge from the analysis was the increased risk of relapse for patients who had a severe event or difficulty with their own physical health during follow-up, hazard ratio 3.06 (95 per cent confidence interval 1.29 to 7.31, *p* value 0.01). Own-health events and difficulties had been analysed separately for two reasons. Firstly, they might influence the outcome of breast cancer by some direct physiological mechanism, as distinct from any effect mediated by emotional stress. Secondly, however, some of them might actually have been unrecognized manifestations of recurrent breast cancer, in which case any association would be spurious.

As only a limited duration of follow-up had been possible within the time-frame of the original study, a case-note review of the cohort at five years after diagnosis has since been carried out, revealing a further 18 cases of relapse. Statistical analysis showed a continuation of the same trends found in the original study, with similar five-year survival curves for patients who had, and those who had not, reported severe life events at interview (28).

In summary, this large and detailed clinical study detected no increase in risk of breast cancer relapse following a severe life event. Its negative result may be regarded as surprising in view of the widespread belief in a link between stress and cancer growth, and laboratory findings which might explain such a link in terms of hormonal or immunological changes. A critical look at our own methodology is called for. The strengths of the project included a reasonably large and representative patient sample; a comprehensive and well-established measure of life events; and a prospective design which enabled well over 90 per cent of interviews to be conducted with both parties blind to the outcome of the breast cancer. However it had several limitations.

Was the sample large enough to detect what we were looking for? If life event stress was a major risk factor, comparable in importance to axillary lymph node involvement, the study would have had sufficient power to detect this but a larger sample would have been required to make certain that a more modest effect was not missed.

Were the patients followed-up for a long enough period? This is an important point, since breast cancer is often a slow-growing tumour and it might conceivably take several years for any influence of life events to become apparent. Patients were only assigned to the 'relapse' category if they had histological or radiological confirmation of recurrence, but several others must have had occult metastases which would have become manifest with longer follow-up. The five-year case-note review of the cohort has already gone some way to answering this question, and a ten-year follow-up is planned.

Might awareness of disease status, on the part of patient or interviewer or both, have compromised the validity of the data? 'Effort after meaning' might have encouraged over-reporting of stress by patients who already knew they had relapsed, but only 44 of the 580 interviews (8 per cent) were in this category, and any bias from this source would have led to a false-positive result rather than a false-negative one. The eleven proxy interviews with relatives (only 2 per cent of the total) might have been incomplete as regards minor life events but would almost certainly have covered severe ones.

Was the personal meaning of life events sufficiently considered? The LEDS method places more emphasis on the objective features of life events than on details of the individual's emotional response or attribution of control. Reaction to a divorce, for example, might take the form of guilt, anger, fatalistic acceptance, or a sense of liberation for different people. The nature of the subjective reaction would presumably be of crucial importance in mediating any causal link between life event stress and disease, and the ideal study would have measured this, besides including the many other variables (such as personality, mental attitude to disease, and coping style) which might be relevant to the impact of events and/or directly influence prognosis of the breast cancer. In practice, attempting to do this would involve unacceptably long patient assessments and complex statistical analysis.

Could patients' life event experience be a reflection of their disease status? Definitive diagnosis of relapse is sometimes preceded by vague unrecognized prodromal symptoms, for example tiredness due to anaemia or behavioural change due to cerebral metastases. Such changes might trigger off certain life events, while preventing others from taking place at all, in ways that can only be guessed at. Restricting the analysis to events rated independent of the patients would have avoided the issue, but at the expense of ignoring major stressors such as divorce which, while not independent, are clearly relevant to the inquiry.

Could the process of carrying out a prospective study have changed the phenomena under observation? The purpose of our research interviews was the gathering of information in objective fashion, and no psychotherapeutic function was intended. All the same, talking in depth about personal matters to a detached but sympathetic interviewer might well have been a significant emotional experience for some of our patients. The suggestion that our detailed monitoring of patients' life event stress actually prevented its translation into relapse of breast cancer cannot necessarily be dismissed as grandiose or far-fetched. The finding of a higher relapse rate in the non-participants, who denied themselves the possible benefits of the research interviews, would lend support to this theory!

The contrast between the Southampton results and those of the Guy's study (24) merits comment. Relapsed breast cancer patients at Guy's reported significantly more severe life events and difficulties since diagnosis than did their disease-free controls. Many explanations for the discrepancy have been put forward. Some relate to sampling differences. The Guy's study achieved a 100 per cent rate, in contrast to Southampton's 83 per cent which may have introduced a bias. Guy's patients were younger, a potentially important difference since both life event experience and the natural history of breast cancer vary with age and menopausal status. The type of life events and difficulties may have differed between the two samples, perhaps due to socio-demographic differences between London and the provinces, and/or different referral policies to the hospitals concerned. Breast cancer treatment policies vary over time and between centres, for example none of the Guy's patients received tamoxifen. The most striking difference however lies in the study design, the Southampton one being prospective so that the bulk of interview data was obtained from patients still in clinical remission, and the Guy's one retrospective so that neither patient nor interviewer could be blind to diagnosis of relapse.

## 4   A personal comment

Most investigators in this field probably set out, as I did myself, expecting and perhaps hoping to demonstrate that emotional stress does promote breast cancer growth. Positive results are intuitively more interesting; more likely to be accepted for publication in a medical journal and to attract notice in the popular media; and often lead on to further research projects, in this case clarifying the mechanism of stress–cancer links, or evaluating psychosocial interventions to improve cancer prognosis.

Negative findings from a clinical project such as this do not necessarily mean that life event stress has no influence at all on the breast cancer process. Maybe an effect exists only in some subgroups of patients, or maybe there is a complex mixture of conflicting effects which tend to cancel each other out in large samples. However, the results of this and other work do weigh against the likelihood of an important link for the majority of patients, so casting doubt on the relevance of further clinical studies, and on the ethics of laboratory experiments which involve inflicting stress on animals.

Emotional responses to the negative results of this project have been some-what polarized. Many people, including a number of my own patients and friends with personal histories of breast cancer, have been relieved to learn that life event stress may not be such a bad prognostic factor as is commonly thought. After all, life events form an unavoidable part of human experience. Some of them can be readily construed as the subject's own fault, whereas others are entirely outside her control; and an unpleasant event is bad enough in itself, without the added worry that it will cause recurrence of cancer. Other people, including some professionals, have responded to the negative findings with disappointment or incredulity. Deeply held, emotionally based con-victions that stress causes cancer should not, of course, interfere with the scientific evaluation of research; but in practice they probably do. Psychosocial influences on breast cancer growth may be considered 'fascinating but clinically unimportant' (32); exaggerating their importance can burden patients with worry and guilt (33). Human nature is such, however, that interest in this topic will continue to flourish, at least until the biological causes of breast cancer are better understood.

4.1 ACKNOWLEDGEMENTS

I wish to thank all the colleagues who helped with the research project described here, in particular Pamela Pinder, Marie Cruddas, and Clive Osmond; and the Medical Research Council for funding the work.

# 5   References

1. Andrews, G. and Tennant, C. (1978). Life event stress and psychiatric illness. *Psychol. Med.*, **8**, 545–549.
2. Paykel, E. S. (1983). Methodological aspects of life event research. *J. Psychosom. Res.*, **27**, 341–352.
3. Newberry, B. H., Gordon, T. L., and Meehan, S. M. (1991). Recent animal studies of stress and cancer. In *Cancer and Stress* (ed. C. L. Cooper, and M. Watson) Wiley, Chichester.
4. Holmes, T. H. and Rahe, R. H. (1967). The Social Readjustment Rating Scale. *J. Psychosom. Res.*, **11**, 213–218.
5. Brown, G. W. and Harris, T. O. (1989). *Social Origins of Depression*. Tavistock, London.
6. Brown, G. W. and Harris, T. O. (1989) *Life Events and Illness*. Unwin Hyman, London.
7. Muslin, H. L., Gyarfas, K., and Pieper, W. J. (1966). Separation experience and cancer of the breast. *Ann. N.Y. Acad. Sci.*, **125**, 802–806.
8. Greer, S. and Morris, T. (1975). Psychological attributes of women who develop breast cancer: a controlled study. *J. Psychosom. Res.*, **19**, 147–153.
9. Schonfield, J. (1975). Psycholosical and life-experience differences between Israeli women with benign and cancerous breast lesions. *J. Psychosom. Res.*, **19**, 229–234.
10. Cheang, A. and Cooper, C. L. (1985). Psychosocial factors in breast cancer. *Stress Med.*, **1**, 61–66.
11. Priestman, T. J., Priestman, S. G. and Bradshaw, C. (1985). Stress and breast cancer. *Br. J. Cancer*, **51**, 493–498.
12. Hughes, J. E., Royle, G. T., Buchanan, R., and Taylor, I. (1986). Depression and social stress among patients with benign breast disease. *Br. J. Surg.*, **73**, 997–999.
13. Cooper, C. L., Cooper, R., and Faragher, E. B. (1989). Incidence and perception

of psyshosocial stress: the relationship with breast cancer. *Psychol. Med.*, **19**, 415–422.

14. Geyer, S. (1991). Life events prior to manifestation of breast cancer. *J. Psychosom. Res.*, **35**, 355–363.

15. Hughes, J. E. (1990). Psychological manifestations of benign breast disease. In *Benign Breast Disease*, (ed. J. A. Smallwood and I. Taylor) Edward Arnold, London.

16. Schwarz, R. and Geyer, S. (1984). Social and psychological differences between cancer and non-cancer patients; cause or consequence of the disease? *Psychother. Psychosom.*, **41**, 195–199.

17. Edwards, J. R., Cooper, C. L., Pearl. S. G., de Paredes, E. S., O'Leary, T., and Wilhelm, M. C. (1990). The relationship between psychosocial factors and breast cancer: some unexpected results. *Behav. Med.*, **16**, 5–14.

18. Jones, D. R., Goldblatt, P. O., and Leon, D. A. (1984). Bereavement and cancer; some data on deaths of spouses from the longitudinal study of the Office of Population Censuses and Surveys. *Br. Med. J.*, **289**, 461–464.

19. Ewertz, M. (1986). Bereavement and breast cancer. *Br. J. Cancer*, **53**, 701–703.

20. Greer, S., Morris, T., and Pettingale, R. W. (1979). Psychological response to breast cancer; efrect on outcome. *Lancet*, **ii**, 785–787.

21. Dean, C. and Surtees, P. G. (1989). Do psychological factors predict survival in breast cancer? *J. Psychosom. Res.*, **33**, 561–569.

22. Funch, D. P. and Marshall, J. (1983). The role of stress, social support and age in survival from breast cancer. *J. Psychosom. Res.*, **27**, 77–83.

23. Cassileth, B. R., Lusk, E. J., Miller, D. S., Brown, L. L., and Miller, C. (1985). Psychosocial correlates of survival in advanced malignant disease? *N. Engl. J. Med.*, **312**, 1551–1555.

24. Ramirez, A. J., Craig, T. J. K., Watson, J. P., Fentiman, I. S., North, W. R. S., and Rubens, R. D. (1989). Stress and relapse of breast cancer. *Br. Med. J.*, **298**, 291–293.

25. Ramirez, A. J., Richards, M. A., Gregory, W., and Craig, T. K. J. (1990) Psychological correlates of hormone receptor status in breast cancer. *Lancet*, **335**, 1408.

26. Mulder, C. L., van der Pompe, G., Spiegel, D., Antone, M. H., and de Vries, M. (1992). Do psychosocial factors influence the course of breast cancer? *Psycho-oncol.*, **1**, 155–167.

27. Barraclough, J., Pinder, P., Cruddas, M., Osmond, C., Taylor, I. and Perry, M. (1992). Life events and breast cancer prognosis. *Br. Med. J.*, **304**, 1078–1081.

28. Barraclough, J., Osmond, C., Taylor, I., Perry, M., and Collins, C. (1993). Life events and breast cancer prognosis (letter). *Br. Med. J.*, **307**, 325.

29. American Psychiatric Association (1980). *Diagnostic and Statistical Manual of Mental Disorders*. American Psychiatric Association, Washington DC.

30. Cox, D.R. and Oakes, D. (1984). Time-dependent covariates. In *Analysis of Survival Data*. Chapman and Hall, London.

31. Harris, J. R., Lippman, M. E., Veronesi, U., and Willett, W. (1992). Breast

cancer (a review in three parts). *N. Engl. J. Med.*, **327**, 319–328, 390–398, 473–480.

32. Chen, C. C. and Fahy, T. (1992). Life events and breast cancer prognosis (letter). *Br. Med. J.*, **304**, 1632.

33. Angell, M. (1985). Editorial: Disease as a reflection of the psyche. *N. Engl. J. Med.*, **312**, 1570–1572.

# 8

# Does psychological status influence cancer patient survival? A case still in need of evidence

## J. L. RICHARDSON, H. LANDRINE, AND G. MARKS

## 1 Introduction

Is survival after the diagnosis of cancer influenced by psychological factors such as depression, hostility, locus of control, or anxiety? Does optimism improve the survival of cancer patients, while pessimism cuts it short? Physicians, psychologists, and lay people are aware that occasionally an individual with a poor prognosis survives for an unexpectedly long period while, conversely, those with a good prognosis unexpectedly survive for a short period. Is this because the former had a 'fighting spirit' while the latter a 'helpless and hopeless attitude?' It appeals to an inherent sense of justice if those who fight-to-live in fact survive and those who give up die sooner; but, how often do those with a long life expectancy and fighting spirit surprise others by dying rapidly, while the hopeless and helpless individual continues to survive, albeit without much enjoyment of their extended life?

Some studies examining psychological factors and cancer survival postulate that mood states, coping styles, or personality traits may influence complex endocrinological or immunological pathways, and that these might presumably alter the growth rate of certain tumours. But, survival after a cancer diagnosis is the result of a complex interaction of biological, treatment, behavioural, and social variables. Thus, studies of the role of the psychological effects must be integrated with existing known predictors of cancer patient survival and must demonstrate that other explanations have been ruled out. If a relationship is found, the mechanism for the effect needs to be carefully examined. For example, denial could lead to delay in diagnosis or to non-compliance with one's treatment regimen, thus profoundly influencing survival. On the other side of the coin, an optimistic attitude may promote self-care behaviours that extend life.

In this chapter we review eleven well-known studies of psychological factors in cancer survival. Although this is not an exhaustive review, we focused our analyses on these eleven studies because several are frequently cited as supporting and stimulating the examination of the role of psychological factors in survival with cancer. Reviewing these studies as a whole allows us to evaluate the strength of the collective data. We pay particular attention to the 'within-study variation' in the findings because often a single 'significant' effect is highlighted while pertinent null findings are down-played or ignored. We also scrutinize the studies for design weaknesses and confounding variables. As will be shown below, measurement problems preclude clear interpretation of many results. Furthermore, several studies have not controlled for disease factors, health status at the time psychological data were obtained, social class differences, or behavioural variables known to affect survival after cancer diagnosis. Consequently, the data are open to plausible alternative interpretations. Finally, we discuss the roles of behavioural and social factors such as patient compliance with medication and subject ethnicity as factors affecting survival, and offer suggestions for improving methodological approaches.

## 2 Review of the findings

In chronological order, the studies we examined were conducted by Derogatis *et al.* (1979) (1), Rogentine *et al.* (1979) (2), Greer *et al.* (1979, 1990) (3, 4), Speigel *et al.* (1989, 1991) (5, 6), Funch and Marshall (1983) (7), Temoshok *et al.* (1985) (8), Cassileth *et al.* (1985) (9), Leigh *et al.* (1987) (10), Hislop *et al.* (1987) (11), Jamison *et al.* (1987) (12), and Richardson *et al.* (1990)

**Table 1** Consistency of findings and measurement

| Dimensions | Related to longer survival | No relationship with survival |
|---|---|---|
| Depression | 1. Derogatis *et al.* 1979 (affect Balance Sheet) High scores (1) | 1. Spiegel *et al.* 1981 (POMS) (35) <br> 2. Jamison *et al.* 1987 (Zung) (12) <br> 3. Greer *et al.* 1979 (Hamilton) (3) <br> 4. Hislop *et al.* 1987 (own measure) (11) <br> 5. Leigh *et al.* 1987 (Beck) (8) <br> 6. Temoshok *et al.* 1985 (Beck) (8) <br> 7. Richardson *et al.* 1990 (Beck/Zung) (13) |
| Anxiety | 1. Leigh *et al.* 1987 (Spielberger) High Scores (10) <br> 2. Jamison *et al.* 1987 (Spielberger) Low Scores (12) | 1. Spiegel *et al.* 1981 (POMS) (35) <br> 2. Hislop *et al.* 1987 (own measure) (11) <br> 3. Rogentine *et al.* 1979 (SCL90-R) (2) <br> 4. Derogatis *et al.* 1979 (SCL90-R) (1) <br> 5. Derogatis *et al.* 1979 (Affect Balance Scale) (1) <br> 6. Temoshok *et al.* 1985 (MMPI) (8) <br> 7. Jamison *et al.* 1987 (S-R Anxiousness) (12) |
| Anger/Hostility | 1. Hislop *et al.* 1987 (own measure) Low anger (11) <br> 2. Derogatis *et al.* 1979 (SCL90-R) High anger (1) | 1. Spiegel *et al.* 1981 (POMS) (35) <br> 2. Greer *et al.* 1979 (HDHQ Scale) (3) <br> 3. Rogentine *et al.* 1979 (SCL90-R) (2) <br> 4. Derogatis *et al.* 1979 (Affect Balance Scale) (1) <br> 5. Jamison *et al.* 1987 (Multiple Affect Adjective Checklist) (7) <br> 6. Jamison *et al.* 1987 (MAACL) (12) |
| HLOC-Chance | 1. Jamison *et al.* 1987 (MHLOC Walston) Low chance (12) | 1. Spiegel *et al.* 1981 (MHLOC-Walston) (35) <br> 2. Richardson *et al.* 1990 (MHLOC-Walston) (13) |
| HLOC-Powerful others | | 1. Spiegel *et al.* 1981 (MHLOC-Walston) (35) <br> 2. Jamison *et al.* 1987 (MHLOC-Walston) (12) <br> 3. Richardson *et al.* 1990 (MHLOC-Walston) (13) |
| HLOC-Internal | | 1. Spiegel *et al.* 1981 (MHLOC-Walston (35) <br> 2. Jamison *et al.* 1987 (MHLOC-Walston) (12) <br> 3. Richardson *et al.* 1990 (MHLOC-Walston) (13) |
| Rotter's Locus of Control | | 1. Hislop *et al.* 1987 (Rotter) (11) <br> 2. Rogentine *et al.* 1979 (Rotter) (2) |
| Self esteem | | 1. Spiegel *et al.* 1981 (Janis-Fields) <br> 2. Hislop *et al.* 1987 (Rosenberg Scale) (11) |

**Table 1**   (*continued*)

| Dimensions | Related to longer survival | No relationship with survival |
|---|---|---|
| | | 3. Jamison *et al.* 1987 (Cooperstein measure) (12) |
| Extraversion | 1. Hislop *et al.* 1987 (Eysenck Personality Inventory) High extraversion | 1. Greer *et al.* 1979 (Eysenck Personality Inventory) (3) |
| Neuroticism | | 1. Greer *et al.* 1979 (Eysenck Personality Inventory) (3) |
| | | 2. Hislop *et al.* 1987 (Eysenck Personality Inventory) (11) |
| Stress | 1. Funch and Marshall 1983 (Own measure) Low stress (7) | 1. Greer *et al.* 1979 (own measure) (3) |
| | | 2. Hislop *et al.* 1987 (Holmes and Rahe) (11) |
| Coping/Personality | 1. Temoshok *et al.* 1985 (Own measure) High Faith non-verbal type C, Low histrionic—narcissistic (8) | 1. Spiegel *et al.* 1981 (coping—own measure) (35) |
| | 2. Greer *et al.* 1979 (Own measure) High fighting spirit, Low hopeless/helpless, High denial (3) | 2. Spiegel *et al.* 1981 (denial—own measure) (35) |
| | 3. Derogatis *et al.* 1979 (Own measure) low scores overall adjustment (1) | 3. Greer *et al.* 1979 (own measure) (3) |
| | 4. Rogentine *et al.* 1979 (Own measure) High scores on subjective life change required (2) | 4. Hislop *et al.* 1987 (own measure) (3) |
| | | 5. Richardson *et al.* 1990 (MOOS Coping style—behavioural, cognitive avoidance, information seeking, emotional, logical affective, problem solving) (13) |
| | | 6. Cassileth *et al.* 1985 (Hopeless/helpless Beck Scale) (9) |
| | | 7. Greer *et al.* 1979 (overall adjustment—own measure) (3) |
| | | 8. Cassileth *et al.* 1985 (Rogentine's scale) (9) |
| | | 9. Temoshok *et al.* 1985 (Seven coping scales—own measure) (8) |
| Somatization | | 1. Rogentine *et al.* 1979 (SCL90-R) (2) |
| Obsession | | 1. Rogentine *et al.* 1979 (SCL90-R) (2) |
| Sensitivity | | 1. Rogentine *et al.* 1979 (SCL90-R) (2) |
| Paranoia-psychoticism | 1. Derogatis *et al.* 1979 (SCL90-R) High scores on paranoia-psychoticism (1) | 1. Rogentine *et al.* 1979 (SCL90-R) (2) |
| Severity index | | 1. Rogentine *et al.* 1979 (SCL90-R) (2) |
| | | 2. Derogatis *et al.* 1979 (SCL90-R) (1) |
| Total symptom scores | | 1. Spiegel *et al.* 1981 (POMS) (35) |
| | | 2. Rogentine *et al.* 1979 (SCL90-R (2) |
| | | 3. Derogatis *et al.* 1979 (SCL90-R) (1) |

(13). Table 1 summarizes the psychological variables assessed, the measures used to assess them, and the results found in these studies. Most often, no relationship between psychological factors and survival was found; the null results listed in column 3 far outweigh the positive findings in column 2.

For example, only two (10, 12) of nine investigations found a relationship between anxiety and survival, and those two investigations had opposite findings. Only one (1) of seven studies that examined depression found a relationship with survival and this one found that higher depression levels related to longer survival. Only one (12) of five studies that examined locus of control found a relationship, and that was for higher chance control and shorter survival, and none of the three studies that examined self esteem found a relationship. Likewise, only two (1, 11) of nine investigations found a relationship between anger/hostility and survival, and again, these two had opposite findings. For each significant relationship found between a measure of psychological status and survival at least one other study found no relationship between that same psychological factor and survival. Indeed, out of more than 70 tests of relationships between various psychological factors and survival, only 13 found significant relationships. These constructs have generally been measured using standardized psychological measurement tools with known validity and reliability such as the Beck Depression Inventory, the Speilberger State/Trait Anxiety Scales, and the Multidimensional Health Locus of Control Scale. The results from these studies do not provide strong support for the hypothesis that psychological factors play a significant role in cancer survival (14).

On the other hand, several studies that indicate an association between psychological status and survival utilize a measurement tool developed by the respective authors specifically for the study purposes (see 'own measure' notation given in Table 1). Unfortunately, these do not measure the same constructs, are often classifications from structured interviews, are difficult to grasp from the published articles and even more difficult to replicate, and have unknown validity and reliability. Consequently, a strong and consistent body of evidence does not emerge. Such assessments are also more susceptible to (conscious or unconscious) experimenter expectations and biases. We compared the number of significant results found when using standardized instruments (7 of 59) versus 'own measures' (6 of 15) of psychological factors, by using the entries in Table 1. A chi-square for the association of these variables was calculated ($\chi^2 = 5.6$, df = 1, $p = .02$) indicating a significant relationship between type of assessment used and finding a significant result. Thus, these studies usually did not find a relationship between psychological factors and cancer survival (61 of 74 tests), but when a relationship did emerge (13 of 74 tests) it was more likely to appear when researchers used their own measures than when they used standardized measures. Despite the lack of evidence from the standardized scales and the inconsistent evidence from the non-standard scales, more attention has been paid to the positive results than to the negative.

The eleven studies reviewed present information on 1149 patients. Most researchers conducted a large series of univariate significance tests (one for each independent variable). Such analyses increase the probability of finding a significant relationship that might not hold up in a multivariate analysis or on repeat studies. Totalling across these studies, 204 significance tests were conducted, with only 32 of these being significant. This number (15.7 per cent) is only slightly better than would appear by chance.

These studies also varied in their operational definition of outcomes examined. In some studies, survival was defined as a dichotomy such as death or recurrence at a specific point of assessment. In other studies, survival was defined as the time period between diagnosis and death but in some studies the time since the start of treatment or, even more problematic, since psychological assessment was used. If the investigators base their length of survival on time from assessment to death, the study presents a distorted assessment of true survival time because the lead time prior to assessment is ignored. If the elapsed time from diagnosis to assessment is longer for the short-term survivors (6, 10), and they also exhibit psychological factors predictive of short-term survival (from the time of assessment) this may indicate that the short-term survivors had experienced more treatment failures, heard more bad news, and felt more resigned to the often relentless progression of the disease at the time of assessment. Most studies fail to use statistical methods developed specifically to examine differences in survival assessed as a continuous time variable (such as Kaplan Mier plots and Cox regression).

Further difficulties in interpretation are raised because psychological factors may have been assessed at a time that would have been emotionally charged by either the diagnosis or the treatment. In some studies psychological assessments occurred at diagnosis, after surgery, or after and during chemotherapy and other therapies. Psychological test scores acquired at the point of diagnosis may allow an analysis of the relationship between initial response and later survival but may not reflect psychological reactions or coping styles after the initial shock has worn off. Psychological assessments conducted after surgery are problematic, because post-surgery outcome and psychological factors are confounded; patients' psychological test scores (for example hopelessness) acquired at this point are likely to be a reflection of post-surgical prognosis and disfigurement. We cannot know if higher post-treatment depression scores are related to poor survival because of depression or because of poor prognosis. There are reasons to believe that poor post-surgery

**Table 2**  Characteristics of individual studies

| Study | Subjects | Cancer type | Definition of survival | When assessed | No. of sig. tests/No. of sig. findings |
|---|---|---|---|---|---|
| Derogatis et al. (1979) (1) | 35 women | Metastatic breast | Discrete | Second out-patient visit | 13/7 |
| Rogentine et al. (1979) (2) | 64 women and men | Melanoma | Later recurrence | 1 week post-surgery | 15/1 |
| Greer et al. (1979, 1990) (3, 4) | 69 women | Stage I and II breast | Continuous | Prior to and after surgery | 13/2 |
| Spiegel et al. (1981, 1989) (35, 5) | 86 women | Metastatic breast | Continuous | Before and during study | 13/1 |
| Funch and Marshall (1983) (7) | 208 white women | Stage I and II breast | Continuous | At diagnosis | 6/1 |
| Temoshok et al. (1985) (8) | 59 men and women | Melanoma (49 stage I, 10 stage II) | Continuous measure of thickness | Close to time of diagnosis | 38/9 |

**Table 2** *(continued)*

| Study | Subjects | Cancer type | Definition of survival | When assessed | No. of sig. tests/No. of sig. findings |
|---|---|---|---|---|---|
| Cassileth *et al.* (1985) (9) | 204 women and men | Various types | Recurrence and continuous | 2–8 weeks post-diagnosis | 9/0 |
| Leigh *et al.* (1987) (10) | 101 women and men | Various types | Discrete | Unknown | 20/2 |
| Hislop *et al.* (1987) (11) | 135 women | Breast | Continuous | Within 3 months of diagnosis | 14/4 |
| Jamison *et al.* (1987) (12) | 49 women | Metastatic breast | Discrete | Unknown | 20/2 |
| Richardson *et al.* (1990)' (13) | 92 men and women | Haematological | Continuous | At diagnosis and 6 months | 20/1 |
| | 47 men and women | Rectal | Continuous | 6 weeks and 6 months post-surgery | 23/2 |

outcome rather than psychological factors *per se* accounted for poor survival in studies where psychological factors were assessed post-surgery. For example, Greer assessed psychological responses in 69 patients pre-and post-surgery and while there was no relationship between survival and psychological responses before surgery there was a significant relationship with post-surgery expressions of hopelessness (3). Poor surgery outcome, rather than the poor psychological attitude with which it is correlated, may account for these differences.

Most studies failed to control for age of subjects, stage of disease at entry into the study, health status at the start of the study, characteristics of tumour, and length and type of treatment patients had received; any and/or all of which would relate to both emotional reactions and prognosis. Failure to control for disease characteristics or treatment characteristics can be problematic. In most studies the investigators did not control for the length and type of treatment that patients received. In several studies, significant differences in the treatment received by survivors and non-survivors were found with these differences favouring the surviving group. In one case, short-term survivors had received significantly more chemotherapy (1). In another case, short-term survivors were older, experienced more pain, and had a longer elapsed time from diagnosis to assessment (10). Moreover, in another case after controlling for biological risk factors and delay in diagnosis, psychological variables had no effect on melanoma tumour progression (thickness or level) (8).

## 3   Behavioural and social issues that require further study

From the preponderance of null findings in Table 1, we cannot conclude that there is a reliable relationship between psychological factors and cancer survival. Although we believe that studying psychological states in survival can provide important information, we also have concerns that very important behavioural and social mechanisms have been overlooked in this pursuit. We address three issues: the extent to which patients in these studies complied with their cancer treatment; the mechanism by which psychological factors ostensibly play a role in survival; and the sociocultural context and implications of this line of research.

### 3.1   COMPLIANCE AND SURVIVAL

Poor compliance has been shown to be the cause of poor disease control among patients with hypertension (15–17), epilepsy (18), childhood asthma (19–21), post-chemotherapy fever (22), affective disorders (23), heart disease

(24), and other health problems (25). However, there are very few studies that have examined the level of compliance with long-term chemotherapy regimens for the treatment of cancer (26–29). We have previously shown, that adult patients with haematological cancers are on average, non-compliant with oral self-administered allopurinol more than 70 per cent of the time, and miss scheduled appointments more than 30 per cent of the time (28, 29). A study of pediatric leukaemia and lymphoma patients indicated that 33 per cent of the children and 59 per cent of the adolescents did not comply with oral prednisone (26). Another study of children with haematologic malignancy showed that there was an increase from 19 per cent non-compliance at two weeks from diagnosis to 39 per cent non-compliance at 20 weeks (27).

Given the considerable variance in, and the significant role of compliance in treatment outcome, it is reasonable to raise questions about the relationship between compliance and cancer survival. Surprisingly, very few studies have examined this relationship. We examined the role of compliance with oral medication and clinic appointments in the survival of 94 newly diagnosed patients with haematologic malignancies (30). Patients were assigned at entry either to a control condition or an intervention condition designed to improve compliance. Significant increases in compliance with allopurinol were found for patients in the intervention groups (45 per cent) as compared with the control group (21 per cent). Control patients attended clinic an average of 64 per cent of the time, whereas intervention group patients attended between 82 per cent and 93 per cent of the time.

Most importantly, survival was significantly higher for those in the intervention group, for those with higher allopurinol compliance, and for those with less severe disease. It is probable that allopurinol served as a surrogate marker for other daily self-administered medications which have a direct impact on the tumour (for example melphelan, hydroxyurea, chlorambucil, 6-mercaptopurine) as shown by the significant correlation between allopurinol and prednisone levels. The relationship between compliance with allopurinol and survival times provides evidence for the substantial impact of compliance with self-administered medication on survival.

## 3.2 COMPLIANCE, SELF-CARE, AND THE MECHANISM OF EFFECT

Although compliance clearly influences the therapeutic response to an effective pharmacological agent, a few studies have shown that the effect of compliance on treatment outcome is independent of whether the patient was taking drug or placebo (22, 31–34). In the afore-mentioned study, membership in the intervention group continued to have an independent and significant effect on survival, even when compliance is controlled, although the mechanism was unclear (30). These studies suggest that other factors related to medication compliance may act independently to produce a treatment response.

We speculate that at least three mechanisms are possible: behavioural, psychological/neurological/immunological pathways, and quality of care. The intervention programmes emphasized the importance of keeping appointments, monitoring side-effects, coming to the hospital for fever or bleeding, drinking liquids, maintaining daily activities, talking honestly with the doctor or nurse to facilitate problem solving, and including the patient's family in the care-giving team. It may be that compliance is a marker for improved self-care in several dimensions. It is also possible that the programmes trained the patients to be responsible for their own care, allowing them a greater sense of control resulting in less fear and anxiety. It is also possible that the health care providers developed a more supportive relationship with their intervention group patients and paid more attention to them, in effect provided them with better medical care.

Support for this interpretation is provided by the Speigel *et al.* study (5, 6, 35). Speigel randomly assigned patients to a group therapy or control group and the former showed better survival than the latter. The psychotherapy group focused on issues chosen by its members; foremost among these were discussions of how to interact with physicians and other medical staff to increase the quality of care received. The psychotherapy group (who had superior survival) had better initial health status, shorter average length of time from recurrence to study entry, and were of higher social class; thus their superior survival is open to question. Nevertheless, the sessions avoided the pitfalls of the vagaries of 'fighting cancer with your mind' and emphasized mutual patient support, manipulating the system, and other factors that may have led to their longer survival. In a similar way to our own study however, Speigel *et al.* did not collect data on potential moderators of survival (diet, exercise, demanding better care) to help clarify the mechanism by which patients may have helped themselves to survive. Thus, the behavioural, the psychological/neurological/immunological, and the quality of care hypotheses are all potential explanations for the effect.

When examining the role of psychological factors in cancer survival, patient compliance with treatment, self-care, and the quality of care received must be assessed and controlled. Furthermore, the psychological factors investigated must be demonstrated to be independent of compliance, self-care, and care received; if the factor is a cause, a correlate, or a consequence of any of these three variables, then these variables rather than psychological factors could account for survival differences. Obviously, many of the psychological factors investigated (for example depression, hopelessness) can decrease these three variables and result in poor survival, while others (for example hostility, optimism, extraversion, anxiety) could increase these variables and lead to better survival. Again, the question is one of the mechanisms of effect of psychological factors on survival. If that mechanism is compliance, self-care, and quality of care received, then psychological factors are ancillary to these patient and patient-physician interaction variables. This suggests that patient survival is accounted for, and may be improved by, assuring equality of care. Social class and ethnic differences in cancer survival underscore these points.

## 3.3 SOCIAL CLASS, ETHNICITY, AND SURVIVAL

Failure to control for the social class of subjects in a given study is a great source of concern because social class is a strong and reliable predictor of survival and there are reasons to suspect that the survivors and non-survivors (or, long-versus short-term survivors) in some studies differed by social class (5, 7). Funch and Marshall (7) found a significant relationship between patients' ratings of their subjective stress, in part consisting of their perception that their family income was inadequate, and poorer outcomes. These findings may have more to do with lower social class than with stress. The failure of these studies to acknowledge the importance of social class in cancer patient survival and to control for social class differences raises serious questions about whether psychological differences or underlying social class differences account for their findings.

Survival times for almost all types of cancer are shorter among African–American than white-American men and women (36), and shorter among those with lower socio-economic status (SES) as compared with those with higher status (37–39). Although some of this disparity is due to later stage at diagnosis of cancer (36, 40–42), with few exceptions (43), the poorer survival of African–Americans persists within stage of disease (36). Because racial differences in survival persist after controlling for prognostic variables such as stage at diagnosis, histology, and age, aspects of the treatment process need to be explored. Differences between ethnic groups may exist in access to care and quality of care, even after controlling for age and stage.

While reliable ethnic differences in cancer survival are well documented, rarely does anyone suggest that psychological factors account for these differences. Where ethnic differences in survival are concerned, attention has focused instead on differences in social class between African–Americans and whites, on the poor nutritional (44) and initial health status associated with lower social class, on ethnic differences in stage at diagnosis and oestrogen receptor status, and on differences in care received as explanations for differential survival. Several studies suggest that such variables account for much of the difference in survival including two studies, indicating that African–American women with breast cancer receive less adequate medical care than their white counterparts (45, 46). Thus, when ethnically diverse patients are included in studies of cancer survival, treatment, status, and biological variables are highlighted and analysed. Yet, when ethnically homogeneous samples are studied, these important objective variables are ignored in favor of non-objective and often ambiguous psychological factors whose mechanism of effect on survival is not readily discerned. The need to assess and control these variables in studies of ethnically homogenous samples is clear. When all of these variables are assessed simultaneously, the role of psychological factors in survival also will also be clear. That is, when differences in survival that are accounted for by social class, ethnicity, compliance, treatment, self-care, care received, initial health status, and tumour characteristics are controlled, whatever variance remains may be attributable directly to psychological factors; we suspect this will be minimal.

## 4 Potential pitfalls in the study of psychological factors in cancer patient survival

There are many implications of the tenet that psychological factors are involved in cancer survival; put crudely, that patients die sooner because of their attitudes and personalities. Serious social, medical, ethical, and political implications can accompany this conclusion. For example, a plethora of economic, biological, behavioural, social, and treatment variables have been suggested as causes for ethnic differences in cancer mortality. Is it reasonable to claim that minorities and the poor die, while whites and the wealthy survival because of their attitudes and personalities unless these other variables have been ruled out? If survival is primarily dependent on access to care as assessed by early detection of disease and enrollment in up-to-date treatment protocols, then access to care is the primary issue and to suggest otherwise is, in a sense, to 'blame the victim' of an expensive and often inaccessible health care system.

The design of interventions to improve survival must be based on an understanding of which mechanism(s) are important. For example, the objective of the interventions could be to elevate mood, improve compliance, improve self-care, improve immune function, or improve medical care. It is dangerous to indicate that it is how a person copes or thinks that is a problem, it is hard to change one's coping style in the best of circumstances, how much more unlikely is this when faced with cancer? In addition, if a person's 'style of coping' is a learned and relatively stable personality construct, especially by the age of most cancer diagnoses, how reasonable is it to expect changes in this style when a person is undergoing cancer treatment? Furthermore, what assurance is there that these changes would result in better immune function and in improved survival? But there are specific behaviours that patients can control such as delay, compliance, dietary intake, and others that will likely have a positive effect on survival.

## 5  Additional issues to consider in the further study of psychological factors in cancer patient survival

In the process of writing this chapter we have attempted to identify guidelines for the further exploration of the relationship between psychological status and cancer patient survival. First, it is possible that psychological factors are important only for certain types of cancers, or only when the disease is in the early stages. Subsequent studies could be designed to test groups that are homogeneous, not solely on disease site but on stage as well. Misguided attempts to treat cancer as a single disease and to expect homogeneity in the role of psychosocial factors in survival should be avoided. It is probable that any hypothesized relationship between psychological status and survival after cancer diagnosis would constitute a small component of a very complex causal chain dominated by the biological basis of the disease. The most important determinants of patient survival are cancer site, stage, and histology and these need to be controlled either in the design or the analysis. Treatment, access to care, compliance, and self-care also need to be carefully measured as important determinants of survival.

Second, a major limitation in any study of this issue is the sensitivity of available measures. Although studies err when they focus on the single significant finding even though many measures may not be significant, standardized scales tap only a small component of psychological states. Although the standardized scales chosen represent measures of the constructs involved and have been used before in research relevant to these questions, they may nevertheless be inadequate to tap the ways in which a person copes with the cancer diagnosis. Careful psychometric development and validation of scales to measure personality constructs such as 'fighting spirit' or 'hopeless and helpless' as a response to the diagnosis of cancer (or any serious disease) might help lead to a reproducible test of this construct. Measurement of psychological status in cancer patients is further complicated because it may vary to some extent from day to day and since it is often measured at clinic appointments for treatment it may be an unstable indicator. The disease and/or the treatment may alter psychological functioning; understanding of the prognosis also may influence psychological states. A more serious illness that is explained in those terms by a medical practitioner may in fact reduce the expression of optimism on the part of the patients. Furthermore, the exhibition of a coping style such as 'fighting spirit' may in fact indicate a coping style that leads to compliance, better self-care, maintenance of better diet and exercise patterns, and a demand for high quality medical care.

The role of psychological characteristics in complex immunological pathways should be investigated and understood in healthy subjects under stress. We should try to understand the relationship between emotions, coping style, health and illness in the healthy person rather than in the person with cancer where the immune system is already compromised by the disease, by the treatment, or by both. Immunologic function is a consequence and indicator of the disease and its progression, as well as an indicator of response to cytotoxic treatment.

## 6  Summary and conclusion

When we suggest that patients die because of their attitudes and personalities rather than because of the biological characteristics of their disease and their current and historical access to quality care, we ignore the factors that, by and large, produced these survival differences and maintain them. We also ignore the self-care behaviors so often linked to developing cancer and dying or surviving. Although we cannot conclude that psychological factors are unrelated to cancer survival, it is appropriate to suggest that the case for psychological factors in cancer survival has not yet been adequately tested; whether such factors are involved in survival or not is a question that remains open, awaiting well-designed studies in which the many variables highlighted here are controlled, and the alternative explanations of the findings that they entail are ruled-out. We conclude that the empirical case for psychological factors in cancer survival has not been made and that the increasingly popular belief in the role of these factors is premature. Nevertheless, these results should not be taken to mean that patients themselves have no role in determining the length of survival after the diagnosis of cancer. It may well be that such studies are pointing to coping styles that lead patients to better self-care behaviour. Our previous research has shown that compliance with medication taken by the patient and the number of appointments kept, are important predictors of survival (30) Spiegel's (5, 6) work also indicates that group support aimed especially at utilizing the health care system to maximum advantage and focusing on their own self-care behaviours may also influence survival. An analysis of differences in self-care and compliance, in the context of access to care will need to be explored empirically, and further attention needs to be given to the ways in which psychological status or coping style influence these behaviours.

# 7 References

1. Derogatis, L. R., Abeloff, M. D., and Melisaratos, N. (1979). Psychological coping mechanisms and survival time in metastatic breast cancer. *JAMA*, **242**, 1504–1508.
2. Rogentine, G. N., Van Kammen, D. P., Fox, B. H., Docherty, J. P., Rosenblatt, J. E., Boyd, S. C. *et al.* (1979). Psychological factors in the prognosis of a malignant melanoma: A prospective study. *Psychosom. Med.*, **41**, 647–655.
3. Greer, S., Morris, T., and Pettingale, K. W. (1979). Psychological response to breast cancer: Effect on outcome. *Lancet*, **ii**, 785–787.
4. Greer, S., Morris, T., Pettingale, K. W., and Haybittle, J. L. (1990). Psychological response to breast cancer and 15-year outcome. *Lancet*, **335**, 49–50.
5. Spiegel, D., Bloom, J. R., Kraemer, H. C., and Gottheil, E. (1989). Effect of psychosocial treatment on survival of patients with metastatic breast cancer. *Lancet*, **2**, 888–901.
6. Spiegel, D. (1991). A psychosocial intervention and survival time of patients with metastatic breast cancer. *Advances*, **7**, 10–19.
7. Funch, D. P. and Marshall, J. (1983). The role of stress, social support and age in survival from breast cancer. *J. Psychosom. Res.*, **27**, 77–83.
8. Temoshok, L., Heller, B. W., Sagebiel, R. W. Blois, M. S., Sweet, D. M., DiClemente, R. J. *et al.* (1985). The relationship of psychosocial factors to prognostic indicators in cutaneous malignant melanoma. *J. Psychosom. Res.*, **29**, 139–153.
9. Cassileth, B. R., Lusk, E. J., Miller, D. S., Brown, L. L., and Miller, C. (1985). Psychosocial correlates of survival in advanced malignant disease?. *N. Engl. J. Med.*, **312**, 1551–1155.
10. Leigh, H., Percarpio, B., Opsahl, C., and Ungerer, J. (1987). Psychological predictors of survival in cancer patients undergoing radiation therapy. *Psychother. Psychosom.*, **47**, 65–73.
11. Hislop, T. G., Waxler, N. E., Coldman, A. J., Elwood, J. M., and Kan, L. (1987). The prognostic significance of psychosocial factors in women with breast cancer. *J. Chronic Dis.*, **40**, 729–735.
12. Jamison, R. N., Burish, T. G., and Wallston, K. A. (1987). Psychogenic factors in predicting survival of breast cancer patients. *J. Clin. Oncol.*, **5**, 768–772.
13. Richardson, J. L., Zarnegar, Z., Bisno, B., and Levine, A. (1990). Psychosocial status at initiation of cancer treatment and survival. *J. Psychosom. Res.*, **34**, 189–201.
14. Berkowitz, L. (1992). Some thoughts about conservative evaluations of replications. *PSPB*, **18**, 319–324.
15. Sackett, D. L., Haynes, R. B., Gibson, E. S., and Johnson, A. (1976). The problem of compliance with antihypertensive therapy. *Pract. Cardiol.*, **2**, 35–39.
16. Caldwell, J. R., Cobb, S., Pawling, M. D., and deJongh, D. (1981). The dropout problem in antihypertensive therapy. *J. Chronic Dis.* **22**, 579–592.

17. Wagner, E. H., Truesdale, R. A., and Warner, J. R. (1981). Compliance treatment practices and blood pressure control: Community and survey findings. *J. Chronic Dis.*, **34**, 519–525.

18. Stanaway, L., Lambie, D. G., and Johnson, R. H. (1985). Noncompliance with anti-convulsant therapy as a cause of seizures. *N. Z. Med, J.*, **98**, 150–152.

19. Witek, T. J., Schacter, E. N., and Dean, N. L. (1983). A review of the hospital course of asthmatic children and adults. *Ann. Allergy*, **50**, 236–240.

20. Eney, R. D. and Goldstein, E. O. (1976). Compliance of chronic asthmatics with oral administration of theophylline as measured by serum and salivary levels. *Pediatrics*, **57**, 513–517.

21. Sublett, J. L., Pollard, S. J., Kadlec, G. J., and Karibo, J. M. (1979). Non-compliance in asthmatic children: A study of theophylline levels in a pediatric emergency room population. *Ann. Allergy*, **43**, 95–97.

22. Pizzo, P. A., Robichaud, K. J., Edwards, B. K., Schumaker, C., Kramer, B. S., and Johnson, A. (1983). Oral antibiotic prophylaxis in patients with cancer: A double-blind randomized placebo controlled trial. *J. Pediatr.*, **102**, 125–133.

23. Jamison, K. R. and Akiskal, H. S. (1983). Medication compliance in patients with bipolar disorder. *Psychiatr. Clin. North Am.*, **6**, 175–192.

24. Lipid Research Clinics Coronary Primary Prevention Trials Results. II. (1984). The relationship of reduction in incidence of coronary heart disease to cholesterol lowering. *JAMA*, **251**, 365–374.

25. Haynes, R. B., Taylor, D. W., and Sackett, D. L. (1979). *Compliance in Health Care*. Johns Hopkins University Press. Baltimore.

26. Smith, S. D., Rosen, D., Trueworthy, R. C., and Lowman, J. T. (1979). A reliable method for evaluating drug compliance in children with cancer. *Cancer*, **43**, 169–173.

27. Tebbie, C. Cummings, K. M., Smith, L., Richards, M., and Mallon, J. (1986). Compliance of pediatric and adolescent cancer patients. *Cancer*, **58**, 1179–1184.

28. Levine, A. M., Richardson, J. L., Marks, G., Chan, K., Graham, J., Selser, J. N. *et al.* (1987). Compliance with oral drug therapy in patients with hematologic malignancy. *J. Clin. Oncol.*, **5**, 1469–1476.

29. Richardson, J. L., Marks, G., Johnson, C. A., Graham, J. W., Chan, K. K., Selser, J. N. *et al.* (1987). Path model of multidimensional compliance with cancer therapy. *Health Psychol.* **6**, 183–207.

30. Richardson, J. L., Shelton, D. R., Krailo., M., and Levine, A. M. (1990). The effect of compliance with treatment on survival among patients with hematologic malignancies. *J. Clin. Oncol.*, **8**, 356–364.

31. Epstein, L. H. (1984). The direct effect of compliance on health outcome. *Health Psych.*, **3**, 385–393.

32. Hogarty, G. E., Goldberg, S. C., and the Collaborative Study Group. (1973). Drug and sociotherapy in the aftercare of the schizophrenic patient: One year relapse rates. *Arch. Gen. Psychiatry*, **28**, 54–64.

33. Fuller R., Roth, H., and Long, S. (1983). Compliance with disulfiram treatment of alcoholism. *J. Chronic Dis.*, **36**, 161–170.

34. Coronary Drug Project Research Group (1980). Influence of adherence to treatment and response of cholesterol on mortality in the Coronary Drug Project. *N. Engl. J. Med.*, **303**, 1038–1041.

35. Spiegel, D., Bloom, J. R., and Yalom, I. (1981). Group support for patients with metastatic cancer. *Arch. Gen. Psychiatry*, **38**, 527–533.
36. NCI, Cancer Statistics Review 1973–87. (1990). (Eds Gloeckler, L. A., Hankey, B. F., and Edwards, B. K.) *USDHHS, NCI NIH Pub* © *90-2789*. Bethesda, Maryland.
37. Berg, J., Ross, R., and Latourette H. (1977). Economic Status and Survival of Cancer Patients. *Cancer*, **39**, 467–477.
38. Farley, T. A. and Flannery, J. T. (1989). Late-stage diagnosis of breast cancer in women of lower socioeconomic status: public health implications. *AJPH*, **79**, 1508–1512.
39. Karjalainen, S. and Pukkala, E. (1990). Social Class as a Prognostic Factor in Breast Cancer Survival. *Cancer*, **66**, 819–826.
40. Dayal, H., Power, R., and Chiu, C. (1982). Race and Socioeconomic Status in Survival from Breast Cancer. *J. Chronic Dis.*, **35**, 675–683.
41. Mandelblatt, J., Andrews, H., Kerner, J., Zauber, A., and Burnett, W. (1991). Determinants of late stage diagnosis of breast and cervical cancer: the impact of age, race, social class, and hospital type. *AJPH*, **81**, 646–649.
42. Richardson, J. L., Langholz, B., Bernstein, L., Burciaga, C., Danley, K., and Ross R. K. (1992). Stage and delay in breast cancer diagnosis by race, socioeconomic status, age and year. *Br. J. Cancer*, **65**, 922–926.
43. Sutherland, C. M. and Mather, E. J. (1986). Long-term survival and prognostic factors in breast cancer patients with localized (no skin, muscle, or chest wall attachment) disease with and without positive lymph nodes. *Cancer*, **57**, 622–629.
44. Coates R. K., Clark, W. S., Eley, J. W., Greenberg, R. S., Huguley, C. M. Jr., and Brown, R. L. (1990). Race, nutritional status, and survival from breast cancer. *J. Natl. Cancer Inst.*, **82**, 1684–1692.
45. McWhorter, W. P. and Mayer, W. J. (1987). Black/White Differences in Type of Initial Breast Cancer Treatment and Implications for Survival. *AJPH*, **77**, 1515–1517.
46. Diehr, P., Vergan, J., Chu-J., Feigl, P., Glaefke, G., Moe, R. *et al.* (1989). Treatment modality and quality differences for black and white breast-cancer patients treated in community hospitals. *Med. Care*, **27**, 942–958.

# 9

# The role of psychological factors in cancer onset and progression: a critical appraisal

J. L. LEVENSON, C. BEMIS, AND B. A. PRESBERG

## 1 Introduction

Many professionals and laypeople believe that psychological factors play a major role in cancer onset and progression. The media have promoted popular ideas of overcoming cancer through 'mind over body', and there are self-help books and retreat centres where patients can learn imagery and relaxation techniques to fight their cancer. Guided imagery (visualizing white cells attacking cancer cells), cognitive restructuring (thinking positive thoughts), and assertiveness training have all been promoted alongside traditional health care for the cancer patient to 'combat' the disease.

Enthusiasm for these optimistic theories and practices should be tempered by acknowledgement of the fact that scientific evidence supporting a relationship between psychological factors and cancer lags far behind. In part, this may be due to the complexities involved in studying cancer, for a host of factors may contribute to onset and progression. This chapter reviews the scientific evidence pertaining to the major psychological factors that have been studied. The flawed research design and analysis of many existing reports will also be discussed.

From a historical perspective, the 1950s witnessed a surge in public interest in psychosomatic medicine and in research linking psychological, social, and environmental factors to disease onset and progression. A major finding was the association between smoking and lung cancer. In the following decade, personality traits, conflicts, and affects were examined as possible contributors to the onset and promotion of many diseases, including cancer. Exposure to certain environmental and occupational toxins were also linked to several types of cancer. The 1960s likewise witnessed the growth of experiments using animals in the hope of better understanding the effects of psychological and behavioural factors on cancer, while controlling confounding variables. Extrapolating conclusions from these studies which apply to human cancer remains problematic and will be discussed later. The 1970s saw rapid advances in immunology and neurochemistry, and psychiatry became more involved with the biological basis of mental disorders. Intriguing associations between certain affective states and the neuroendocrine system were demonstrated. Further research in psychoneuroimmunology in the 1980s explored the relationship between immunological and psychosocial variables, as well as the implications for cancer vulnerability and progression (1).

In this chapter, we will look at two hypotheses, along with the positive and negative studies associated with them: (1) cancer onset and progression are affected by psychosocial variables; and (2) psychological factors affect the immune system, which in turn can contribute to cancer onset and progression. Psychosocial variables examined here include affective states, coping/defensive styles and personality traits, behaviours, and stressful life events. The impact of psychosocial interventions on cancer outcome will also be discussed.

While extensive research in psycho-oncology has appeared over recent decades, much of it is methodologically flawed (for a review see ref (2)). Flaws have included use of small and biased samples, heterogeneous sample groups of mixed patients with very different cancer types and/or cancers at different stages, limited or no statistical analysis, poor controls, and retrospective sub-ject recall bias. Several studies that seemed to show significant effects were inconclusive because of non-equivalence in groups at baseline, either in disease severity or in the therapy received (many studies did not even monitor this possibility). Some studies failed to attend to important potential confounding factors such as smoking or diet. A number of studies measured too many psychological variables and then overly emphasized the few 'discovered' posi-tive associations in published results. Failure to standardize measures of initial psychological factors and measures of medical outcome has also been frequent.

Extensive reviews of this topic are available to the reader (1, 3, 4) and we have supplemented these with reports from Index Medicus and MEDLINE searches through to the end of 1992. Studies were not included in the present review if they were judged to be seriously flawed methodologically (according to the criteria noted above). Very few studies met the full set of criteria. Given the limitations of reviewing a very small number of studies, we also included other studies that, based on our qualitative judgment, had methodological strengths that outweighed their flaws.

# 2   Affective states

## 2.1   EPIDEMIOLOGICAL STUDIES OF DEPRESSION

The linking of affective states, particularly depression, with the onset of cancer has been an active area of study. One large epidemiologic study of 2020 male employees of Western Electric reported that depressive symptoms on the Min-nesota Multiphasic Personality Inventory (MMPI) were associated with twice the risk of death from cancer 17 years later and with a higher-than-normal incidence of cancer for the first 10 years (5). This finding persisted at 20-year follow-up (6). The Western Electric study has been cited for many years as supporting the association between depressive symptoms and increased cancer risk. On critically re-examining these data, however, Bieliauskas and Garron (7) found that the depression scores that were reported to be 'high' were not in the pathological range.

More recent epidemiological studies have demonstrated negative findings. In a prospective cohort study of 9832 women over a period of 10–14 years follow-up, Hahn and Petitti (8) failed to find an association between MMPI-Depression (MMPI-D) scores and breast cancer in women who were initially cancer-free. Severe depression reflected by MMPI-D scores of ≥70 also showed no correlation. Kaplan and Reynolds (9) studied 688 healthy subjects prospectively over 17 years for the development of cancer. Subjects completed an 18-item self-rating depression index. No association was found between the development of cancer and depression. Weissman *et al.* (10) followed 515 randomly selected subjects over 6 years and found that depressive symptoms (on the Self-Assessment Depression Scale) did not predict subsequent mortality. Datore *et al.* (11) found significantly *lower* MMPI-D scores in men who subsequently developed any type of cancer. A study by Zonderman *et al.* (12) with a 10-year follow-up from the National Health and Nutrition Examination Survey found no significant depressive symptoms (using the Cheerful vs. Depressed subscale from the General Well-Being Schedule and the Center for Epidemiologic Studies Depression Scale) that could be seen as predictors of cancer morbidity or mortality.

In general, most studies examining depressive states are flawed by their lack of specification. Most investigators have not differentiated between various depressive disorders and have not examined depressions from the perspective of past history, duration, chronicity, or treatment pursued. Whether or not differences in depressive states might influence cancer outcome (for example characterologic depressions vs. melancholic depressions) remains unknown. Many reports have regarded feelings of hopelessness and helplessness as equivalent to the presence of depression. Additionally, it is problematic to compare studies that use different instruments to measure the presence of depression. Instruments vary in whether they are designed to measure depressive states, traits, or clinical depression, which further confounds cross-comparison of studies. Another problem is that studies often do not control for other relevant psychosocial variables. For example, depression precipitated by loss of a significant other may be confounded by changes in coping/defensive styles or changes in habits such as excessive alcohol intake, poor diet, or increased social isolation. A more complete review of depression and cancer can be found in Bieliauskas and Garron (7).

Few studies have systematically examined the prevalence of psychiatric disorders among cancer patients, and, of these, many have been limited by biased samples and instruments that measure symptoms rather than diagnoses. In contrast, Derogatis *et al.* (13) assessed 215 cancer patients using explicit (DSM-III) diagnostic criteria. The results indicated that 47 per cent of the patients received a DSM-III diagnosis, including 44 per cent with an Axis I disorder and 12 per cent with a personality disorder. Approximately 68 per cent of the psychiatric diagnoses consisted of adjustment disorders, while 13 per cent represented major affective disorders, that is major depression and/or dysthymic disorder (6 per cent of the entire sample). This prevalence rate is close to the 6-month prevalence rate for major affective disorders in the general population found in the Epidemiologic Catchment Area study (14). Psychiatric symptoms in cancer patients are not static and can be expected to be affected by both disease course and treatment (15, 16), and even by their physicians' affect (17).

## 2.2 CLINICAL STUDIES OF DEPRESSION

Besides epidemiological studies, other research has focused on the impact of affective states on outcome in cancer patients. Studies examining the effect of depression on cancer outcome in clinical samples most often have focused on breast cancer. Much of the data have been retrospective and can be criticized not only for lack of controls, but also for the bias that exists when patients who know their diagnosis are queried about lifestyle and affective states. Another problem with most studies of depression and cancer has been that few studies have measured lifetime prevalence of depression. In a report by Greer *et al.* (18), breast cancer patients who demonstrated a 'fighting spirit' or who used denial had a higher survival rate than those with stoic acceptance or expressed hopelessness and helplessness. This study has been criticized, however, for not controlling for stage of disease. Although recent clinical studies also have not found a relationship between depression and cancer outcome (19, 20), one study in radiation therapy patients actually found high anxiety or depression predictive of *lower* mortality three years later (21).

Anecdotal reports have long noted that depression is sometimes the presenting symptom of pancreatic cancer, occurring well before symptoms of the tumour begin (22–25). Whether this represents a prodrome or a form of paraneoplastic syndrome remains controversial. Recent studies have confirmed that depression occurs with greater frequency and severity in pancreatic cancer than in other gastrointestinal cancers, although the underlying mechanism remains obscure (26).

## 2.3 BEREAVEMENT

Bereavement has been recognized as a significant stressor and often has been assumed to be a risk factor in cancer onset and progression. An early retrospective study showed that the onset of haematologic malignancy appeared to be preceded by significant losses in children and young adults (27). Recent studies have not shown bereavement to be a factor in the development or progression of cancer (18, 28, 29). Epidemiological studies are lacking in this area. Bereavement is associated with a significant increase in mortality in the first year in men younger than 75 years of age. However, an examination of the causes of death has shown that accidents, cardiovascular disease, some infectious diseases, and cirrhosis, but not cancer, contributed to the increase. In addition, bereaved women do not show an increase in mortality due to cancer. Thus, bereavement has not been shown to be a factor in cancer onset and progression.

New interest in bereavement has been triggered by studies showing depressed immune function during acute grief (30, 31). However, depressed levels of immune function were not pathologically low in these studies. Irwin *et al.* (32)

examined natural-killer-(NK) cell activity and T-cell subpopulations in three groups of women: those experiencing bereavement, those anticipating their husband's death from lung cancer, and a control group. NK-cell activity was significantly lower in both groups compared with controls, with the most depressed subjects demonstrating the most reduced NK-cell activity and changes in the ratio of T helper to T suppressor cells. These studies provide intriguing data, but it is premature to draw conclusions about whether depressed immune function can influence cancer onset and/or progression.

## 3 Coping/defensive style and personality traits

A large body of literature has described the cancer patient's degree of emotional expressiveness and its purported effect on prognosis. Descriptive case reports began appearing in the 1950s, noting shorter survival in patients with depressed, resigning characteristics compared with patients who were able to express more negative emotions, such as anger. However, many studies were flawed by a failure to control for staging and other confounding variables. In a 30-year follow-up study of 972 physicians, it was reported that 'loners' were much more likely to develop cancer than the group characterized by 'acting-out' and emotional expression, though potential confounding variables were not examined (33). Temoshok and Heller (34) conceptualized 'expressive vs. repressive' variables in terms of a type C behaviour pattern. The type C individual was described as a cooperative, unassertive patient who suppresses negative emotions, particularly anger, and who accepts/complies with external authorities. The type C behaviour pattern contrasts with the type A behaviour pattern studied as a factor in the development of coronary artery disease. In an investigation of the relationship between type C and melanoma tumour thickness and invasion; tumour thickness and measures of type C personality correlated, particularly in subjects under the age of 55 (35). Kneier and Temoshok also found that melanoma patients were more 'repressed' on self-report measures of repressiveness than were both cardiovascular patients and disease-free controls (36). The Melbourne Colorectal Cancer Study found that cancer cases are more likely to have certain personality traits (very similar to the type C pattern) than controls (37). As mentioned earlier, a study by Greer *et al.* showed that breast cancer patients who used denial or who possessed a 'fighting spirit' survived longer than those patients who demonstrated hopelessness and helplessness, although the stage of disease was not controlled (18). Support for similar ideas about lower cancer rates being correlated with high emotional expressivity has also been found in China as well (38).

Negative studies have also appeared, such as that by Cassileth *et al.* (19), showing that none of the multiple psychosocial factors thought to be predictive of health (including hopelessness/helplessness) predicted cancer survival (see also Holland (1) and Jamison *et al.* (20)). Cassileth's study has been criticized because it used melanoma patients with primarily advanced disease, at which point the role of psychological factors would be likely to be less influential. Other studies have demonstrated no difference in coping styles between breast cancer patients vs. controls (39), head and neck cancer patients vs. controls (40), and the absence of a relationship between coping style and breast cancer course (41). Epidemiological studies have not supported a relationship between emotional repression and cancer incidence or mortality (5, 6, 42).

# 4   Interpersonal variables

Relatively fewer studies have examined the effects of interpersonal variables on cancer. One prospective study of former medical students reported that lack of closeness with their parents and less satisfactory relationships were associated with later development of cancer (43). A prospective study of breast cancer patients found a number of positive relationship variables predictive of increased survival (44). Social relations and support and their effects on cancer patients (as with other diseases) are complex phenomena, and may vary with cancer site and extent of disease (45).

# 5   Stressful life events

Interest in this area has been particularly stimulated by animal studies that have shown that stress in animals can hasten the onset of viral-induced cancer (mainly using susceptible mouse strains). Other studies have shown that stress can enhance the carcinogenic potential of several known mutagens in animal subjects. Animal studies demonstrating negative findings also exist and have shown that under certain conditions stress can reduce susceptibility or delay the 'take' of implanted tumours. Fox has extensively critiqued both the positive and negative findings in animal studies (4) (see also Chapter 1 of this volume).

   A number of human studies have shown an increased incidence of stressful life events preceding the onset of cervical, pancreatic, gastric and lung cancer (46–50), and more recently in colorectal (51) and breast (52, 53) cancer. Some research links life stresses with cancer recurrence or progression, but the samples are small and the results not unequivocal (53–55). Many other studies have failed to find any association between preceding stressful life events and cancer onset (56–60). Keehn *et al.* (61) found no excess in cancer during a 24-year follow-up of World War II veterans who were discharged with a diagnosis of (war-related) psychoneurosis. In addition, no increase in cancer rate was demonstrated in POWs from three wars (62). In 1983, on the basis of the sum of human and animal studies, Fox (4) concluded that if stressful events and/or other psychological factors do have an effect on cancer incidence, it is small. We believe that this conclusion is just as valid today.

# 6 Psychosocial intervention and cancer outcome

Recent studies have shown improvement in the quality of life in cancer patients receiving group therapy, including improved mood and vigour, decreased pain, and better adjustment (63–67). However, not until recently has systematic research supported a finding of increased survival time in cancer patients receiving psychotherapy. We discuss here some illustrative examples and refer the reader elsewhere for a more detailed consideration (63, 64) (see also Chapter 4).

Grossarth-Maticek *et al.* (65) studied women with metastatic breast cancer, including one group receiving chemotherapy and a group who had declined it. Within each of these two groups, women were randomly assigned to receive or not to receive psychotherapy. Survival time was extended in patients who received psychotherapy alone or chemotherapy alone compared with patients who received no treatment; survival was longest in those who received both psychotherapy and chemotherapy, with apparent synergistic effects.

Spiegel and colleagues (67–69) randomly assigned metastatic breast cancer patients to a 1-year regimen of psychosocial treatment consisting of weekly supportive group therapy with training in self-hypnosis for pain control. The control group had routine oncological care. At 1 year, the psychotherapy treatment group had less mood disturbance, fewer phobic responses (68), and they complained of half as much pain (69). At 10-year follow-up, the mean survival time had been 34.8 months for the group randomized to psychotherapy as opposed to 18.9 months for the control group. The authors had expected to, and did, find a beneficial effect of treatment on mood and vigour but had not expected that psychosocial treatment would affect survival. Greater longevity in their sample was associated with less mood disturbance and higher ratings on vigour (67). Spiegel *et al.* speculated on how the benefits of group psychotherapy for cancer patients can be explained. They hypothesized that patients received social support through the group, which provided an atmosphere in which they could express their feelings and feel accepted. The group may also have allowed patients to problem-solve more effectively and thereby to achieve better compliance with their medical programmes. Better pain control and control of anxiety and depression may also have contributed to better self-care habits such as diet and exercise. The finding of increased longevity in therapy group members requires prospective replication since Spiegel's re-analysis was conducted years after the original experiment, and with the expectation that the null hypothesis would be true.

Fawzy *et al.* (66) evaluated the immediate and prolonged effects of a 6-week structured psychiatric group intervention for postsurgical patients with malignant melanoma. Patients who received the intervention had higher vigour than controls at 6 weeks and less depression, fatigue, and total mood disturbance at a 6-month follow-up. Experimental subjects demonstrated more active coping than controls, both at the conclusion of the intervention and at follow-up.

# 7  Mechanisms explaining the effects of psychological factors on cancer

## 7.1 PSYCHOLOGICAL FACTORS, THE IMMUNE SYSTEM, AND CANCER

Behavioural immunology is the study of the interaction between psychosocial variables and the immune system. Do psychosocial variables act via the immune system to influence cancer onset and progression? Two separate lines of research shed light on such a postulated relationship, corresponding to two linked hypotheses: (1) psychosocial variables influence the immune system; and (2) the immune system influences cancer onset and progression.

Bereavement as a psychological response to the loss of a relationship has been shown in many studies to alter aspects of immune function (see Holland for an extensive review of this literature (1)). Kiecolt-Glaser *et al.* (70, 71) have demonstrated that NK-cell activity varies with stress and lack of social support. More recently Levy *et al.* (72) have found an association between perceived level of social support and NK-cell activity in 120 Stage I and II breast cancer patients.

The complex relationships between various components of the immune system, as well as the immune components that may serve as markers of clinical significance in cancer development and outcome are largely unknown. NK cells are a subclass of lymphocytes which are thought to serve in malignant cell surveillance by recognizing and destroying mutant cells that may have precancerous programmes.

Studies that have demonstrated altered immune function associated with psychosocial factors have *not* been able to demonstrate a further connection to cancer onset and progression. Confounding variables, such as genetic make-up, that may influence immune efficiency and susceptibility to stresses (both psychological and physiological) have not been taken into account in human studies demonstrating psychosocial influences on immune function.

The hypothesis that immune function is involved in cancer surveillance has been demonstrated in animal studies showing that immunosuppressed rodents develop tumours not specific to a given site. Humans who are immunosuppressed can also develop tumours at multiple sites. However, it is still too early to discuss an integrative model for cancer onset and progression that acts via the immune system under the influence of psycho-social variables.

Recent research has illuminated psychosocial/immune interactions and outcome in individuals who already have cancer. Levy *et al.* (73, 74) examined NK-cell activity and three distress indicators in women with breast cancer at the time of mastectomy and 3 months after. They found that adjustment level, lack of social support, fatigue, and depressive symptoms accounted for 30 per cent of the NK-cell variance seen at 3 months. In this group, more metastatic nodes were also associated with depressive features and decreased NK-cell activity. This group's research continues to reveal complex rather than simple causal relationships between psychological factors, social support, NK-cell activity, and development of metastatic disease (75). The sustained beneficial psychological outcomes with psychiatric group intervention in postsurgical patients with malignant melanoma recently reported by Fawzy *et al.* (66) have been described above. They also found that experimental subjects had significant increases in particular NK-cell types and increased NK-cytotoxic activity at 6-month follow-up (76) (see chapter 11 for further details).

Consider another illustration of the complexity in trying to establish clear, causal links between psychological factors and cancer, mediated via immune system effects. This chapter has cited a variety of studies examining effects of depression on cancer incidence or outcome, and some effects of depression on immune function. Most studies have not noted whether depressed subjects were taking antidepressants, which have been shown in rodents to depress NK-cell function (77) and to stimulate malignant growth (78).

## 7.2 ANIMAL MODELS

Many experiments examining psychological factors affecting cancer have used animal models, particularly in studying the relationship between stress and cancer onset and progression. Extrapolation of these results to humans can be dangerously misleading. Key differences between cancer in experimental animals and cancer in humans should be noted: rodent strains that are highly inbred may be more susceptible to developing cancers; and many spontaneous cancers in animals are viral, contrasting with only 2–3 per cent of known cancers that are viral in humans. Potentially confounding variables include: (i) external factors such as the quality, quantity, and time course of the stressor; (ii) coexisting factors such as the diet, parity, and housing of animals; and (iii) factors of the internal milieu such as pre-existing viral invasion, genetic susceptibility, and immunocompetence of the organism. Heavy doses of carcinogens are typically used in animal experiments, yielding tumours with strong antigens that may facilitate detection by the immune system. By contrast, in most forms of human cancer, carcinogens are low-dose and long-acting, presumably yielding weaker antigens which might escape immune surveillance.

The human paradigm for cancer cell surveillance is less well known but, in addition to the immune system, DNA repair may contribute additional protection. Animal studies will continue to help us understand many of the complex variables involved with cancer onset and progression only if we are careful not to draw premature conclusions from them about human cancers. As noted earlier, depending on the animal model and experimental paradigm chosen, stress has been shown to increase and decrease cancer development and progression.

## 7.3 NON-IMMUNOLOGICAL MECHANISMS

Non-immunological explanations could also account for the effects of some psychological factors on cancer development and outcome. The effect of some psychological factors on mortality (for example cynicism) may be mediated by smoking and alcohol (79), although these relationships may be interactive rather than simple (80) (see chapter 5). Psychological factors have been shown to affect whether and when patients seek medical attention for their initial cancer symptoms in some (81), but not all studies (82). High anxiety has been directly related to poor attendance at a breast examination clinic and poor adherence to breast self-examination in high risk patients (83). Psychological factors contribute to patients' choices of treatment options (84), which in turn impact on psychological status (15, 85).

# 8 Clinical implications

Depression and anxiety remain common but relatively underdiagnosed and undertreated in cancer patients. We believe that the question of whether mood or anxiety disorders affect the incidence, course, or clinical outcomes of cancer has yet to be definitively answered by systematic research. Nevertheless, depression and anxiety warrant clinical attention because of their clear adverse effects on the quality of life of cancer patients. Behaviour with obviously harmful effects for cancer patients (smoking, alcohol abuse, non-compliance with treatment) should also be targeted for intervention.

Psychotherapeutic interventions may be of great benefit to cancer patients. If it is suggested, however, in an overly optimistic manner that psychological therapies will actually deliver cure or remission, there is a risk of deeply disappointing patients and their families and distracting from the direct benefits of psychiatric treatment to enhance the quality of life. *Psychiatrists and psychologists should keep in mind that psychosocial interventions are more likely to contribute to quality than to quantity of life in cancer patients.* Psychiatric interventions are primarily justified if they reduce distress and dysfunction, such as when depressive or anxiety disorders are diagnosed in the context of oncological illness. Studies showing that psychotherapeutic interventions can reduce anxiety and depression in cancer patients have been cited above (63–67). A smaller number of studies have demonstrated the benefits of anti-anxiety and antipdepressant medications in oncology (86, 87).

## 9  Alternative therapies and the popular literature

This book summarizes many intriguing findings on the relationship between mind and body in cancer. To most investigators, these relationships appear complex and resistant to facile explanation. This chapter supports a cautious, rational, and sceptical approach toward the clinical applications of this work. In contrast, a large and growing popular literature of 'mind/body medicine' (88) has taken inspiration from the scientific literature and made the leap to specific interventions.

The popular treatments in existence propose to act on some or all of the psychosocial factors addressed in this chapter: affective state, coping style and personality, life stress and anxiety, and immune mechanisms. We here cite some examples, and outline potential risks (full discussion of the popular literature is beyond the scope of this chapter).

A number of authors promote approaches to improve mood states. Advocates of positive thinking (89, 90), humour and laughter (91), and cognitive reframing (92) see these as enabling cancer patients to combat depressive states that may accompany cancer, and thereby not only improve quality of life but also directly combat the cancer itself. Other approaches aim to change personality and coping style. Borysenko teaches patients to change the way they view their cancer, to see cancer as a personal challenge rather than a threat (92). The Simontons encourage their patients to 'be a different kind of person' (93). They see cancer as giving the individual 'permission' to change their behaviour and personality; options are opened up and the individual is able to take more control over life. The common thread in these approaches is the attempt to help the individual get as much control as possible over their inner reactions and outer lives.

Various behavioural approaches are also advocated to deal with life stresses and anxiety. Borysenko and others prescribe yoga, meditation, and relaxation techniques. Chopra is an advocate of Transcendental Meditation used within a program of Ayurvedic medicine (94).

While all of these interventions, in addition to their primary benefits, have been claimed by some proponents to boost immune system performance, other alternative therapies are directly intended to improve immune function. Specific visualization techniques are taught that involve mental imagery of the immune system at work (93, 95). Proper visualization is claimed to improve the ability of the immune system to fight cancer.

While these approaches may be helpful for some, their efficacy in combating cancer has yet to be objectively demonstrated. Furthermore, a prescription to change one's life or one's attitude is not without potential risks or harms. Foremost among these is guilt. Popular literature may lead some patients to feel responsible for their disease (or relapse) because they were unable to develop the 'right attitude' or personality characteristics to 'beat' cancer. People may feel an inordinate amount of responsibility to heal themselves, and may feel that they have not loved enough or visualized correctly if their efforts fail. A number of proponents of 'mind/body medicine' do address the issue of whether their approach induces guilt (90, 91), but it is generally minimized as a concern. Furthermore, it is ironic that such 'low tech' alternative therapies often prove to be quite expensive.

Another potential harm of alternative therapies is their pursuit in place of conventional medical treatment. This is less relevant in cases where conventional treatment also has little proven benefit (and unpleasant side-effects), but becomes a concern when patients forego effective chemotherapy, surgery, or radiation therapy. Similarly, alternative therapies may be counterproductive if they are used instead of potentially helpful conventional psychiatric treatment for treatable conditions such as major depression or anxiety disorders.

More subtle concerns arise when proponents of interventions that are appealing and benevolent make them universal prescriptions. A focus on personality change may provide a constructive form of re-direction for one patient, whilst generating frustration and alienation for another. The scientific literature attempts to delineate various psychological factors and confounding variables affecting cancer, while the popular literature draws sweeping conclusions that generally ignore the differences. Clinicians should be open to discussing patient's reactions to the popular literature and to giving guidance and support on what may or may not be helpful to the individual patient.

## 10 Summary

In summary, a number of studies have lent some support to the relationship between a variety of psychological factors and the onset, exacerbation, and/or outcome of neoplastic disease. At the present time, no clear associations (let alone causal relationships) have been proven, both because of methodological limitations in the positive studies and because of other studies of comparable methodology that have failed to find such relationships.

Compared with other known risk factors, psychosocial factors may by themselves (other than via cigarette smoking or alcoholism) make a small contribution to cancer onset. However, more recent methodologically sounder studies have suggested that cancer progression, rather than onset, is influenced by psychosocial factors. Better, systematically designed research is needed to further elucidate the impact of psychological factors on cancer. Future studies will need to control for staging, the type of cancer and treatment, and confounding variables such as smoking and other risk-associated behaviors. They also will need to include well-matched controls.

The gap that currently exists between our scientific knowledge base and popular beliefs about cancer onset and progression can be problematic for individuals with cancer and their health care providers. How can cancer patients distinguish between the popular ideas based on fact and those founded on myth? Are cancer patients responsible for their disease because they didn't have the 'right attitude' or personality characteristics that would have enhanced their disease resistance? Does seeking a cure for cancer in 'love and miracles' complement or undermine standard cancer care? There are some beliefs that exist about cancer onset and progression that may not be empirically supported but that nevertheless can contribute to a patient's sense of well-being and control, while others may have an adverse impact.

While psychosocial interventions are more likely to contribute to the quality, rather than the quantity of life of cancer patients, their proper scope of application remains to be worked out. Scarce resource allocation needs to be directed at psychosocial interventions that have empirical support. With the application of improved, systematic studies, it is hoped that we will obtain a clearer understanding of where resources should be directed in the future.

# 11 References

1. Holland, J. C. (1989). Behavioural and psychosocial risk factors in cancer: human studies. In *Handbook of Psychooncology*, (ed. J. C. Holland and J. H. Rowland), pp. 705–726. Oxford University Press, New York.
2. Jensen, A. B. (1991). Psychosocial factors in breast cancer and their possible impact upon prognosis. *Cancer Treat. Rev.*, **18**, 191–210.
3. Spiegel, D. and Sands, S. H. (1994). Psychological influences on metastatic disease progression. In *Progressive States of Malignant Neoplastic Growth*, (ed. H. E. Kaiser), Martinus Nijhoff, Dordrecht, The Netherlands. In press.
4. Fox, B. H. (1983). Current theory of psychogenic effects on cancer incidence and prognosis. *J. Psychosoc. Oncol.*, 1, 17–31.
5. Shekelle, R. B., Raynor, W. J. Jr., Ostfeld, A. M., Garron D. C., Bieliauskas, L. A., Liu S. C., Maliza, C., and Paul, O. (1981). Psychological depression and 17-year risk of death from cancer. *Psychosom. Med.*, **43**, 117–125.
6. Persky, V. W., Kempthorne-Rawson, J., and Shekelle, R. B. (1987). Personality and risk of cancer: 20-year follow-up of the Western Electric Study. *Psychosom. Med.*, **49**, 435–449.
7. Bieliauskas, L. A. and Garron, D. C. (1982). Psychological depression and cancer. *Gen. Hosp. Psych.*, **4**, 187–195.
8. Hahn, R. C. and Petitti, D. B. (1988). Minnesota Multiphasic Personality Inventory-rated depression and the incidence of breast cancer. *Cancer*, **61**, 845–848.

9. Kaplan, G. A. and Reynolds, P. (1988). Depression and cancer mortality and morbidity: prospective evidence from the Alameda County study. *J. Behavioral Med.*, **11**, 1–13.

10. Weissman, M. M., Myers, J. K., Thompson, W. D., and Belanger, A. (1986). Depressive symptoms as a risk factor for mortality and for major depression. In *Life-Span Research on the Prediction of Psychopathology*, (ed. L.Erlenmeyer-Kimling and N. E. Miller), pp. 251–260. Lawrence Erlbaum, Hillsdale, N. J.

11. Dattore, P. G., Shontz, F. C., and Coyne, L. (1980). Premorbid personality differentiation of cancer and noncancer groups: a test of the hypothesis of cancer proneness. *J. Consult. Clin. Psychol.*, **48**, 388–394.

12. Zonderman, A. B., Costa, P. T. Jr., and McCrae, R. R. (1989). Depression as a risk for cancer morbidity and mortality in a nationally representative sample. *JAMA*, **262**, 1191–1195.

13. Derogatis, L. R., Morrow, G. R., Fetting, J., Penman, D., Piasetsky, S., Schmale, A. M., Henrichs, M., and Carnicke, C. L. J. (1983). The prevalence of psychiatric disorders among cancer patients. *JAMA*, **249**, 751–757.

14. Myers, J. K., Weissman, M. M., Tischler, G. L. Holzer, C. E. 3d., Leaf, P. J., Orvaschel, H., Anthony, J. C., Boyd, J. H., Burke, J. D. Jr., and Kramer, M. (1984). Six-month prevalence of psychiatric disorders in three communities (1980–1983). *Arch. Gen. Psych.*, **41**, 959–967.

15. Lasry, J. C. and Margolese, R. G. (1992). Fear of recurrence, breast-conserving surgery, and the trade-off hypothesis. *Cancer*, **69**, 2111–2115.

16. Goldberg, J. A., Scott, R. N., Davidson, P. M., Murray, G. D., Stallard, S., George, W. D., and Maguire, G. P. (1992). Psychological morbidity in the first year after breast surgery. *Eur. J. Surg. Oncol.*, **18**, 327–331.

17. Shapiro, D. E., Boggs, S. R., Melamed, B. G., Graham-Pole, J. (1992). The effect of varied physician affect on recall, anxiety, and perceptions in women at risk for breast cancer: an analogue study. *Health Psychol.*, **11**, 61–66.

18. Greer, S., Morris, T., and Pettingale, K. W. (1979). Psychological response to breast cancer: effect on outcome. *Lancet*, **2**, 785–787.

19. Cassileth, B. R., Lusk, E. J., Miller, D. S., Brown, L. L. and Miller, C. (1985). Psychological correlates of survival in advanced malignant disease? *N. Engl. J. Med.*, **312**, 1551–1555.

20. Jamison, R. N., Burish, T. G., and Wallston, K. A. (1987). Psychogenic factors in predicting survival of breast cancer patients. *J. Clin. Oncol.*, **5**, 768–772.

21. Leigh, H., Percarpio, B., Opsahl, C., and Ungerer, J. (1987). Psychological predictors of survival in cancer patients undergoing radiation therapy. *Psychother. Psychosom.*, **47**, 65–73.

22. Pomara, N. and Gershon, S. (1984). Treatment resistant depression in an elderly patient with pancreatic carcinoma: case report. *J. Clin. Psych.*, **45**, 439–440.

23. Yaskin, J. C. (1931). Nervous symptoms as earliest manifestations of carcinoma of the pancreas. *JAMA*, **96**, 1664–1668.

24. Savage, C. and Noble, D. (1954). Cancer of the pancreas: two cases simulating psychogenic illness. *J. Nerv. Ment. Dis.*, **120**, 62–65.

25. Fras, I., Litin, E. M., and Bartholomew, L. G. (1968). Mental symptoms as an aid in the early diagnosis of carcinoma of the pancreas. *Gastroenterology*, **55**, 191–198.

26. Shakin, E. J. and Holland, J. (1988). Depression and pancreatic cancer. *J. Pain and Symptom Management*, **3**, 194–198.
27. Greene, W. A., Young, L. E., and Swisher, S. N. (1956). Psychological factors and reticuloendothelial disease. *Psychosom. Med.*, **18**, 284–303.
28. Klerman, G. L. and Clayton, P. (1984). Epidemiologic perspectives on the health consequences of bereavement. In *Bereavement: Reactions, Consequences, and Care* (report of the Committee on Health Consequences of the Stress of Bereavement), (ed. M. Osterweis, F. Soloman, and M. Green). Institute of Medicine, National Academy of Sciences, National Academy Press, Washington, DC.
29. Helsing, K. J. and Szklo, M. (1981). Mortality after bereavement. *Am. J. Epidemiol.*, **114**, 41–52.
30. Bartrop, R. W., Lazarus, L., Luckhurst, E., Kiloh, L. G., and Penny, R. (1977). Depressed lymphocyte function after bereavement. *Lancet*, **1**, 834–836.
31. Schleifer, S. J., Keller, S. E., Camerino, M., Thornton, J. C., and Stein, M. (1983). Suppression of lymphocyte stimulation following bereavement. *JAMA*, **250**, 374–377.
32. Irwin, M., Daniels, M., and Weiner, H. (1987). Immune and neuroendocrine changes during bereavement. *Psych. Clin. North Am.*, **10**, 449–465.
33. Shaffer, J. W., Graves, P. L., Swank, R. T., Pearson, T. A. (1987). Clustering of personality traits in youth and the subsequent development of cancer among physicians. *J. Behav. Med.*, **10**, 441–447.
34. Temoshok, L. and Heller, B. (1981). Stress and 'type C' versus epidemiological risk factors in melanoma. Proceedings of the 89th Annual Convention of the American Psychological Association, Los Angeles.
35. Temoshok, L., Heller, B. W., Sageviel, R. W., Blois, M. S., Sweet, D. M., DiClemente, R. J., and Gold, M. L. (1985). The relationship of psychological factors of prognostic indicators in cutaneous malignant melanoma. *J. Psychosom. Res.*, **29**, 139–153.
36. Kneier, A. W. and Temoshok, L. (1984). Repressive coping reactions in patients with malignant melanoma as compared to cardiovascular patients. *J. Psychosom. Res.*, **28**, 145–155.
37. Kune, G. A., Kune, S., Watson, L. F., and Bahnson, C. B. (1991). Personality as a risk factor in large bowel cancer: data from the Melbourne Colorectal Cancer Study. *Psychol. Med.*, **21**, 29–41.
38. Guo, G. N. (1992). A correlation study of psychologic stress factors and cancer by stepwise and logistic regression analyses. *Chung Hua Chung Liu Tsa Chih*, **13**, 416–418.
39. Buddeberg, C., Wolf, C., Sieber, M., Riehl-Emde, A., Bergant, A., Steiner, R., Landolt-Ritter, C., and Richter, D. (1991). Coping strategies and course of disease of breast cancer patients. Results of a 3-year longitudinal study. *Psychother. Psychosom.*, **55**, 151–157.
40. Yamagiwa, M., Harada, T., Kubo, M., Miyahara, Y., Amesara, R., and Sakakura, Y. (1991). Psychological states and personality as factors in the morbidity of head and neck malignant tumors. *Nippon Jibiinkoka Bakkai Kaiho*, **94**, 67–73.
41. Edwards, J. R., Cooper, C. L., Pearl, S. G., de Paredes, E. S., O'Leary, T., and

Wilhelm, M. C. (1990). The relationship between psychosocial factors and breast cancer:some unexpected results. *Behav. Med.*, **16**, 5–14.

42. Ragland, D. R., Brand, R. J., and Fox, M .B. H. (1987). Type A behavior and cancer mortality in the Western Collaborative Group Study (abstract). *Psychosom. Med.*, **49**, 209.

43. Graves, P. L., Thomas, C. B., and Mead, L. A. (1991). Familial and psychological predictors of cancer. *Cancer Detect. Prev.*, **15**, 59–64.

44. Waxler-Morrison, N., Hislop, T. G., Mears, B., Kan, L., (1991). Effects of social relationships on survival for women with breast cancer:a prospective study. *Soc. Sci. Med.*, **33**, 177–183.

45. Ell, K., Mishimoto, R., Mediansky, L., Mantell, J., and Hamovitch, M. (1992). Social relations, social support and survival among patients with cancer. *J. Psychosom. Res.*, **36**, 531–541.

46. Ernster, V. L., Sacks, S. T., Selvin, S., and Petrakis, N. L. (1979). Cancer incidence by marital status: US Third National Cancer *Survey. J. Natl. Cancer Inst.*, **63**, 567–585.

47. Fras, I., Litin, E. M., and Pearson, J. S. (1967). Comparison of psychiatric symptoms in carcinoma of the pancreas with those in some other intra-abdominal neoplasms. *Am. J. Psych.*, **123**, 1553–1556.

48. Horne, R. L. and Picard, R. S. (1979). Psychosocial risk factors for lung cancer. *Psychosom. Med.*, **43**, 431–438.

49. Leherer, S. (1980). Life change and gastric cancer. *Psychosom. Med.*, **42**, 499–502.

50. Schmale, A. H. and Iker, H. P. (1965). The psychological setting of uterine cervical cancer. *Ann. N.Y. Acad. Sci.*, **125**, 807–813.

51. Kune, S., Kune, G. A., Watson, L. F., and Rahe, R. H. (1991). Recent life change and large bowel cancer. Data from the Melbourne Colorectal Cancer Study. *J. Clin. Epidemiol.*, **44**, 57–68.

52. Geyer, S. (1991). Life events prior to manifestation of breast cancer: a limited prospective study covering eight years before diagnosis. *J. Psychosom. Res.*, **35**, 355–363.

53. Forsen, A. (1991). Psychosocial stress as a risk for breast cancer. *Psychother. Psychosom.*, **55**, 176–185.

54. Funch, D. P. and Marshall, J. (1983). The role of stress, social support and age in survival from breast cancer. *J. Psychosom. Res.*, **27**, 77–83.

55. Ramirez, A. J., Craig, T. K., Watson, J. P., Fentiman, I. S., North, W. R., and Rubens, R. D. (1989). Stress and relapse of breast cancer. *Br. Med. J.*, **298**, 291–293.

56. Finn, F., Mulcahy, R., and Hickey, W. (1974). The psychological profiles of coronary and cancer patients, and of matched controls. *Ir. J. Med. Sci.*, **143**, 176–178.

57. Graham, S., Snell, L. M., Graham, J. B., and Ford, L. (1971). Social trauma in the epidemiology of cancer of the cervix. *J. Chronic Dis.*, **24**, 711–725.

58. Snell, L. and Graham, S. (1971). Social trauma as related to cancer of the breast. *Br. J. Cancer*, **25**, 721–734.

59. Greer, S. and Morris, T. (1975). Psychological attributes of women who develop breast cancer: a controlled study. *J. Psychosom. Res.*, **19**, 147–153.

60. Grissom, J., Weiner, B., and Weiner, E. (1975). Psychological correlates of cancer. *J. Consult. Clin. Psychology*, **43**, 113.
61. Keehn, R. J., Goldberg, L. D., and Beebe, G. W. (1974). Twenty-four year mortality follow-up of army veterans with disability separations for psychoneurosis in 1944. *Psychosom. Med.*, **36**, 27–46.
62. Keehn, R. J. (1980). Follow-up studies of World War II and Korean conflict prisoners. *Am. J. Epidemiol.*, **111**, 194–211.
63. Trijsburg, R. W., van Knippenberg, F. C., and Rijpma, S. E. (1992). Effects of psychological treatment on cancer patients: a critical review. *Psychosom. Med.*, **54**, 489–517.
64. Andersen, B. L. (1992). Psychological interventions for cancer patients to enhance the quality of life. *J. Consult. Clin. Psychol.*, **60**, 552–568.
65. Grossarth-Maticek, R., Schmidt, P., Vetter, H., and Arndt, S. (1984). Psychotherapy research in oncology. In *Health Care and Human Behavior*, (ed. A. Steptoe and A. Mathews), pp. 325–341. Academic Press, London.
66. Fawzy, F. I., Cousins, N., Fawzy, N. W., Kemeny, M. E., Elashoff, R., and Mortor, D. (1990). A structured psychiatric intervention for cancer patients. I: Changes over time in methods of coping and affective disturbance. *Arch. Gen. Psych.*, **47**, 720–725.
67. Spiegel, D., Bloom, J. R., Kraemer, H. C., and Gottheil, E. (1989). Effects of psychosocial treatment on survival of patients with metastatic breast cancer. *Lancet*, **2**, 888–891.
68. Spiegel, D., Bloom, J. R., and Yalom, I. D. (1981). Group support for patients with metastatic cancer: a randomized prospective outcome study. *Arch. Gen. Psych.*, **38**, 527–533.
69. Spiegel, D. and Bloom, J. R. (1983). Group therapy and hypnosis reduce metastatic breast carcinoma pain. *Psychosom. Med.*, **45**, 333–339.
70. Kiecolt-Glaser, J. K., Garner, W., Speicher, C., Penn, G. M., Holliday, J., and Glaser, R. (1984). Psychosocial modifiers of immuno competence in medical students. *Psychosom. Med.*, **46**, 7–14.
71. Kiecolt-Glaser, J. K., Glaser, R., Strain, E. C., Stout, J. C., Tarr, K. L., Holliday, J. E., and Speicher, C. E. (1986). Modulation of cellular immunity in medical students. *J. Behav. Med.*, **9**, 5–21.
72. Levy, S. M., Herberman, R. B., Whiteside, T., Sanzo, K., Lee, J., and Kirkwood, J. (1990). Perceived social support and tumor estrogen/progesterone receptor status as predictors of natural killer cell activity in breast cancer patients. *Psychosom. Med.*, **52**, 73–85.
73. Levy, S. M., Herberman, R. B., Maluish, A. M., Schlien, B., and Lippman, M. (1985). Prognostic risk assessment in primary breast cancer by behavioural and immunological parameters. *Health Psychol.*, **4**, 99–113.
74. Levy, S., Herberman, R., Lippman, M., and d'Angelo, T. (1987). Correlation of stress factors with sustained depression of natural killer activity and predicted prognosis in patients with breast cancer. *J. Clin. Oncol.*, **5**, 348–353.
75. Levy, S. M., Herberman, R. B., Lippman, M., d'Angelo, T., and Lee, J. (1991). Immunological and psychosocial predictors of disease recurrence in patients with early-stage breast cancer. *Behav. Med.*, **17**, 67–75.
76. Fawzy, F. I., Kemeny, M. E., Fawzy, N. W., Elashoff, R., Morton, D.,

Cousins, N., and Fahey, J. L. (1990). A structured psychiatric intervention for cancer patients, II: Changes over time in immunologic measures. *Arch. Gen. Psych.*, **47**, 729–735.

77. Eisen, J. N., Irwin, J., Quay, J., and Livnat, S. (1989). The effect of antidepressants on immune function in mice. *Biol. Psychiatry*, **26**, 805–817.

78. Brandes, L. J., Arron, R. J., Bogdanovic, P., Tong, J., Zaborniak, C. L., Hogg, G. R., Warrington, R. C., Fang, W., and LaBella, F. S. (1992). Stimulation of malignant growth in rodents by antidepressant drugs at clinically relevant doses. *Cancer Res.*, **52**, 3796–3800.

79. Almada, S. J., Zonderman, A. B., Shekelle, R. B., Dyer, A. R., Daviglus, M. L., Costa, P. T. Jr., and Stamler, J. (1991). Neuroticism and cynicism and risk of death in middle-aged men: the Western Electric Study. *Psychosom. Med.*, **53**, 165–175.

80. Grossarth-Maticek, R. and Eysenck, H. J. (1990). Personality, smoking, and alcohol as synergistic risk factors for cancer of the mouth and pharynx. *Psychol. Rep.*, **67**, 1024–1026.

81. Vracko-Tusevljak, M. and Kambic, V. (1989). The significance of psychological factors in the early diagnosis of laryngeal and hypopharyngeal tumors. *Laryngorhinootologie*, **68**, 118–121.

82. Keinan, G., Carmil, D., and Rieck, M. (1991–92). Predicting women's delay in seeking medical care after discovery of a lump in the breast: the role of personality and behavior patterns. *Behav. Med.*, **17**, 177–183.

83. Kash, K. M., Holland, J. C., Halper, M. S., and Miller, D. G. (1992). Psychological distress and surveillance behaviors of women with a family history of breast cancer. *J. Natl. Cancer Inst.*, **84**, 24–30.

84. Margolis, G. J., Goodman, R. L., Rubin, A., and Pajac, T. F. (1989). Psychological factors in the choice of treatment for breast cancer. *Psychosomatics*, **30**, 192–197.

85. Holland, J. C. and Rowland, J. H. (eds) (1989). *Handbook of Psychooncology*. Oxford University Press, New York.

86. Costa, D., Mogos, I., and Toma, T. (1985). Efficacy and safety of mianserin in the treatment of depression of women with cancer. *Acta Psychiatr. Scand.*, **72**, 85–92.

87. Holland, J. C., Morrow, G. R., Schmale, A., Derogatis, L., Stefanek, M., Berenson, S., Carpenter, P. J., Breitbart, W., and Feldstein, M. (1991). A randomized clinical trial of alprazolam versus progressive muscle relaxation in cancer patients with anxiety and depressive symptoms. *J. Clin. Oncol.* **9**, 1004–1011.

88. Can your mind heal your body? (1993). *Consumer Reports*, **58**, 107–115.

89. Siegel, B. S. (1986). *Love, Medicine, and Miracles*. Harper and Row, New York.

90. Jampolsky, G. G. (1983). *Teach Only Love*. Bantam Books, Toronto.

91. Cousins, N. (1989). *Head First: The Biology of Hope*. E. P. Dutton, New York.

92. Borysenko, J. (1987). *Minding The Body, Mending The Mind*. Bantam Books, Toronto.

93. Simonton, O. C., Matthews-Simonton, S., and Creighton, J. (1980). *Getting Well Again*. Bantam Books, New York.

94. Chopra, D. (1989). *Quantum Healing: Exploring the Frontiers of Mind/Body Medicine*. Bantam Books, New York.

95. Achterberg, J. (1985). *Imagery in Healing*. New Science Library, Boston.

# PART III

Psychoimmune mechanisms in the cancer
patient. Possible links between
psychosocial factors and cancer
progression: their therapeutic
potential/limitations

# 10
# Anti-tumour immune mechanisms

## B. SOUBERBIELLE AND A. DALGLEISH

## 1 Introduction

The immune system is a complex network of cells and cellular messengers (cytokines) whose primary role is to police the human body against foreign antigens, that is infectious agents (1, 2) and thus it is a system which is programmed to distinguish non-self from self antigens (3). Most tumour immunologists believe that cancer cells are dissimilar enough from normal (self) cells at the molecular level, both qualitatively or quantitatively, to be recognized as foreign by the immune system.

Anti-tumour immunity is multifactorial being mediated by specific and non-specific mechanisms. Some of these mechanisms are more critical than others depending on the type of cancer.

The immune system possesses two fundamental properties which distinguish it from other reactions such as inflammation. Firstly, the ability to differentiate self from non-self even though the differences may be minor and secondly, memory, whereby the immune system can mount an effective and vigorous immune response to an antigen which it has previously encountered. In order for an immune system to function efficiently against foreign antigens it must be programmed not to recognize self, in other words to be tolerant to self antigens, yet at the same time remain capable of responding to similar foreign antigens.

Self-reactive lymphocytes are deleted in the thymus whereas T-cells reactive against foreign antigens are recruited. This process depends upon the affinity of recognition of a self or foreign peptide and it is, therefore, not surprising that this process is not 100 per cent efficient, with some potential self-reactive cells of low affinity surviving. A second mechanism, that of peripheral tolerance ensures that these clones do not react against self antigens under normal circumstances. In autoimmune diseases self-reactive clones are de-tolerized and, in the case of tumours, potential anti-tumour responses are rendered tolerant to the tumour. In order to understand these mechanisms further it will be necessary to describe the immune system in more detail.

## 1.1 THE IMMUNE SYSTEM

The major component of the immune system is the leukocyte population which is subdivided into neutrophils and macrophages which are scavenger cells, and lymphocytes which are subdivided into T- and B-cells which control the cell-mediated and humoral component of the immune response respectively.

### 1.1.1  *The specific arm of the immune system*

Lymphocytes are small resting cells which circulate through the body ready to react specifically with their corresponding antigen. An important feature of the immune system is memory: an individual has first to be primed (sensitized) to a specific antigen in order to be able to mount a more efficient (in duration and in strength) secondary immune response in a subsequent encounter with this antigen. This is achieved through specific recognition of the antigen by the lymphocyte surface receptors which are immunoglobulins (antibodies) for B-cells, and T-cell receptors (TCR) for T-cells. Stimulation of these lymphocytes will generate numerous circulating memory cells increasing the chance of specific antigen recognition during subsequent contact with the antigen. Along with these memory cells, specific effector B and T-cells are also produced.

The production of the huge diversity of specific antigen receptors required by the host would require an enormous number of genes if the 'one-gene-one protein' rule was applied. However, the immune system has overcome the inherent limitations of such a system by deriving immense diversity through the re-arrangement and juxtaposition of a relatively small number of genes. These code for the building blocks of the antigen-specific receptor. Both the B- and the T-cell receptors follow the similar pattern of the variable (V), diversity (D), and joining (J) regions which are re-arranged next to the constant (C) region. For each antigen receptor, the following general scheme applies. One of a limited number of V genes (for example of the order of 300 in the case of immunoglobulin (Ig) V genes) is re-arranged next to a D and/or J gene, both also coming from a family of a limited number of V and J genes. Next to those, one of few C region genes is rearranged (4) (Figures 1 and 2).

Antigen recognition differs between B- and T-lymphocytes. The antibody responses are primarily concerned with the inactivation, or neutralization, of free or soluble antigen. B-cell antibodies directly associate with the antigen and recognize generally the tertiary structure (or native form) of the antigen. The parts of the antigen molecules which are recognized by B-cells are called epitopes and the availability, hydrophilicity, convexity, and flexibility of the antigen molecule are required for good recognition (5). On the other hand, T-cells can only recognize an antigen which has been processed into small peptides of around 8 to 30 amino acids by an antigen-presenting cell (APC) or a target cell (in the case of cytotoxic T-cells). The peptide is presented

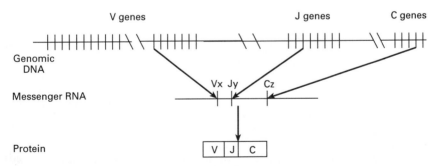

**Figure 1** Schematic representation of the mechanisms which generate the immense diversity seen in the immunoglobins and the T-cell receptors repertoire. This diagram represents the making of a light chain of an immunoglobulin. There are multiple V genes in the genome but one will be translocated near a J gene and a C gene. The same principle applies to the heavy chains of the immunoglobulins and the T-cell receptors.

to a T-cell in association with a major histocompatibility (MHC) molecule expressed on the surface of an APC/target cell—MHC molecules are called human histocompatibility antigens (HLA) in humans. Therefore, MHC/HLA molecules are pivotal for T-cell recognition.

### 1.1.2   The HLA system

There are two types of HLA molecules: Class I and Class II. MHC Class I molecules are formed by a single chain of three immunoglobulin-like domains and a beta-2 microglobulin molecule, whereas Class II HLA molecules are formed by two chains, alpha and beta, each formed by two immunoglobulin-like domains. When expressed on the APC, the different domains of both the HLA Class I and Class II molecules form a pocket where the peptide antigen fits into in order to be presented to T-cells. There are at least 3 loci of Class I genes (A, B, C) and in the same way there are also at least 3 different types of gene-encoded Class II molecules (DR, DQ, DP). Each individual possesses two Class I A, B, and C molecules and two Class II DR, DQ, and DP molecules (as there is one set of genes transmitted by his/her father and one transmitted

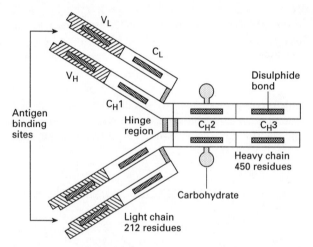

**Figure 2   The basic structure of IgG.** The amino-terminal end is characterized by sequence variability (V) in both the heavy and light chains, referred to as the $V_H$ and $V_L$ regions respectively. The rest of the molecule has a relatively constant (C) structure. The constant portion of the light chain is called the $C_L$ region. The constant portion of the heavy chain is further divided into three structurally discrete regions: $C_H1$, $C_H2$, and $C_H3$. These globular regions, which are stabilized by intrachain disulphide bonds, are referred to as 'domains'. The sites at which the antibody binds antigen are located in the variable domains. The hinge region is a segment of heavy chain between the $C_H1$ and $C_H2$ domains. Flexibility in this area permits the two antigen-binding sites to operate independently.

by the mother) (6). HLA diversity among the general population is provided by different alleles coding for each of these molecules at each locus. The number of different alleles is limited (7) (see Figures 3 and 4 for a representation of the HLA system). On the basis of the large diversity of TCRs recognizing the association HLA and antigen and on the basis of the huge number of possible foreign antigens available in nature, each HLA molecule can bind more than one antigen peptide depending on the contact of the peptide with the different amino acids of the pocket of the HLA molecule (8).

### 1.1.3 T-lymphocyte subsets

There are two main subsets of T-lymphocytes; those which are HLA Class I restricted for the recognition of the antigen, and those which recognize the peptide antigen in association with Class II HLA molecules. The HLA class

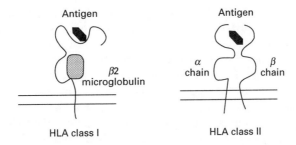

**Figure 3** Schematic representation of a HLA class molecule and a HLA class II molecule. A HLA class I molecule presents an antigenic peptide in the groove formed by the first and the second domain of the molecule. The beta 2 microglobulin molecule makes contact with the third domain of the HLA molecule and contributes to the three-dimensional structure of the HLA molecule. A class II molecule consists of two chains alpha and beta, each of them consists of two domains. The two chains form a groove where the antigenic peptide is presented to the T-cell.

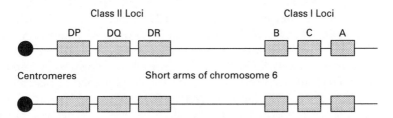

**Figure 4** Schematic representation of the genomic organization of the HLA genes on the short arm of chromosomes 6. An individual possesses two chromosome 6 and therefore expresses two allelic forms of each class II molecule DP, DQ, and DR and two allelic forms of each class I molecule A, B, and C.

restriction is, in part, determined by two different molecules expressed on the T-cell, called CD4 and CD8. Mature T-cells express either CD4 or CD8. The CD8 molecule makes contact with the HLA Class I molecule whereas CD4 makes contact with the Class II molecule. There are different types of T-cells depending on their functions. Cytotoxic T-lymphocytes (CTL) recognize and kill the target cell (for example virally infected cells) and are generally CD8-positive cells and thus Class I restricted. T-helper ($T_h$) cells are involved in controlling the antibody production and the CTL immune response. They also participate in the eradication of microbial infection by inducing delayed type hypersensitivity reactions (DTH lymphocytes) by the secretion of different cytokines. T-helper cells are CD4-positive cells and interact with the Class II molecules presenting the antigen on the APC. A third population of T-lymphocytes are called T-suppressor ($T_s$) cells but their specific existence has been questioned, mainly because it has been difficult to clone and, therefore, characterize them in detail. The effector suppressor cells are part of the CD8-positive T-lymphocyte population although CD4-positive lymphocytes, called T-suppressor inducer cells, are necessary for their induction. $T_s$ cells suppress T- and B-cell responses and may be important in reducing the incidence of autoimmune reactions in the general population. They are likely to be important in cancer immunity (9). The T-cell receptor consists of $\alpha$ and $\beta$ chains which interact with the MHC molecule. A second subset displays $\gamma$ $\delta$ chains and these represent a more primitive T-cell which makes up less than 55 per cent of the total population. Their role, if any, in controlling malignancy is unknown (Table 1).

### 1.1.4   Accessory molecules

The recognition of antigen and subsequent activation of the T-lymphocyte is influenced by molecules other than the TCR, MHC, CD4, or CD8 molecules. Adhesion molecules on T-cells and on the APC/target cell promote and maintain the antigen recognition and the communication between the T-cell and the APC/target cell. For example, the LFA-1 antigen on the T-cell reacts with ICAM on the APC and in the same way CD2 binds to LFA-3 (10). More recently another adhesion molecules called B7 (not to be confused with the HLA Class I molecule named HLA B7) (see Fig. 5) expressed on the APC/target cells interacting with CD28 on T-cells has been shown to be important for tumour T-cell recognition (11, 12). It provides a second signal following the interaction of the TCR, antigen, MHC, CD4 or 8 complex and is clearly important for the first, or specific, signal to register as is demonstrated by experiments blocking or replacing its expression.

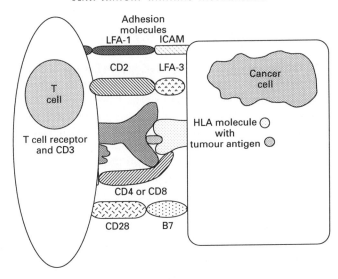

**Figure 5** Schematic representation of the molecules involved in T-cell recognition of an antigen-presenting cell or a tumour cell. The T-cell receptor recognizes the antigen in association with a MHC molecule and the different adhesion molecules promote and maintain this recognition.

### 1.1.5 The natural immune defence system

This immune response consists of many of the responses seen in non-specific inflammation. Natural immune mechanisms are capable of lysing cells without prior sensitization. This immune response is triggered in a non-specific way by many stimuli (for example adherence of a bacteria to a macrophage or activation of the alternative complement pathway by microbial polysaccharide). However, it can also be triggered after the specific recognition of antigens by lymphocytes. Such non-specific triggering of inflammation could, theoretically, lead to pathogenic autoimmune reactions in certain situations. Most of the components playing a role in non-specific inflammation have been implicated in anti-tumour destruction. These include mononuclear phagocytes and resident macrophages, natural killer (NK) cells, polymorphonuclear cells and eosinophils, the complement system and an array of different cytokines secreted after non-specific and specific interaction of antigens with the immune system. Other cells artificially activated by cytokine treatment have been shown to be important in some cancers for example lymphokine activated killer (LAK) cells expanded after IL-2 treatment (13).

## 2  Tumour immunity: historical perspectives

The idea that tumour growth, multiplication, and metastasis could be controlled, or at least influenced, by the immune system came mainly from biologists and experimental pathologists of the second part of the last century. Pathological description of tumours in relation to the immune system were then followed by tumour transplantation experiments in animals; firstly in non-inbred animals (that is with dissimilar genetic background) and then in inbred mice (that is with the same genotype) (14).

There had been early reports of injection of tumour tissue into humans as a form of vaccine a century previously (15), but it is difficult to know if they were carried out on the the basis of an immunological theory or not. One can only presume that the repeated self-innoculation of one of Louis XIV physician's with cancer specimens was due to a desire to prevent developing cancer. In 1895, when bacterial immunity was thought to be entirely serum-mediated, Hericourt and Richet injected 50 patients with anti-tumour antisera raised in dogs and donkeys and claimed some successes which were, at best, both limited and transient. Experiments in animals pioneered by Ludwik Gros and Edward Foley showed that tumour grafts could be rejected in inbred mice which had previously been immunized with the same tumour cells. It was also noticed in animals that chemical- and viral-induced tumours were very immunogenic, whereas spontaneous tumours were rarely immunogenic. The realization that it was T-cell lymphocytes that mediated tumour rejection was an important landmark in the history of tumour immunity.

Towards the end of the last century William B. Coley, a New York surgeon, used a mixture of killed bacteria, known as Coley's toxin, as a treatment for cancer. Coley noticed that in some patients bacterial infection could lead to tumour regression. He, therefore, injected his patients with a mixture of killed bacteria and claimed success with partial and complete regression in some cases for a number of different types of cancers. More recently his granddaughter analysed the case histories of the patients treated by the Coley's toxin and showed that this approach significantly improved the outcome of some patients (16). The mechanism of this treatment is not known but it is thought that the release in the body of soluble factors such as tumour necrosis factor (TNF) and other cytokines induced by killed bacteria could explain part of its efficacy. Coley's work was not easily repeated, and he perfected his treatment over a number of years realizing that the formulation and manufacturer, appropriate dose, and confirmed administration of the toxins at a level which induced systemic symptoms was crucially important. Unfortunately, this approach was buried under the new chemo- and radiotherapeutic approaches which were to follow and was abandoned.

**Table 1** Tumour immunology

---

*EFFECTORS OF THE IMMUNE RESPONSE*

| *Specific* | *Non specific* |
|---|---|
| Cytotoxic T-lymphocytes (CTLs) | Macrophages |
| CD8 | NK cells |
| CD4 | LAK cells |
| B-cells produce antibodies which direct cell-mediated | Complement |
|   cytotoxicity (ADCC) | Cytokines |

Targets they may recognize:

*CELLULAR*
Major and minor histocompatibility genes
Altered histocompatibility antigens
NK determinants
Macrophage determinants
Virus-encoded antigens

*ANTIBODY*
Tissue-specific antigens
Differentiation antigens
Blood-group antigens
Private antigens
Retrogenic or embryonal antigens expressed on tumours;
  $\alpha$ fetoprotein—germ cell tumours and hepatomas
Carcinoma embryonic antigen (CEA) colon and $\beta$ human
  chorionicgonadotrophin ($\beta$HCG)
Ectodermal tumours
Germ-cell tumours

---

2.1 FACTORS IN FAVOUR OF AN EFFECTIVE ANTI-TUMOUR IMMUNE
    RESPONSE IN HUMANS

The presence of a lymphocytic infiltrate on histological examination of some tumours (for example breast carcinomas) suggests that inflammatory reaction could influence tumour growth. Spontaneous tumour regressions have been observed in some instances particularly in melanoma, renal cell carcinoma, neuroblastoma, hypernephroma, and choriocarcinoma, thereby inferring a possible effective immune pressure upon these malignancies (14). However, these regressions are not common. Immunosuppressed individuals have also a higher risk of developing some, but not all, types of malignancy. The risk of cancer in organ allotransplanted patients is at least 100-times higher than in the general population and the cancers are mainly lymphoreticular in origin with a high risk of lymphoma of the central nervous system. The incidence of Kaposi sarcoma and epithelial cancer of the skin is also increased in these patients. These cancers are often associated with oncogenic viruses which are, presumably, held in check by an effective immune system. Examples are Epstein–Barr virus (EBV) and non-Hodgkin's lymphoma, and human papilloma virus (HPV) in skin and urogenital cancers. The same type of cancers are also increased in the acquired immunodeficiency syndrome (AIDS) (17). Effective treatment of renal cell carcinoma and melanoma with inter-feron and interleukin-2 (IL-2), with complete or partial responses reported in up to 30 per cent of patients (although few of the complete responders become long-term survivors), suggests also that effective manipulation of the immune system can induce tumour regression (albeit temporarily in some cases) (18, 19, 20, 21). The recent reports of the use of α-interferon in maintaining remissions in patients with multiple myeloma (following the successful induc-tion by standard chemotherapy) presumably successfully alters the balance between the myeloma and the immune system in the host's favour (22).

## 2.2 CHARACTERIZATION OF TUMOUR-SPECIFIC ANTIGENS

Much time and effort has been spent characterizing tumour antigens which may be recognized as foreign by the immune system (23). These structures appear to be different between murine tumours and human tumours and, (in animal models), between spontaneous arising tumours and induced tumours (for example by UV light or by polycyclic hydrocarbons). Some tumour antigens on induced tumours have already been characterized (for example murine endogeneous leukaemia virus (MLV) antigen in radiation-induced tumours, and altered H-2 antigen (MHC Class I) in UV-induced tumours or a 96 kDa protein in methylcholanthrene (MCA)-induced tumours) (24).

The main problem in tumour immunity is that, despite the fact that tumour cells are thought to arise generally from a single clone, there is an important antigenic diversity amongst tumour cells in a given individual, and between the primary tumour and its metastases. The density of tumour antigens expressed on tumour cells may be more critical than the uniqueness of these antigens to tumour cells (compared with normal cells) in relation to tumour recognition by the immune system and this rule appears to apply to CTL and antibody recognition of tumours.

It has been demonstrated that tumour antigens can fall into three broad categories and this applies both to B-cell antigens (15) and to T-cell antigens (25). The first group, tumour-specific antigens (TSA), are not expressed by normal cells, and are unique to an individual tumour (and thus not expressed by another individual with the same histological tumour type). The second group of tumour antigens are expressed on autologous (that is of the same individual), but are also expressed on allogeneic, tumour cells (that is from different individual). The last group includes antigens which are expressed preferentially by tumour cells but which are also expressed by normal cells. Most of the tumour antigens fall into the last category and are differentiation antigens or cluster determinants (CD) which are expressed at a certain stage of a cell lineage development and arrested by the malignant process. Embryonic/fetal antigens also fall into this third category of tumour antigens as they may be expressed in low quantity in normal adult tissue, and over-expressed in tumour cells (for example carcinoembryonic antigen, which can be found in normal adult colonic mucosa, is often seen in colon cancer). Alpha-feto protein ($\alpha$FP) and $\beta$ human chorionic gonadotrophin hormone ($\beta$HCG) are seen during fetal development but are expressed at high levels in patients with germ cell ($\alpha$FP, $\beta$HCG) or liver tumours ($\alpha$FP).

Another category of tumour antigens is characterized by viral proteins in virally induced tumours (26, 27). These antigens are very important since, in theory, they could act both as targets for vaccine prevention or as targets in already established tumours. Numerous viruses have been shown to induce tumours in animals such as the herpes virus which causes Marek's disease in chickens, and the polyoma viruses and adenoviruses which cause cancer in rodents. RNA oncogenic retroviruses are associated with a variety of leukae-mias, lymphomas, sarcomas, and carcinomas in mice, birds, cats, cattle, and primates.

In many of these animal model systems, the T-cell response is critical for the process of rejection, recognizing the SV40 T antigen (28, 29, 30) and the peptides expressed from the E1A/E1B early region genes which are critical in the adenovirus system (31).

In humans, viral-induced tumours represent up to 20 per cent of all cancers worldwide, although they are not so well represented in the western World. Hepatitis B (HBV) virus is clearly causally associated with hepatocellular carcinoma which is highly prevalent in Africa and S.E. Asia. The Epstein–Barr virus, a DNA herpes virus, is involved in the aetiopathogenesis of Burkitt's lymphoma in Africa, and nasopharyngeal carcinoma (NPC) in China, and immunoblastic lymphoma in immunosuppressed individuals. It has also been implicated as a possible causal agent of Hodgkin's disease (32). The fact that EBV is endemic in western populations which rarely contract these diseases underscores the importance of co-factors in the development of the tumours. Nevertheless, EBV is clearly oncogenic *in vitro* in animal models, and is clonally involved in Burkitt's lymphoma (BL) and nasopharyngeal carcinoma in humans. The immune response to EBV is critical in the development of lymphomas, and the role of polyclonal B-cell stimulation is thought to be important in the development of BL. The development of lymphomas in immunosuppressed individuals underscores the importance of anti-EBV immunosurveillance. The human papilloma viruses (HPVs) are associated with benign warts as well as malignancies of the cervix, vulva, penis, anus, and the human (squamous) skin and may be involved in other cancers such as those of the bladder. Over 60 subtypes of HPVs have been described and these are tumour-type specific, such as the association of HPV 16 (and 18) with cancer of the cervix. The first human retrovirus T-cell lymphotropic virus type 1 (HTLV-1) is the causative agent of the adult T-cell leukaemia-lymphoma (ATLL) which is frequent in Japan. HTLV-1 infects CD4-helper cells and is able to transactivate the gene for the cytokine, IL-2, and its receptor which has the effect of permanently activating the CD4 cells, as IL-2 is theoretically able to autostimulate through the hyperexpressed IL-2 receptor. However, this is only capable of 'setting up' the cell for malignant change which clearly involves other steps, such as chromosomal trans-locations, which is presumably a chance phenomenon as only a small percentage (< 7 per cent) of HTLV-1-infected people develop ATLL over a lifetime. The disease is a clonal one with a randomly integrated HTLV-1 provirus which does not require autologous IL-2 stimulation for growth.

Tumour incidence or progression of some types of tumours has been asso-ciated with HLA status and it is conceivable that this could be explained by the lack of an efficient anti-viral T-cell immunity in those patients who do not possess the HLA restriction elements. This would allow presentation of specific viral epitopes to T-cells. Cervical carcinoma has been linked to DR5 and DQw3 Class II alleles, and nasopharyngeal carcinoma has been linked to HLA A2, Bw46, and B17, as well as the haplotype A2, B16, DR1 (35–35).

Apart from the obvious use of viral antigens for making preventive vaccine (for example an effective anti-hepatitis B vaccine which prevents HBV infec-tion will prevent hepatocellular carcinoma), it is conceivable that some viral proteins could act as targets for the immune system in an attempt to treat established human tumours (for example papilloma antigens in cervical carcinoma or EBV antigens for BL, NPC, or Hodgkin's disease) (32, 36).

It has been proposed that in some cancers the immune response towards viral antigen in tumours could be detrimental rather than protective. Some have suggested that the pathology of Hodgkin's Disease is consistent with a host versus viral reaction similar to chronic graft-versus-host disease in which normal lymphocytes proliferate after recognition of a viral antigen, perhaps expressed by the Reed–Steinberg cells, the latter being specific for HD (37). This would be consistent with the polyclonal proliferation and disturbance of the immune system so often seen in HD patients.

## 2.3 NON-SPECIFIC ARM OF THE ANTI-TUMOUR IMMUNE RESPONSE

Natural immunity is effected by cells which can lyse tumours spontaneously without prior sensitization. These cells include NK cells, mononuclear phago-cytes, and polymorphonuclear phagocytes.

### 2.3.1 *Natural killer (NK) cells*

NK cells are thought to have mainly evolved as anti-viral cells, but also appear to play some role in tumour surveillance. They have neither immunological memory nor MHC restriction. NK cells are mainly large granular lymphocytes (LGL) which express intracytoplasmic azurophilic granules and have a high cytoplasmic nuclear ratio and which bear the antigens CD56, but lack CD3 (marker of commited lymphocytes) in humans. They are CD3 −, NK1.1 +, AsGM1 +. MAC-1 +, Ly 5 +, LFA + in the mouse. In humans at least two populations of NK cells exist: CD3 −, CD56 +, CD16 + (Fc RIII), IL2R − and CD3 −, CD56 +, CD16 −, IL2R + (38). They represent 2–5 per cent of the peripheral blood lymphocytes. The arguments put torward for a possible anti-tumour role for NK cells is that: (1) there is an increased incidence of tumours with age correlating with a decrease in NK activity; and (2) nude mice with intact NK cells, but no T- or B-lymphocytes, are able to kill small tumour inocula.

NK cells (as well as lymphokine-activated killer or 'LAK' cells) do not localize very well in the tumour site and it is clear that NK cells only play a role when tumour burden is small suggesting that they may prevent blood-borne metastases from seeding. They have little effect against established tumours. The antigens recognized by NK cells are thought to be principally sugar-containing molecules, as lectin-binding domains appear to be involved in the recognition process (39). Glycoprotein expression is known to be inadequate in tumour cells (40).

Overall the target epitopes recognized by NK cells appear to fall into two groups; one being ubiquitous and the other more restricted. Interestingly, these targets appear to be more prevalent on tumours adapted to tissue culture. In addition, the targets are more recognizable on cells with no or reduced MHC molecules, where its increased expression renders a cell resistant to cell killing.

The target structure does not involve the Fc receptor of the NK cell even though there is a virtual overlap of the NK population with the K cell population which mediates antibody dependent cell mediated cytotoxicity (ADCC).

NK cell-mediated cytotoxicity or 'NK activity' is enhanced following several hours incubation with interferon-γ and IL-2. The action of these cytokines probably involves both transforming non-cytopathic NK precursors into a lytic state, and enhancing the cytolytic capacity of already active cells. NK cells can themselves produce IFN-γ and IL-2.

### 2.3.2 *Lymphokine-activated killer cells (LAK) cells*

LAK cells are cells activated *in vitro* or *in vivo* by IL-2 treatment. They are non-MHC restricted in their tumour killing unlike CTL. Early clinical studies using infusion of LAK cells expanded *in vitro* and high doses of IL-2 was associated with a number of spectacular remissions in patients with malignant melanoma and renal cell carcinoma. However, the treatment was very toxic (13). Subsequently, it has been demonstrated that LAK-cell treatment did not add to the efficacy of IL-2 treatment alone and that lower doses of IL-2 are as effective as the more toxic higher doses (20, 41). Moreover, the activity of the LAK cells and IL-2 does not correlate with measurable immunological parameters (42). It may be then that the responses seen with these treatments are due to cytotoxic T-cells induced by the treatment, which recognize a still unknown tumour-associated antigen. Cytotoxic T-lymphocytes generated by IL-2, from tumour-infiltrating lymphocytes (TIL), have been shown to selectively kill autologous tumours cells and have been reported to be effective in some melanoma patients (43, 44).

## 2.3.3   Macrophages

Macrophages may be involved in tumour control at several levels. They are clearly involved in the surveillance stage of tumours in murine systems as macrophage poisons reduce the latent period of skin tumours induced by ultraviolet light in mice, and macrophage growth stimulants increases the latent period in the same system. Although macrophages directly invade tumour tissues, the degree of invasion rarely correlates with the spread of the tumour. Macrophages are not cytotoxic until activated, whereupon they demonstrate enhanced bacterial and tumour killing potential. They are activated by a number of agents including endotoxin, immune complexes, and cytokines such as interferon-$\gamma$. The mechanism of tumour cell killing involves both cytolytic and cytostatic components, which include a non-phagocytic process involving the secretion of lysosomal enzymes aimed at the cell membrane as well as phagocytosis of antibody-sensitized cells (45).

In addition to their anti-tumour activity, macrophages also secrete tumour-promoting factors such as fibroblastic growth factor (FGF), lytic enzymes (which can promote tumour invasion), as well as immunosuppressive factors such as prostaglandin E which can suppress T and NK cell-mediated responses. In addition, they can secrete both tumour-growth factors and tumour-hibiting factors such as PDGF, EGF, and TGF-$\beta$ (47). Eosinophils can also modulate an anti-tumour response and be predominant in some tumour inflammatory responses (48).

The complement system and neutrophils also appear to be critical in (ADCC) against some tumours (see also Section 2.3). It has been recently reported that in breast cancer there is a persistent complement activation seen by immunocytochemistry on breast cancer cells, and activation of the alternative complement pathway in small cell lung cancer has been reported (49). The significance of this phenomena is unknown. It appears that individuals suffering from complement deficiency do not develop more tumours than the general population. On the other hand, Janssen and colleagues have reported that a pre-operative high level of C1-inhibitor (C1-INH) strongly correlates with recurrence of gastric carcinoma after surgery (50).

## 2.3.4 Cytokines

Cytokines can be described as a densely interconnected system of protein messengers involved in the regulation of the cellular activities associated with inflammation, tissue repair, and the immune response. They are secreted by cells of the immune system (for example macrophages, NK, T and B-cells) but also other cells in the body, for example endothelial cells or fibroblasts. The term includes such overlapping peptide groups as interleukins, lymphokines, monokines, and miscellaneous growth factors. Cytokines elicit a broad range of paradoxical effects; they can be both proliferative and anti-proliferative and it is possible that when used therapeutically either response could be seen depending on the net balance of these factors. Cancers are disorders of cell growth and differentiation and, therefore, cytokines are, by definition, implicated in carcinogenesis. They also determine the immune response by inducing macrophage, T- and B-cell activation, in addition to modulating HLA and adhesion molecule expression. This potential for enhancing an anti-tumour response has led to several clinical trials. In addition, some cytokines show a direct anti-tumour effect in some systems (murine), for example tumour necrosis factor (TNF) and more recently IL-4.

Because the effects of cytokines are so numerous, widespread, and interactive, it is not surprising that the administration of non-physiological doses is associated with widespread systemic side-effects. Cytokines associated with an anti-tumour response at some level(s) include the interleukins 1, 2, 4, 6, 7, 10, and 12, TNF $\alpha$ and $\beta$ (lymphotoxin), and interferon $\alpha$, $\beta$ and $\gamma$. Some also have potential for treatment of immunodeficiency states like granulocyte–macrophage colony-stimulating factor (GM-CSF), G-CSF, and interleukins 1, 3, 6 and 11. (For a recent overview of cytokine actions the reader is referred to ref. 51). In the clinic, interferons showed disappointing results for most of the solid tumour types, but unexpected responses in hairy cell leukaemia, Kaposi's sarcoma, and as a maintenance treatment for multiple myeloma. IL-2 showed limited response in melanoma and renal cell carcinoma but occasional long-term remissions have been reported,and TNF has, so far, been shown to be inactive and toxic at the doses used. Phase I clinical trials of IL-1 and IL-4 have recently commenced and Phase II studies alone and in combination are planned.

Early studies in murine tumour models showed that some tumours which were resistant to both high dose IL-2 treatment, as well as to IL-2 expanded cells *in vitro*, were exquisitely sensitive when both treatments were given together. This led to clinical studies where LAK cells were given with high-dose bolus IL-2 to a number of patients with advanced malignancy, as discussed previously in Section 2.2.2.

Studies with IL-2 (and the interferons) have highlighted the discrepancy between murine and human responses to such immunomodulation. This might suggest that the LAK targets are more dominant in mice than in humans. The fact that murine models may represent a poor model for human tumours needs to be borne in mind in assessing the clinical potential of the numerous other cytokines now being reported.

IL-1 appears to have direct, anti-proliferative effects on a number of tumour cell lines, some of which regress *in vivo* when IL-1 is administered in mice. Synergy has been observed between IL-1 and IL-2 in mice. Clinical studies in man suggest that dose-limiting toxicities are similar to those of IL-2 and TNF. Combination therapy with IL-2 is under investigation.

IL-4 has a wide range of actions on immune and haemopoietic cells. It is secreted mainly by activated T-cells and NK cells. Many of the actions of IL-4 appear to depend on co-stimuli, although independent anti-tumour effects on cell lines and murine models have been reported. Phase I studies indicate some clinical activity in humans, and Phase II studies are in progress. IL-4 may be synergistic with other cytokines, and the combination of IL-4 with IL-2 is under study at present.

IL-6 stimulates acute-phase proteins, promotes the growth of B and T-cells and enhances NK, LAK, and TIL activity. It has direct anti-tumour activity against weakly immunogenic early murine tumours, but not more advanced tumours.

IL-7, IL-10, and IL-12 act as T-cell growth factors, but none have proved useful in clinical trials to date. IL-7 induces LAK and CTL activity in mice. IL-10 augments the effect of IL-2 and IL-4 on T-cells and IL-2-induced CTL development. However, IL-10 is also immunosuppressive and hence it is hard to predict the likely clinical effect of this cytokine *in vivo*. IL-12 is a cytotoxic T-cell stimulant, NK-cell maturation factor, and can enhance CTL responses against allogeneic cells. (See ref. 52 for a more detailed review of these cytokines).

The role of cytokines in tumours is most impressive when cytokines genes are transfected into tumour cells and re-infused back into the host. IFN-$\alpha$, TNF, IL-2, IL-4, and IL-7 have all been shown to induce a strong, local immune response which leads to the regression of not only the transfected tumour cells, but also some untransfected tumour cells (via a bystander effect). This approach has important implications for the treatment of human cancers. Combinations of cytokines (for example INF-$\alpha$ + IL-2 or IL-2 and IL-4) are particularly attractive and studies using this approach are currently being designed for clinical use. TNF-$\alpha$ has also been transfected into TILs in an attempt to arm these tumour-homing lymphocytes with the tumouricidal actions of such a cytokine. Unfortunately, the process of introducing the cytokine gene may destroy the homing potential of such lymphocytes, as clinical studies using the approach are not as successful as had been hoped.

2.4 SPECIFIC FACTORS INVOLVED IN TUMOUR IMMUNITY

## 2.4.1 *Humoral immunity*

ADCC is mediated by antigen-specific antibodies whose Fc portion becomes attached to the Fc receptors of different killer cells (macrophages, neutrophils, NK cells, eosinophils). There are at least three types of Fc receptors for IgG: FcγRI (CD64), FcγRII (CD32) and FcγRIII (CD16) (23). These activate the complement system which induces cell lysis. The density of tumour-associated antigen expression is critical for an effective ADCC response as lysis only occurs when the tumour cell expresses high levels of tumour associated antigen (TAA). The ADCC response (as well as LAK-cell activity) is influenced by numerous soluble factors and/or hormones, in addition to the previously mentioned cytokines, such as indomethacin, which enhances ADCC activity as does GM-colony-stimulating factor (GM-CSF) (54, 55).

The humoral immune response against non-Hodgkin's lymphoma (NHL) is important *in vivo*, and it is likely that the idiotype on clonal tumoural NHL B-cells can act as a target for the immune system (56). Less specific antigens expressed on B and T-cells can act as targets. For example treatment of NHL patients with a monoclonal antibody, CAMPATH, which recognizes a differentiation antigen CDw52, expressed on all lymphocytes and monocytes, has shown some therapeutic activity (57). Apart from the anti-tumour response to NHL, the humoral immune response does not appear to correlate with demonstrable resistance of the host to solid tumours in animal models or in human situations (58). In MCA-induced sarcoma, tumour-specific antibodies do not provide *in vivo* protection despite the fact that cells are lysed *in vitro* in the presence of complement plus antibodies. Morever, antibodies could be harmful in some situations as they could mask tumour antigens from the immune system or modulate the expression of tumour antigens on the cell surface.

There have been many attempts to use monoclonal antibodies to target tumours. Apart from the lack of tumour-specific antigens, they have not proven effective as less than 1 per cent of monoclonal antibodies actually bind to the tumour. Direct killing by passive infusion of antibodies (such as CAMPATH-1) has led to some impressive responses in lymphomas, and similar studies using antibodies to more specific CD markers (such as CD19, CD36, CD38) are in progress. However, unless humanized and made as a mouse human chimera the anti-mouse response renders them ineffective. The problem of variability of the immunoglobulin idiotype on lymphomas may not be as great as originally thought as there are only a limited number of dominant idiotypes used by most B-cell lymphomas. This means that a panel of antibodies could be used to select highly specific monoclonal antibodies to target one or more dominant epitopes, or that the idiotypes could be used as a vaccine (as opposed to a passive therapy) to induce an active specific immune response against the idiotype. Occasional and rare responses have been claimed using this approach. Recently antibodies have been linked to cytokine genes to increase the anti-tumour potential of this approach. Although the majority of human tumour control is undoubtedly T-cell mediated, lymphomas and other B-cell neoplasms (such as multiple myeloma) may be most effectively targeted at the level of their Ig idiotypes.

### 2.4.2   Cellular immune response by T-cells

There is now an almost general consensus that T-cell mediated immunity is of critical importance for rejection of solid tumours (59). This is most clearly demonstrated against virally induced tumours (31, 60). Cytotoxic T-cells are believed to be critical in tumour rejection. Unlike HLA Class II molecules which are expressed only on antigen-presenting cells. HLA Class I molecules are expressed on most cells in the body and, therefore, induction of an HLA Class I restricted T-cell response specific for tumour antigens is likely to be beneficial against tumour cells which are mostly derived from cell lineages other than those of APC. CTL recognize peptide fragments as short as eight amino acids and the potential for expression of tumour-specific antigens is great in tumour cells. This could be generated by a mutation of a gene, or activation of a gene that is silent in normal tissues and these peptides could bypass the natural immune tolerance against autoantigen (61). Recently, a gene encoding an antigen recognized by CTL has been cloned in human melanoma (62). It has also been consistently shown that HLA Class I A2 molecule is critical for T-cell recognition of melanoma and this HLA restriction allelic element could be critical for the recognition of a tumour-specific melanoma antigen, (63, 64).

Compared with Class I HLA molecules, Class II HLA molecules are only expressed on APC (macrophages, dendritic cells, activated B-cells, and activated T-cells) as well as an array of other cells treated by cytokines, for example endothelial cells. The hyperexpression of Class II HLA molecules is thought to be a triggering factor for some autoimmune diseases (65). Some tumour cells express MHC Class II such as metastatic melanoma and melanoma cell lines [our own unpublished observation] as do other cancer cell lines especially when treated with cytokines (66). Interestingly, Class II restricted CTL form a major part of the CTL response in some viral systems (for example herpes simplex virus and measles) (67, 68). It appears that Class II restricted response(s) may mediate tumour destruction in some animal models.

In some animal tumour systems, for example AKR leukaemia, transfection of Class II MHC molecules in AKR cells induces rejection of these cells when they are injected into the animal whereas transfection of Class I molecules is without effect (69). However, in most other systems, such as experimental B16 melanoma, the contrary is true with an anti-tumour effect promoted after Class I transfection (70). The immunological explanation of this experiment is probably that increased expression of MHC molecules could enhance the presentation of tumour-specific antigens. Other explanations include the ability to present endogeneous proteins more effectively than non-transfected cells, as well as having an effect on the expression of adhesion molecules (71). Adhesions molecules are critical for T-cell recognition as well as for the ability of a tumour cells to metastasize (10, 72). Defects in a single adhesion molecule, such as CD44, may allow a tumour cell to metastasise.

Aberrant expression of different molecules (HLA, adhesions molecules) may allow the tumour to escape from the immune system. Both MHC Class I and Class II molecules are reduced in different cancers (73–76). The same phenomenon has been observed for adhesion molecules such as the decreased expression of LFA-1 seen on Burkitt's lymphoma cells or of LFA-3 on bladder transitional cell carcinoma. These studies have important implications. Although HLA molecules may be detected in normal quantity in some tumours (as with broadly reactive monoclonal antibodies) undetectable specific epitopes may not be functional.

Early studies in human tumour immunology focused solely on the possibility of targeting TAAs. Many of the more recent studies suggest the search for elusive TAAs *per se* is not as important as correcting the *presentational defects* of these molecules. Replacement of MHC molecules into highly tumourogenic cell lines renders them non-tumourogenic and capable of inducing an immune response in a tumour-bearing animal that will not only attack the MHC transfected tumour cells but also the non-transfected cells via a bystander effect. This has exciting implications for solid tumour vaccine strategies against human cancers.

## 3 Summary and conclusions

The immune network is, to some extent, self regulating but is influenced by hormonal and neural signals, as are all biological systems (77). There is evidence that communication between the brain and the immune system is important for both systems (78). It is thus possible that psychological factors, such as stress, could influence the capacity of the immune system to respond to antigenic stimuli, which, in turn, could influence the capacity of the body to fight tumour growth.

There are few controlled epidemiological studies to support the theory that stress significantly influences the incidence or the prognosis of cancers (79). With regards to breast cancer, for example, Ramirez and colleagues found that stress was related with first relapse in a retrospective study of 50 women. However, Barraclough and colleagues did not find such a link in a prospective study of 204 patients (80). Comments on methodology or the lack of good methodology about these types of studies have been made to favour both camps—those who believe a link exists between stress and cancer and those who think that it is far from proven.

The question of whether or not psychological factors could have an effect on tumour growth influences not only research on cancer but also the clinical management of cancer patients. Most patients with cancer are aware of the effects of stress on many illnesses, for example cardiovascular disease, irritable bowel syndrome, and depression, and often suspect a link between stress and cancer; it is a question often asked of their cancer physician or general practitioner.

Over the next decade, a number of new anti-tumour approaches based on the understanding of how the immune system interacts with tumours which have been discussed here will be tried. It is hoped that the lessons learned from these clinical studies will allow us to harness the enormous potential power of the immune system to control cancer—which has learnt to evade it so effectively.

# 4   References

1.  Roitt, I., Brostoff, J., and Male, D. (1989). *Immunology*, Gower, London.
2.  Randall, R. E. R. and Souberbielle, B. E. (1990). Presentation of virus antigens for the induction of protective immunity. In *Control of Virus Diseases*, (ed. N.J. Dimmock *et al.*) S.G.M. **45**, pp. 21–51. Cambridge University Press.
3.  Nossal, G.J . V. (1987). The basic components of the immune system. *N. Eng. J. Med.*, **316**, 1320–1325.
4.  Male, D., Champion, B., and Cooke, A. (1987). *Advanced Immunology*, pp. 2.1–3.11. J. B. Lippincott Company, Philadelphia.
5.  Novotny, J., Handschumacher, M., and Bruccoleri, R. E. (1987). Protein antigenicity: a static surface property. *Immunol. Today*, **8**, 26–31.
6.  Trowsdale, J., Ragoussis, J., and Campbell, R. D. (1991). Map of the human MHC. *Immunol. Today*, **12**, 443–446.
7.  Bodmer, J. G., Marsh, S. G. E., Albert, E. D. *et al.* (1991). Nomenclature for factors of the HLA system, 1990. *Tissue antigens*, **37**, 97–104.
8.  Rudensky, A. Y., Preston-Hurbburt, P., Hong, S. C., Barlow, Janeway Jr. C. A. (1991). Sequence analysis of peptides bound to MHC Class II molecules. *Nature*, **353**, 622–627.
9.  Dorf, M. E., Kuchroo, V. K., and Collins, M. (1992). Suppressor T-cells: some answers but more questions. *Immunol. Today*, **13**, 241–243.
10. Springer, T. A. (1990). Adhesions molecules of the immune system. *Nature*, **346**, 425–434.
11. Townsend, S. and Allison, J. P. (1993). Tumour rejection after direct co-stimulation of CD8 T-cells by B7 transfected melanoma cells. *Science*, **259**, 368–370.

12. Chen, L., Ashe, S., Brady, W. A. *et al.* (1992). Co-stimulation of the anti-tumour immunity by the B7 counter receptor for the T-cell molecule CD28 and CTL A-4. *Cell,* **71**, 1093–1102.

13. Rosenberg, S. A. (1988). Immunotherapy of cancer using interleukin 2: Current status and future prospects. *Immunology Today,* **9**, 58–62.

14. Currie, G. A. (1974). Cancer and the immune response. In *Current Topics in Immunology Series.* (ed. J. Turk) Edward Arnold, London.

15. Oettegen, H. F. and Old, L. J. (1991). The history of cancer immunotherapy. In *Biologic Therapy of Cancer,* (eds V. T. Jr. De Vita, S. Hellman, and S. A. Rosenberg). J. B. Lippincott, Philadelphia.

16. Nauts, H. C. ans McLaren, J. R. (1990). Coley's toxins—the first century. *Adv. Exp. Med. Biol.,* **267**, 483–500.

17. Groopman, J. E. and Broder, S. (1989). Cancer in AIDS and other immuno-deficiency states. In *Cancer: Principle and Practice of Oncology,* (3rd edn), (eds V. T. Jr. DeVita, S. Hellman, S. and S. A. Rosenberg) pp. 1953–1959. J. B. Lippincott Company, Philadelphia.

18. Rosenberg, S. A., Lotze, M. T., Yang, J. C., Aebersold, P. M., Lineham, W. M., Seipp, C. C. *et al.* (1989). Experience with the use of high-dose interleukin-2 in the treatment of 625 cancer patients. *Ann. Surg.,* **210**, 474–85.

19. Atzpodien, J., Korfer, A., Franks, C., Poliwodea, H., and Kichner, H. (1990). Home therapy with IL-2 and interferon alpha2B in advanced human malignancies. *Lancet,* **335**, 1509–1513.

20. Stein, R. C., Malkovska, V., Morgan, S. *et al.* (1991). The clinical effects of prolonged treatment of patients with advanced cancer with low-dose subcutaneous interleukin-2. *Br. J. Cancer,* **63**, 275–278.

21. Dalgleish, A. G. and Sikora, K. (1992). Melanoma. In *Interleukin-2,* (ed. Jonathan Waxman) pp. 132–144. Blackwell Scientific Publications, Oxford.

22. Mandelli, F., Tribalto, M., Avvisati, G. *et al.* (1988). Recombinant interferon alfa-2b (intron-A) as post-induction therapy for responding multiple myeloma patients. M84 protocol. *Cancer Treatment Reviews,* **15**, suppl. A 43–8.

23. Carney, W. (1988). Human tumor antigens and specific tumor therapy. *Immunol. Today,* **9**, 363–364.

24. Srivastava, P. K. and Old, L. (1988). Individually distinct transplantation antigens of chemically induced mouse tumors. *Immunol. Today,* **9**, 78–83.

25. Anachini, A., Fossati, G., and Parmiani, G. (1978). Clonal analysis of the cytolytic T-cell response to human tumours. *Immunol. Today,* **8**, 385–389.

26. Dalgleish, A. G. (1991). Viruses and cancer. *Br. Med. Bull.,* **47**, 21–46.

27. zur Hausen, H. (1991). Viruses and Cancer. *Science,* **254**, 1167–1173.

28. Tevethia, S. S., Tevethia, M. J., Lewis, A. J., Reddy, V. R., and Weissman, S. M. (1983). Biology of simian virus 40 (SV40) transplantation antigen (TrAg). Analysis of TrAg in mouse cells synthetizing truncated SV40 large antigen. *Virology,* **128**, 319–330.

29. O'Connell, K. A. and Gooding, L. R. (1984). Cloned cytotoxic T-lymphocytes recognize cells expressing discrete fragments of SV40 tumour antigen. *J. Immunol.,* **132**, 953–985.

30. Lathe, R., Kieny, M. P., Gerlinger, P., Clertant, P., Guizani, I., Cuzin, F. *et al.* (1987). Tumour prevention and rejection with recombinant vaccinia. *Nature,* **326**, 878–80.

31. Kast, W. M., Offringa, R., Peters, P. J., Voordovw, H., Melven, R. H., Van der Eb, A. J. *et al.* (1989). Eradication of adenovirus E1-A induced tumours by E1-A specific cytotoxic T-lymphocytes. *Cell*, **59**, 603–14.

32. Rickinson, A. B., Murray, R. J., Brooks, J., Griffin, H., Moss, D. J., and Masucci, M. G. (1992). T-cell recognition of Epstein Barr virus associated lymphoma. In A new look at tumor immunology. In *Cancer Surveys*, (eds A. J. McMichael and W. F. Bodmer). ICRF, Cold Spring Harbor Laboratory Press.

33. Wank, R., Schendel, D. J., and Thomssen, C. (1991). HLA antigen and cervical cancer. *Nature*, **356**, 22–23.

34. Lu, S. J., Day, N. E., Degos, L. *et al.* (1990). Linkage of a nasopharyngeal carcinoma susceptibility locus to the HLA region. *Nature*, **326**, 470–1.

35. Wu, S. B., Huang, S. J., Chang, A. S., Hsieh, T., Hsu, M. M., Hsieh, P. P. *et al.* (1989). Human leukocyte antigens (HLA) frequency among patients with nasopharyngeal carcinoma in Taiwan. *Anticancer Research*, **9**, 1649–1653.

36. Davies, D. H., McIndoe, G. A., and Chain, B. M. (1991). Cancer of the cervix: prospect for immunological control. *Int. J. Exp. Pathol.*, **72**, 239–251.

37. Order, S. E. and Hellman, S. (1972). Pathogenesis of Hodgkin's disease. *Lancet*, **1**, 571–573.

38. Kärre, K., Hansson, M., and Kiessling, R. (1991). Multiple interactions at the natural killer workshop. *Immunol. Today*, **12**, 343–345.

39. Hofer, E., Duchler, M., Fuad, S. A., Houchins, J. P., Yabe, T., and Bach, F. H. (1992). Candidate natural killer cell receptors. *Immunol. Today*, **13**, 429–30.

40. O'Brien, M. E. R., Souberbielle, B., Cowan, M. E. *et al.* (1991). Glycoproteins synthesis in normal and malignant cervical tissue. *Cancer Letters*, **58**, 247–254.

41. Palmer, P. A., Vinke, J., Evers, P., Pourreau, C., Oskam, R., Roest, G. *et al.* (1992). Continuous infusion of recombinant interleukin-2 with or without autologous lymphokine activated killer cells for the treatment of advanced renal carcinoma. *Eur. J. Cancer*, **28A**, 1038–1044.

42. Boldt, D. H., Mills, B. J., Gemlo, B. T. *et al.* (1988). Laboratory correlates of adoptive immunotherapy with recombinant interleukin-2 and lymphokine-activated killer cells in human. *Cancer Res.*, **48**, 4409–4416.

43. Topalian, S. L., Solomon, D., and Rosenberg, S. A. (1992). Tumour-specific cytolysis by lymphocytes infiltrating human melanomas. *J. Immunol.*, **142**, 3714–3725.

44. te Velde, A. A. and Figdor, C. G. (1992). Monocyte mediated cytotoxic activity against melanoma. *Melanoma research*, **1**, 303–309.

45. Rosenberg, S. A., Aebersold, P., Cornetta, K. *et al.* (1990). Gene transfer into human: Immunotherapy of patients with advanced melanoma using tumour-infiltrating lymphocyte modified by retroviral gene transduction. *N.E.J.M.*, **323**, 570–578.

47. Mantovani, A., Bottazi, B., Colotta, F., Sozzani, S., and Ruco, L. (1992). The origin and function of tumour-associated macrophages. *Immunol. Today*, **13**, 265–270.

48. Tepper, R. I., Coffman, R. I., and Leder, P. (1992). An eosinophil-dependent mechanism for the anti tumor effect of interleukin-4. *Science*, **257**, 548–551.

49. Nicolescu, F., Rus, H. G., Retegau, M., and Vlaicu, R. (1992). Complement activation on tumor cells in breast cancer. *Am. J. Pathol.*, **140**, 1039–1043.

50. Janssen, C. W. Jr., Lie, R. T., Mocartmann, M., and Matre, R. (1990). Who gets a second primary cancer after gastric cancer surgery? *Eur. J. Surg. Oncol.*, **165**, 195–199.

51. Balkwill, F. R. (1991). *Cytokines in Cancer Therapy*. Oxford University Press.

52. Stein, R. (1993). The cytokine treatment of cancer. *Curr. Opin. Invest. Drugs*, **2**, 195–203.

53. Fanger, M. W., Shen, L., Graziano, R. F., Guyre, P. M. (1987). Cytotoxicity mediated by human $F_c$ receptor for IgG. *Immunol. Today*, **10**, 92–99.

54. Eisenthal, A. (1990). Indomethacin up regulate the generation of lymphokine-activated killer cell activity and antibody-dependent cellular cytotoxicity mediated by IL-2. *Cancer Immunol. Immunotherapy*, **31**, 342–348.

55. Kushner, B. H. and Cheung, N. K. (1989). GM-CSF enhances 3F8 monoclonal antibody-dependent cellular cytotoxicity against human melanoma and neuroblastoma. *Blood*, **73**, 1936–1941.

56. George, A. J. and Stevenson, F. K. (1990). Humoral effector mechanisms in the immunity to cancer. *Immunol. Today*, **11**, 348–349.

57. Hale, G., Dyer, M. J., Clark, M. R., Phillips, J. M., Marcus, R., Richmann, L. *et al.* (1988). Remission induction in non-Hodgkin's lymphoma with reshaped human monoclonal antibody Campath-1H. *Lancet*, **2**, 1394–1399.

58. Brown, J. P., Klitzman, J. M., Hellstrom, I., Nowinski, R. C., and Hellstrom, K. E. (1978). Antibody response of mice to chemically induced tumours. *Proc. Nat. Acad. Sci. (USA)*, **75**, 955–958.

59. Lotze, M. T. and Finn, O. J. (1990). Recent advances in cellular immunology: implication for immunity to cancer. *Immunol. Today*, **11**, 190–193.

60. Leclerc, J. C., Gomard, E., Plata, F., and Levy, J. P. (1973). Cell mediated immune reaction against tumours induced by oncornavirus. II nature of the effector cells in tumour cell cytolysis. *Int. J. Cancer*, **11**, 426–432.

61. Boon, T., De Plaen, E., Lurquin, C. *et al.* (1992). Identification of tumour rejection antigens recognised by T-lymphocytes. In *A New Look at Tumour Immunology*, (eds A. J. McMichael and W. F. Bodmer) pp. 23–37. Cold Spring Harbor Laboratory Press, ICRF.

62. Van der Bruggen, P., Traversari, C., Chomez, P. *et al.* (1991). A gene encoding an antigen recognised by cytolytic T-lymphocyte on a human melanoma. *Science*, **254**, 1643–1647.

63. Crowley, N. J., Slugluff, C. L. Jr., Darrow, T. L., and Seigler, H. L. (1990). Generation of human autologous melanoma-specific cytotoxic T-cell using HLA-A2 matched allogeneic melanoma. *Cancer Res.*, **50**, 492–498.

64. Pandolfi, F., Boyle, L. A., Trentin, L., Kurnick, J. T., Isselbacher, K. J., and Gattoni-Celli, S. (1991). Expression of HLA-A2 antigen in tumour melanoma cell lines and its role in T-cell recognition. *Cancer Research*, **51**(12), 3164–3170.

65. Bottazo, G. F., Todd, I., Mirakian, R., Belfiore, A., and Pujol-Borrel, R. (1986). Organ specific autoimmunity: a 1986 overview. *Immunol Rev.*, **94**, 137–169.

66. Lundin, K. E. A., Sollid, L. M., Bosnes, V., Gaudernack, G., and Thorsby, E. (1990). T-cell recognition of HLA Class II molecules by gamma interferon on a clonic adenocarcinoma cell line (HT29). *Scand. J. Immunol.*, **31**, 469–472.

67. Schmid, D. S. (1988). The human MHC-restricted cellular response to herpes

simplex virus type 1 is mediated by CD4+, CD8− T-cells ands is restricted to the DR region of the MHC complex. *J. Immunol.*, **140**, 3610–3616.

68. Jacobson, S., Richert, J. R., Biddison, W. E., Satinsky, A., Hatzman, R. J., and McFarland, H. F. (1984). Measles virus-specific T4+ human cytotoxic T-cell clones are restricted by Class II HLA antigens. *J. Immunol.*, **133**, 754–757.

69. Hui, K., Grosveld, F., and Festenstein, H. (1984). Rejection of transplantable AKR leukaemic cells following MHC DNA-mediated cell transformation. *Nature*, **311**, 750–752.

70. Tanaka, K., Gorelik, E., Nozumi, N., and Jay, G. (1988). Rejection of Bl6 melanoma induced by the expression of a tranfected MHC Class I gene. *Mol. Cell. Biol.*, **8**, 1857–1861.

71. Gorelik, E., Jay, G., Kim, M., Hearing, V. J., DeLeo, A., and McCoy, Jr. J. P. (1991). Effect of H-2Kb gene on expression of melanoma-associated antigen and lectin binding sites on B16 melanoma cells. *Cancer Res.*, **51**, 5212–5218.

72. Hart, I. and Saini, A. (1992). Biology of tumour metastasis. *Lancet*, **2**, 1453–1457.

73. Festenstein, H. and Schmidt, W. (1987). Variation in MHC antigenic profiles of tumour cells and its biological effects. *Immunol. Rev.*, **60**, 85–127.

74. Cordon-Cardo, C., Fuks, Z., Drobnjak, M., Moreno, C., Eisenbach, I., and Feldman, M. (1991). Expression of HLA-A, B, C antigens on primary and metastatic tumour cell populations of human carcinomas. *Cancer Res.*, **51**, 6372–6380.

75. Pantel, K., Schlimok, G., Kutter, D., Scaller, G., Genz, T., Wiebecke, B. *et al.* (1991). Frequent down-regulation of major histocompatibility Class I antigen expression on individual micrometastatic carcinoma cells. *Cancer*, **51**, 4712–4715.

76. Momburg, F., Ziegler, A., Harprecht, J., Moller, A., Moldenhauer, G., and Hammerling, G. (1989). Selective loss of HLA-A or HLA-B antigen expression in colon carcinoma. *J. Immunol.*, **142**, 352–358.

77. Khansari, D. N., Murgo, A. J., and Faith, R. E. (1990). Effect of stress on the immune system. *Immunol. Today*, **11**, 170–175.

78. Goezl, E. J., Adelman, D. C., and Sreedharan, S. P. (1990). Neuroimmunology. *Advances in Immunology*, **48**, 161–190.

79. Barraclough, J. (1993). Life events and breast cancer. *Cancer Topics*, **9**, 51–52.

80. Barraclough, J., Pinder, P., Cruddas, M., Osmond, C., Taylor, I., and Perry, M. (1992). Life events and breast cancer prognosis. *Br. Med. J.*, **304**, 1078–1081.

# 11

# Short-term psychiatric intervention for patients with malignant melanoma: effects on psychological state, coping, and the immune system

## F. I. FAWZY, N. W. FAWZY, AND C. S. HYUN

# 1  Introduction

This chapter will review cancer patients' most common psychological responses to their diagnosis, the relationship between coping behaviour and affective states, and the effects of minor, major, and chronic stress as well as affective state and coping behaviour on the immune system. It will also review the effects of psychosocial interventions on levels of distress, coping, and various aspects of the immune system. Finally, the effects of a specific structured psychiatric group intervention on the above variables will be discussed.

# 2  Review of the literature

## 2.1 PSYCHOLOGICAL RESPONSES TO CANCER

The newly diagnosed cancer patient may experience a number of profound psychological reactions. The most common of these are shock and disbelief (1, 2). Denial is also frequently seen at this stage and may prevent overwhelming anxiety. Minimizing the implications of the disease may allow the patient to comprehend the painful news more gradually (3). Anger, possibly directed toward the physician or family members (4) and a combination of sadness, depression, and personal grief may follow (5–8). Most patients then gradually accept reality. At this point anxiety, helplessness, hopelessness, guilt, insomnia, anorexia, irritability, and inability to concentrate often manifest themselves (9). The question 'Why me?' is asked and feelings of persecution are common (10).

## 2.2 COPING AND THE RELATIONSHIP BETWEEN COPING AND AFFECTIVE STATE

How patients cope with these psychological problems may have important implications for their emotional, social, and physical health. Researchers have identified three general coping *methods*:

1.  *Active-behavioural methods* deal directly with the problem and its events by such active means as exercising, use of relaxation techniques, and dietary changes, as well as relying on others for emotional, informational, and instrumental support.

2.  *Active-cognitive methods* deal with the manner in which the patient tries to understand the illness and accepts its effect on his or her life, such as by focusing on positive changes that have occurred since the onset of illness.

3.  *Avoidance methods* attempt to avoid thinking about or behaving in direct response to the illness and include self-medication with alcohol and drugs.

   These behaviours and cognitions may be further organized into eight coping *strategies*. These strategies are as follows:

(1)  *Active-positive strategy* (increasing involvement, planning action, enjoying life 'one day at a time');

(2)  *Active-expressive strategy* (talking with others to gain information or to offer support to others with cancer);

(3)  *Active-reliance strategy* (seeking a friend or relative for help or a physician for intervention);

(4)  *Cognitive-positive strategy* (understanding the illness, creating meaning, thinking about positive changes);

(5)  *Distraction strategy* (being preoccupied with other matters, for example going out more socially);

(6)  *Cognitive-passive strategy* (ruminating, daydreaming);

(7)  *Passive-resignation strategy* (preparing for 'the worst', keeping feelings secret from others);

(8)  *Avoidance-solitary strategy* (avoiding others, taking drugs, or smoking more than usual) (11).

These methods and strategies show differing associations with psychological state. In general, the first five of these appear to be correlated with improvement in psychological well being while the last three tend to be associated with greater psychological distress. Patients who have used active-behavioural methods of coping have reported more positive affective states, higher levels of self-esteem, and fewer physical symptoms (12–14). Billings and Moos (14) found that their physically ill subjects who used active-cognitive methods were less anxious and the women, in particular, were less depressed and reported fewer physical symptoms. Another study found that cognitive restructuring (an active-cognitive method) was positively correlated with greater positive affect and higher self-esteem (15). Namir et al. (11) found that one kind of active-cognitive coping methods (that is cognitive-positive strategies such as praying, thinking about positive meaning and changes), were positively related with positive mood states, self-esteem, concerns about one's condition, and lower physical fatigue levels while cognitive-passive strategies, such as day-dreaming and ruminative thoughts, were negatively associated with such variables. A positive association between avoidance coping, which involves avoidance, denial, escape, and psychological distress has also been noted. Billings and Moos (14) and Namir et al. (11) found an association between avoidance and greater depression, anxiety, and lower quality of life. Namir et al. (11) also found that patients who used distraction had fewer concerns over health, less mood disturbance, lower anxiety, more vigour, and less fatigue. They perceived themselves as healthier than patients who did not use this strategy and actually had fewer medical symptoms. In summary, when a coping behavior succeeds, positive emotions are felt; when it proves to be inadequate or inappropriate, negative emotions of grief, anxiety, anger, and panic are felt. In other words, as the use of these positive and active coping strategies increases negative mood states decrease.

2.3 STRESS AND THE IMMUNE SYSTEM

Research studies have demonstrated a relationship between various forms of stressful life experience and changes in the immune system in both animal and human models. Studies in man have measured the effects of both artificially created and naturally occurring stressors on the immune system. Changes in measures of immune function have been detected following exposure to *major* stressful events such as spousal bereavement or marital disruption. Bartrop et al. (16) reported significantly decreased *in vitro* cell proliferation in response to stimulation by the mitogens, phytohemagglutinin (PHA) and concanavalin A (CON A), in bereaved spouses at six weeks. In a prospective study of 15 spouses of women with advanced breast cancer, Schleifer et al. (17) showed that there was a significant depression in response to PHA, CON A, and pokeweed mitogens (PWM) during the first two months following the death of a spouse compared with prebereavement levels. Irwin *et al.* (18) reported that bereaved women showed reduced natural killer (NK) cell activity and hypercortisolaemia as compared with controls. Two other studies looked at marital disruption and immunity. In the first (19), marital disruption among women was associated with significantly poorer proliferation response to PHA and CON A, significantly lower percentages of NK cells and helper T-cells, and significantly higher antibody titres to Epstein–Barr virus (EBV). In the second study (20), separated/divorced men were more distressed and lonely. They also reported significantly more recent illnesses than married men. These individuals showed significantly poorer values on antibody titres to two herpes viruses. Individuals experiencing more *minor* stresses such as medical student examinations have been found to have significantly lower levels of NK-cell activity, fewer NK cells, and lowered production of gamma interferon (21). Dorian *et al.* (22) showed a transiently elevated number of T- and B-lymphocytes and impaired plaque-forming cells and mitogen responsiveness in a highly stressed group of trainees prior to their exams. These values normalized shortly after the exams were over. One notable study (23) on the family caregivers of Alzheimer's Disease victims, showed that the *chronically* stressed caregivers had significantly lower percentages of total and CD4 (helper/inducer) T-lymphocytes than controls, as well as lower CD4/CD8 (suppressor/cytotoxic) T-cell ratios. They also had higher antibody titres to Epstein–Barr virus (EBV) while the percentages of NK cells and CD8 (cytotoxic) T-lymphocytes were not significantly different. Subjects exposed to experimentally induced combat-like stress (77-hour vigil) showed a heightened ability of their lymphocytes to produce interferon in response to Sendai virus but reduced phagocytosis (24). In another example of induced stress (elective inguinal herniorrhaphy), Linn and Jensen (25) reported that responses to PHA and CON A were significantly lower than controls at five days following operation and response to CON A were still significantly decreased 30 days postoperatively.

## 2.4 AFFECTIVE STATE AND THE IMMUNE SYSTEM

A number of studies investigating affective states (for example depressed mood) and affective disorders (for example major depression) in relation to immune status have been performed (26–32). For example, Schleifer *et al.* (33) found that hospitalized patients with a diagnosis of major depressive disorder (MDD) had lymphocytes with a diminished capacity to proliferate in response to mitogens such as PHA, when compared with matched controls. However, this group of investigators was unable to replicate these findings in a larger, more heterogeneous sample (34). Overall, studies have failed to provide consistent evidence of immunological changes associated with major depression. A few studies have reported associations between normal affective states such as depressed mood and/or loneliness and such aspects of the immune system as decreased CD8 cells (35) and NK-cell activity (36, 37).

## 2.5 COPING AND THE IMMUNE SYSTEM

There is considerable interest in the effect of coping processes on the influence of stressful life experience on immune parameters. Animal studies suggest that having control over a stressor may protect the immune system from stress-induced immune alterations (38). However, only a few studies have been done to examine this relationship in humans. One study of individuals with genital, herpes showed that low use of problem-oriented coping and high use of more passive avoidant strategies to deal with adverse life situations over a six-month period were associated with low CD8 levels and a high rate of herpes recurrence (35). In an experimental study, writing about (that is expressing) emotionally traumatic events that had not previously been disclosed to others was associated with increased proliferative capacity of lymphocytes in response to PHA (39). Consistent with this, Pettingale, Greer, and Tee (40) Found that women with both benign and malignant breast tumors who habitually suppressed anger had higher levels of serum IgA. This parameter has been associated with metastatic spread.

## 2.6 EFFECTS OF PSYCHOLOGICAL INTERVENTIONS ON AFFECTIVE STATE AND COPING

A number of individual therapeutic interventions (for example psychotherapy, psychoanalysis, hypnosis, guided imagery, education, and relaxation training) have been implemented to help cancer patients deal with their psychological reactions. Many of these studies reported improvement in both coping and affective distress (41–47).

Group therapy with cancer patients has also been used for some time but the early literature was largely descriptive. The groups in these studies were described as 'education' and/or 'supportive', and were led by a wide variety of people ranging from experienced group therapists with several years' training to self-help groups conducted by the patients themselves. Such group interventions have been credited with helping patients in a number of ways such as improved self-concept and adjustment to illness (48), decline of anxiety, hostility, depression (49), sharing of problem-solving skills and hope (50), and ventilation of emotions (51).

More recently, several randomized prospective group studies have been reported. Spiegel *et al.* (52) studied patients with metastatic breast cancer and relatively poor prognoses. These patients met weekly in psychological support groups for up to a year. Assessment was made of mood states and maladaptive coping responses. At 12 months, the support group showed significantly less tension, less fatigue, less confusion, and more vigour than those in the control group. They also showed a trend toward having less depression, fewer maladjusted coping responses, and fewer phobias. At ten-year follow-up, only three of the patients were alive and death records were obtained for the other 83. Survival from time of randomization and onset of the intervention was, somewhat to the author's surprise, significantly different with means of 36.3 (S.D. 37.6) months in the intervention group compared with 18.9 (S.D. 10.8) months in the control group. Lower mood disturbance and higher ratings of vigour on the Profile of Mood States at the end of the intervention period were thus significantly associated with greater longevity (53).

A prospective randomized study by Greer *et al.* (54) looked at the effects of adjuvant psychological therapy on anxiety, depression, and adjustment in 174 patients with primary diagnosis or first recurrence of cancer. The experimental patients scored significantly higher in fighting spirit and significantly lower in anxiety, anxious preoccupation, helplessness, and fatalism than the controls. Some of those effects were still seen at the four month follow-up point.

Another randomized prospective group study investigated the impact of an intervention programme immediately following diagnosis versus an intervention started four months later in newly diagnosed cancer patients. Patients were then followed-up for 12 months (55). The intervention consisted of five one-hour sessions with a nurse in which problem-solving techniques, goal setting, cognitive reappraisal, relaxation training, and effective use of resources were taught. Goals of the intervention were to decrease distress in cancer patients by reducing emotional arousal, increasing knowledge, enhancing personal control, and strengthening coping skills. No significant differences were found between the early and later interventions until eight months follow-up. The later intervention group ($n = 102$) were showed significantly less depression, anxiety, and worry, and felt more in control than the early intervention group ($n = 103$). The later intervention group continued to worry less at the 12 month follow-up.

## 2.7 EFFECTS OF PSYCHOLOGICAL INTERVENTIONS ON THE IMMUNE SYSTEM

Few studies have been carried out to assess the effect of a psychosocial intervention on the immune system. One such study (56) assessed the effect of relaxation training or social contact versus no contact in a group of 45 geriatric residents in independent-living facilities. The relaxation group showed a significant increase in NK-cell activity and a significant decrease in antibody titres to herpes simplex virus. The other two groups showed non-significant changes. Another study measured immune processes in first year medical students one month prior to exams and on the first day of a three-day exam period. One half of the students met in a hypnotic/relaxation group between blood draws. Both intervention and control groups showed significant decreases in the percentage of CD4 lymphocytes and NK-cell activity at the exam time point. Frequency of relaxation practice in the intervention group was a significant predictor of the percentage of CD4 cells, but not of CD8 cells or NK-cell activity (57).

Gruber *et al.* (58), in a pilot study of relaxation and imagery for cancer patients, found increases in mitogen response, NK-cell activity, interleukin-2, erythrocyte-rosette assay activity, and serum levels of IgG and IgM.

Several other studies involving hypnotic suggestion, guided imagery, and/or conditioning suggest possible psychological modulation of delayed hypersensitivity reactions in humans. Delayed hypersensitivity (sometimes referred to as a Type IV reaction) is primarily a T-cell-mediated response. Cutaneous testing in previously sensitized individuals is a well-established method for monitoring the Type IV reaction (59). Black *et al.* (60) showed that the Mantoux (purified protein derivative of tuberculin) reaction may be inhibited by suggestions given during hypnosis. Smith and McDaniel (61) gave tuberculin-positive volunteers monthly injections of tuberculin from a coloured vial in one arm and saline from a different coloured vial in the other arm. For five months the contents of the coloured vials were held constant. In the sixth month the colours of the vials were switched and the tuberculin reaction was significantly reduced but saline did not produce a false positive. Zachariae *et al.* (62), in a well-controlled study, were the first to show that the Type IV reaction could be enhanced as well as diminished by the use of guided imagery during hypnosis. All of these studies suggest a connection between the central nervous system and the immune system.

# 3  A structured psychiatric intervention for cancer patients

Based on this review of the literature and clinical experience we developed and implemented a structured psychiatric intervention to study the immediate and long-term effects of such an intervention on affective state, coping, adjustment to the diagnosis of cancer, quality of life, and the immune system in cancer patients. An attempt was also made to examine whether or not any relationships exist between these variables (63, 64).

## 3.1  SUBJECTS AND METHODS

Patients with malignant melanoma being seen at the UCLA John Wayne Cancer Clinic were deemed eligible for the study if: (i) they were Stage I (no metastasis) or Stage II (local node metastasis); (ii) their primary tumour as well as any positive metastatic nodes were surgically excised; (iii) they had no previous psychiatric history; (iv) they were 18 years or older; and (v) they could read and speak English. Patients receiving any treatment which might effect their immunological function were not included in the study.

Originally, 80 patients agreed to participate. Patient drop out, death, and incomplete data resulted in a final number ($N$) of 38 intervention patients and 28 control patients.

### 3.2 ASSESSMENT

The psychological and immunological data were collected prior to the beginning of the intervention groups, six weeks later (after completion of the intervention groups), and six months later. The following assessment techniques were used.

### 3.2.1  *The Profile of Mood States (POMS) (65)*

This 65-item assessment consists of six scales that measure tension–anxiety, depression–dejection, anger–hostility, vigour–activity, fatigue–inertia, and confusion–bewilderment. These scales can be summed to generate a total mood disturbance score (TMD). Higher POMS subscales and TMD scores indicate higher levels of mood disturbance during the previous seven days.

### 3.2.2  *Psychosocial Adjustment to Illness Scale (PAIS) (66)*

The PAIS is designed to assess the quality of a patient's psychosocial adjustment to a current medical illness or its restricting effects. There are seven primary domains of adjustment: health care orientation, vocational environment, domestic environment, sexual relationships, extended family relationships, social environment, and psychological distress. A total psychological adjustment to illness score is also generated.

### 3.2.3  *Quality of Life Scale (67)*

The Quality of Life assessment is a visual analogue scale which results in a measure of 1 to 100, with 1 being the poorest quality of life and 100 being the highest quality of life. This scale provides a more global assessment of how the patient perceives his/her quality of life.

### 3.2.4   Dealing with Illness-Coping Inventory (11)

This 48-item inventory assesses cognitive and behavioural responses made in efforts to cope with the illness (described earlier).

### 3.2.5   Immune parameters

Immunological assessment included immunophenotypic assessment of NK cells and large granular lymphocytes as well as functional assessment of NK-cell activity. Peripheral blood was drawn from control subjects on the same days as intervention subjects between 8 a.m. and 10 a.m. to control for circadian rhythms. We chose to emphasize testing of the NK population as there is evidence that: (1) NK cells may be responsive to such psychological interventions as relaxation; (2) NK cells may be more susceptible than other immune cell populations to external influences, such as cytokine (for example Interleukin-2) administration; (3) NK populations in animal systems play a role in resistance to viral infections; and (4) large granobar lymphocytes (LGLs) with high NK-cell activity are involved in *in vivo* resistance to tumours (68).

It is possible that intervention-induced changes in the NK system could be relevant to the health status of cancer patients, but it should be emphasized that this was not the object of the study.

### 3.3   TREATMENT

The intervention and control patients underwent standard surgical treatment of their tumours and completed the same schedule of assessments by means of the aforementioned scales. The control patients did not participate in any psychiatric or educational intervention. The intervention patients, however, participated in the following psychiatric group intervention.

Groups of seven to ten intervention patients met for one and half hours weekly for six weeks. The group met again six months later for two sessions. The group meetings were structured and supportive. This structured model of group intervention consisted of the following four components.

### 3.3.1   Health education

This consisted of information about health care promotion and maintenance (for example nutrition and the hazards of sun exposure), as well as a series of informal talks about engendering hope and determination and mobilizing coping resources.

### 3.3.2   Stress management

In each group session, according to a pre-established format, the patients were taught specific stress management techniques (for example stress awareness and relaxation training).

### 3.3.3   Enhancement of illness-related coping skills

The method used in this study was modelled after Project Omega (Sobel and Worden 1982 (69); Weisman, Worden, and Sobel 1980 (70)) which focuses primarily on problem solving as a way of diminishing stress and enhancing coping. This approach includes learning an approach to problem solving, practising the approach theoretically, and then applying the approach to personal problems via a series of pictures (one positive and one negative picture for each situation). However, a new series of pictures illustrating ten common problems or situations encountered by cancer patients were developed specifically for this project. Similar to Project Omega, the illustrated problems include loneliness and isolation, fear and apprehension, physician-patient relationships, changes in body image, sexuality and personal contact, communication, social alienation, and depression. Patients were encouraged to apply what they have learned from these pictured situations to their own specific real-life situations.

### 3.3.4   Psychological support

The groups were specifically designed to be supportive in nature, thereby fostering a high degree of cohesion and mutual sharing of concerns and experiences. Members discussed many topics, including illness-related concerns, family problems, and communication with physicians.

### 3.4   RESULTS

### 3.4.1   Profile of Mood States (POMS)

There was a trend showing that the intervention group exhibited better affective state than the control group at six weeks. By six months, these differences had become significant. The intervention group now showed significantly less depression–dejection, fatigue–inertia, confusion–bewilderment, and TMD (total mood disturbance) while showing significantly more vigour–activity (Table 1).

**Table 1**  Mean POMS scores comparing control and intervention groups at six months[a]

|             | Control (n = 28) | S.E.M. | Intervention (n = 38) | S.E.M. | F (1, 61) | p       |
|-------------|------------------|--------|-----------------------|--------|-----------|---------|
| Anxiety     | 8.30             | 0.91   | 6.04                  | 0.77   | 3.30      | .074    |
| Depression  | 7.44             | 1.10   | 3.76                  | 0.93   | 5.99      | .017*   |
| Anger       | 6.67             | 1.16   | 4.92                  | 0.98   | 1.22      | .274    |
| Lack of vigor | 14.33          | 0.85   | 10.39                 | 0.73   | 11.64     | .001*** |
| Fatigue     | 7.77             | 0.91   | 4.88                  | 0.77   | 5.48      | .022*   |
| Confusion   | 5.69             | 0.55   | 3.76                  | 0.47   | 6.55      | .013**  |
| TMD         | 50.30            | 4.29   | 33.67                 | 3.63   | 8.05      | .006**  |

[a] = ANCOVA adjusted treatment means; S.E.M. = Standard error of the mean; $*p < .05$, $**p < .01$, $***p < .001$ with respect to control group; TMD = Total mood disturbance.

### 3.4.2  Coping

At six weeks, the intervention group was using significantly more active-behavioural coping than the control group. Six months after the completion of the intervention schedule the intervention group continued to use significantly more active-behavioural coping and had begun to use significantly more active-cognitive coping methods than the control group. The intervention group was also using significantly more of the effective coping strategies (that is active-positive, active-expressive, active-reliance, cognitive-positive, and distraction), than the control group at both six weeks and at six months. In addition, they were also using the ineffective passive-resignation strategy less often than the control group at six months (Table 2).

### 3.4.3  Psychosocial Adjustment to Illness Scores (PAIS)

Control patients showed slight decreases in five (and increases in three) of the eight PAIS scales at six weeks. Decreases in PAIS scores indicated that less psychological adjustment was required as time went on. The experimental patients had decreases in every category with the amount of decrease being greater than the control in every case. These differences reached significance in the areas of social environment, psychological distress, and total PAIS score at six months (see Table 3).

### 3.4.4  Quality of Life

Experimental patients had an increase of 7.60 points at six weeks and 8.34 points at six months indicating improved Quality of Life compared with

**Table 2** Mean coping scores comparing control and intervention groups at six months [a]

|  | Control (n) | Intervention (n) | F (df) | p-value for treatment effect |
|---|---|---|---|---|
| **COPING METHODS** | | | | |
| Active-Behavioural | 49.59 (28) | 59.88 (38) | 20.86 (1.61) | .0001**** |
| Active-Cognitive | 49.18 (28) | 52.19 (38) | 4.96 (1.61) | .030* |
| Avoidance | 20.53 (28) | 20.68 (37) | 0.03 (1.60) | .860 |
| **COPING STRATEGIES** | | | | |
| Active-Positive | 18.07 (28) | 21.37 (38) | 15.11 (1.61) | .0001**** |
| Active-Expressive | 7.85 (28) | 9.14 (38) | 6.36 (1.61) | .014** |
| Active-Reliance | 6.35 (28) | 8.56 (38) | 7.98 (1.61) | .006** |
| Cognitive-Positive | 22.10 (28) | 24.19 (38) | 6.03 (1.61) | .017* |
| Cognitive-Passive | 7.22 (28) | 7.37 (38) | 0.08 (1.61) | .777 |
| Avoidance-Solitary | 4.02 (28) | 4.04 (37) | 0.00 (1.60) | .971 |
| Distraction | 16.41 (28) | 18.46 (38) | 11.20 (1.61) | .001*** |
| Passive-Resignation | 9.93 (28) | 8.81 (38) | 9.54 (1.61) | .003** [b] |

[a] = ANCOVA adjusted treatment means; [b] = assumption for equality of slopes not met; $^*p < .05$, $^{**}p < .01$, $^{***}p < .001$, $^{****}p < .0001$ with respect to control group.

decreases of 1.65 and 0.23 points, respectively, in the scores of the control patients. These were significant differences.

### 3.4.5 Immune system

The control and intervention groups had immunological values in the range observed for normal healthy individuals and did not differ from each other at baseline. At the end of the intervention (that is at six weeks), the intervention patients showed an increase in CD57 (Leu7[+]) large granular lymphocytes (LGLs) in comparison with controls (see Table 4). Large granular lymphocytes (LGLs) can be found among the CD8 T-cell sub-population and

Table 3 PAIS changes over time between control and intervention groups[a]

| Psychosocial Adjustment to Illness Scale (PAIS) | Baseline | | 6 months | | Interaction | |
|---|---|---|---|---|---|---|
| | Control (n = 28) | Intervention (n = 36) | Control (n = 36) | Intervention (n = 36) | F | P |
| Health care orientation | 50.21 | 52.61 | 50.29 | 50.28 | 1.39 | 0.2437 |
| Vocational environment | 49.93 | 53.64 | 48.29 | 50.97 | 0.48 | 0.4932 |
| Domestic environment | 40.86 | 46.03 | 38.29 | 41.25 | 1.45 | 0.2330 |
| Sexual relationships | 43.61 | 46.58 | 43.96 | 44.72 | 1.09 | 0.3008 |
| Family relationships | 48.82 | 49.97 | 48.75 | 49.67 | 0.02 | 0.8948 |
| Social environment | 29.50 | 41.06 | 32.39 | 33.89 | 13.13 | 0.0006*** |
| Psychological distress | 45.61 | 52.69 | 44.79 | 47.08 | 5.12 | 0.0272* |
| Total PAIS score | 38.86 | 47.53 | 38.36 | 41.19 | 7.43 | 0.0083** |

[a] = Repeated Measures ANOVA; *p < .05, **p < .01, ***p < .001 with respect to control group.

Table 4   Immune variables at baseline, 6 weeks, and 6 months: adjusted treatment means[a] and significance of difference between control and intervention patients

| | Baseline | | | 6 weeks | | | 6 months | | |
|---|---|---|---|---|---|---|---|---|---|
| | Control patients (n) | Intervention patients (n) | p-value for T-test | Control patients (n) | Intervention patients (n) | p-value of F for treatment[d] | Control patients (n) | Intervention patients (n) | p-value of F for treatment[d] |
| **LARGE GRANULAR LYMPHOCYTES** | | | | | | | | | |
| CD57 (LEU 7) | 10.9[b] (26) | 12.1[b] (35) | .467 | 10.7[b] (26) | 12.7[b] (35) | .025* | 11.5[b] (26) | 13.8[b] (35) | .038* |
| **NK PHENOTYPES** | | | | | | | | | |
| CD16 (LEU 11) | 9.6 (26) | 10.3 (35) | .628 | 10.7 (26) | 10.7 (35) | | 10.0 (26) | 13.0 (35) | .022* |
| CD56 (NKH1+) | 13.0 (21) | 13.2 (24) | .956 | 12.8 (21) | 13.1 (24) | | 9.9 (21) | 14.7 (24) | .006* |
| **NK FUNCTION** | | | | | | | | | |
| Augmented NK | 31.3 (16)[c] | 37.1 (17)[c] | .282 | 42.4 (17) | 45.7 (19) | | 43.4 (17) | 63.1 (17) | .034* |

[a] = Baseline means are not adjusted; [b] = percentage of total lymphocytes; [c] = the reduced sample size for the functional tests results from elimination of certain as described in the procedure section; [d] = F tests from ANCOVA; * $p$ values less than 0.05 are presented except for those at baseline values showing no differences between groups.

among the NK cell population. Dual marker analysis indicated that the LGL (Leu7$^+$) percentage in the CD8 (Leu2$^+$) population was increased substantially but no increase was seen in the population of cells that are LGLs and NK cells (that is Leu7$^+$, Leu11$^+$). Only Leu7$^+$ cells that were Leu11$^-$ were elevated at six weeks. Thus it would appear that the increase in LGLs in the intervention patients took place in the CD8 T-cell subpopulation and not in the NK cells at this time. No other significant changes were detected at six weeks.

Six months after completion of the intervention, LGLs (Leu7$^+$ cells) remained increased (see Table 4). However, at this time point the Leu7$^+$ cell increase was seen in the NK (Leu11$^+$) cells, but not in the CD8 (Leu2$^+$) cells.

NK cells, as determined by both CD16 (Leu11) and CD56 (NKH1$^+$) markers, were also increased at six months in the intervention versus the control group (see Table 4). This change was seen mainly in NK cells carrying both NKH$^+$ and Leu11 antigens.

The alpha interferon-augmented NK response was another factor that increased significantly in the intervention group at the sixth month time point (see Table 4). The mean resting value for NK cytotoxicity although higher in the intervention group was not significantly different from the control group.

In order to determine the number of patients in each group who showed immune alterations over time as well as the extent of these changes, individual patients' immune changes over time were evaluated. Small increases (defined as a change from 1 to 25 per cent) and a large increase (defined as a greater than 25 per cent change) were determined. The data (see Table 5) indicate that the majority of subjects in the intervention group showed increases in LGLs and NK cells while the controls did not. The largest increases were seen in the percentage of NK cells (Leu11) and LGLs (Leu7) in the intervention group. While a majority of the intervention patients also showed a moderate to large increase in NK-cell activity (data not shown) and interferon alpha-augmented NK-cell activity, similar increases were seen in the controls.

Four of the POMS subscales may be considered measures of affective state. These are anxiety, depression, anger, and confusion. One aim of the intervention was to improve affective state so these subscales as well as total mood disturbance (TMD) were chosen for correlation with several of the other psychological and behaviour measures as well as with certain immune parameters. The correlations were done on all patients combined to determine if a relationship exists between changes in affective state and the other variables regardless of whether or not these changes might be attributed to the intervention.

**Table 5** Percentage of subjects (*n*) in control and intervention groups who showed a decrease/no change, a small increase, or moderate-to-large increase in immune parameters from baseline to 6 months

| | Control patients | | | | Intervention patients | | | |
|---|---|---|---|---|---|---|---|---|
| | (*n*) | Decrease/ no change (*n*) | Small increase 1–25% (*n*) | Moderate or large increase 26–100% (*n*) | (*n*) | Decrease/ no change (*n*) | Small increase 1–25% (*n*) | Moderate or large increase 26–100% (*n*) |
| **LARGE GRANULAR LYMPHOCYTES** | | | | | | | | |
| CD57 (LEU 7) | (26) | 61.5% (16) | 30.8% (8) | 7.7% (2) | (35) | 5.7% (2) | 48.6% (17) | 45.7% (16) |
| **NK CELLS** | | | | | | | | |
| CD16 (LEU 11) | (26) | 61.5% (16) | 30.8% (8) | 3.9%[a] (1) | (35) | 0% (0) | 31.4% (11) | 68.6% (24) |
| CD56 (NKH1+) | (21) | 57.1% (12) | 28.6% (6) | 14.3% (3) | (23) | 26.1% (6) | 56.5% (13) | 17.4% (4) |
| **NK FUNCTION** | | | | | | | | |
| Augmented NK | (16) | 12.5% (2) | 31.3% (5) | 56.2% (9) | (17) | 17.6% (3) | 11.8% (2) | 64.7%[a] (11) |

$$\% \text{ increase} = \frac{T_2 \text{ (6 months)} - T_0 \text{ (baseline)}}{T_0} \times 100$$

[a] = one more patient increased but had an undetectable baseline value, so that the percentage of increase could not be calculated.

### 3.4.6   Coping with POMS correlations

For the intervention patients at six months, avoidance coping method was significantly and positively correlated with anxiety, depression, confusion, and TMD and negatively, although non-significantly, with anger. Active-cognitive coping was negatively correlated with anger and TMD (see Table 6).

### 3.4.7   POMS with PAIS correlations

For all patients combined, decreases in five of the seven PAIS subscales, as well as the total PAIS score (indicating that less psychosocial adjustment was necessary) showed positive correlations with most of the four affective scales of the POMS and total mood disturbance (only family relationships and social environment failed to show any significant correlations). Domestic environment, sexual relationships, psychological distress, and total PAIS score were significantly positively correlated with anxiety, depression, confusion, and total mood disturbance. Vocational environment correlated with depression and confusion while health care orientation correlated with all four scales and TMD (see Table 7). In other words as negative affect states decreased, the amount of psychosocial adjustment to illness that was needed by these patients also decreased. Of note is that decreases in psychological distress measured in the PAIS had the strongest correlations with decreases in three of the POMS subscales as well as with total mood disturbance.

### 3.4.8   POMS with Quality of Life correlations

For all patients Quality of Life showed strong negative correlations with the four affective POMS subscales (anxiety, depression, anger, and confusion) and total mood disturbance. This shows that as negative affective state decreased the Quality of Life of these patients improved (see Table 8).

### 3.4.9   PAIS with Quality of Life correlations

Just as most of the POMS scales correlated negatively with Quality of Life, so did the PAIS scales (see Table 9). Only health-care orientation and extended family relationships fail to show a significant correlation. Decreases in psychological distress again show the strongest of these correlations.

### 3.4.10   POMS with Immune Measures correlations

Some immune parameters also showed an association with the affective state subscales as well as with total mood disturbance. CD57 LGLs (Leu7) were

# Chapter 11 (table 6)

Table 6  Pearson correlations between unadjusted mood scores (POMS) and coping scores at 6 months in control and intervention groups combined (n = 66)

| | Anxiety | | Depression | | Anger | | Confusion | | TMD[a] | |
|---|---|---|---|---|---|---|---|---|---|---|
| | r | p | r | p | r | p | r | p | r | p |
| **COPING METHODS** | | | | | | | | | | |
| Active-Behavioural | -0.11 | 0.400 | -0.12 | 0.327 | -0.07 | 0.591 | -0.07 | 0.567 | -0.17 | 0.185 |
| Active-Cognitive | -0.16 | 0.192 | -0.21 | 0.086 | -0.27 | 0.027* | -0.17 | 0.181 | -0.25 | 0.041* |
| Avoidance | 0.43 | 0.0004*** | 0.43 | 0.0003*** | 0.23 | 0.058 | 0.28 | 0.022* | 0.46 | 0.0001**** |
| **COPING STRATEGIES** | | | | | | | | | | |
| Active-Positive | -0.20 | 0.101 | -0.21 | 0.098 | -0.17 | 0.184 | -0.17 | 0.180 | -0.28 | 0.021* |
| Active-Expressive | -0.23 | 0.062 | -0.27 | 0.031* | -0.12 | 0.331 | -0.24 | 0.056 | -0.28 | 0.021 |
| Active-Reliance | -0.13 | 0.301 | -0.04 | 0.758 | 0.01 | 0.933 | 0.01 | 0.965 | -0.10 | 0.424 |
| Cognitive-Positive | -0.17 | 0.182 | -0.28 | 0.023* | -0.33 | 0.007** | -0.21 | 0.096 | -0.31 | 0.012** |
| Cognitive-Passive | 0.30 | 0.014** | 0.28 | 0.022* | 0.06 | 0.608 | 0.32 | 0.008** | 0.29 | 0.019* |
| Avoidance-Solitary | 0.22 | 0.072 | 0.29 | 0.019* | 0.14 | 0.278 | 0.09 | 0.463 | 0.22 | 0.079 |
| Distraction | 0.18 | 0.153 | 0.15 | 0.222 | 0.16 | 0.197 | 0.02 | 0.874 | 0.11 | 0.364 |
| Passive-Resignation | 0.11 | 0.380 | 0.07 | 0.587 | 0.04 | 0.748 | 0.13 | 0.303 | 0.16 | 0.202 |

[a] = Total Mood Disturbance; $*p < .05$, $**p < .01$, $***p < .001$, $****p < .0001$.

**Table 7** Pearson correlations between unadjusted mood scores (POMS) and personal adjustment to illness scale (PAIS) at 6 months in control and intervention groups combined ($n = 66$)

| Psychosocial adjustment to Illness Scale (PAIS) | Anxiety | | Depression | | Anger | | Confusion | | TMD[a] | |
|---|---|---|---|---|---|---|---|---|---|---|
| | r | p | r | p | r | p | r | p | r | p |
| Health care orientation | 0.29 | 0.017* | 0.27 | 0.028* | 0.24 | 0.057 | 0.33 | 0.007** | 0.27 | 0.029 |
| Vocational environment | 0.22 | 0.071 | 0.27 | 0.029* | −0.08 | 0.521 | 0.29 | 0.020* | 0.22 | 0.076 |
| Domestic environment | 0.36 | 0.003** | 0.46 | 0.0001**** | 0.12 | 0.327 | 0.44 | 0.0002*** | 0.39 | 0.001*** |
| Sexual relationships | 0.29 | 0.020* | 0.38 | 0.001*** | 0.08 | 0.535 | 0.28 | 0.022* | 0.34 | 0.005** |
| Extended family relationships | −0.16 | 0.212 | −0.21 | 0.086 | −0.14 | 0.274 | −0.08 | 0.547 | −0.13 | 0.304 |
| Social environment | 0.14 | 0.279 | 0.21 | 0.089 | −0.09 | 0.474 | 0.20 | 0.106 | 0.16 | 0.186 |
| Psychological distress | 0.43 | 0.0003** | 0.55 | 0.0001**** | 0.21 | 0.097 | 0.54 | 0.0001 | 0.49 | 0.0001**** |
| Total PAIS | 0.33 | 0.007** | 0.4 | 0.001*** | 0.03 | 0.802 | 0.41 | 0.001*** | 0.36 | 0.003** |

[a] = Total Mood Disturbance; *$p < .05$, **$p < .01$, ***$p < .001$, ****$p < .0001$.

**Table 8** Pearson correlations ($r$) between unadjusted POMS scores and quality of life at 6 months in control and intervention groups combined ($n = 66$)

| | Quality of life | |
|---|---|---|
| Profile of mood states (POMS) | $r$ | $p$ |
| Anxiety | −0.45 | 0.0001** |
| Depression | −0.53 | 0.0001** |
| Anger | −0.33 | 0.0065* |
| Confusion | −0.55 | 0.0001** |
| Total mood disturbance | −0.51 | 0.0001** |

*$p < .01$, **$p < .0001$.

**Table 9** Pearson correlations between unadjusted personal adjustment to illness scale (PAIS) and quality of life at 6 months in control and intervention groups combined ($n = 66$)

| | Quality of life | |
|---|---|---|
| Personal adjustment to illness scale | $r$ | $p$ |
| Health care orientation | −0.17 | 0.1814 |
| Vocational environment | −0.27 | 0.0322* |
| Domestic environment | −0.55 | 0.0001**** |
| Sexual relationships | −0.43 | 0.0004*** |
| Family relationships | −0.07 | 0.5854 |
| Social environment | −0.31 | 0.0127** |
| Psychological distress | −0.52 | 0.0001**** |
| Total PAIS | −0.52 | 0.0001**** |

*$p < .05$, **$p < .01$, ***$p < .001$, ****$p < .0001$

significantly negatively correlated with anxiety, depression, and TMD, and positively correlated with anger. Interferon alpha augmented NK-cell activity correlated negatively with anxiety and TMD, and positively correlated with anger (see Table 10).

3.5 DISCUSSION

This structured psychiatric intervention, lasting six weeks, proved useful in increasing effective coping and decreasing the affective distress that often accompanies the diagnosis of cancer. It also served to decrease the amount of psychosocial adjustment to illness that was required by these patients as well as increasing their overall quality of life and enhancing some parameters of the immune system (that is LGLs, NK-cells, and augmented NK-cell activity).

**Table 10** Pearson correlations between mood scores (POMS) and immune values at 6 months in intervention and control patients combined

| | CD57 (LEU 7) (n = 61) | | CD16 (LEU 11) (n = 61) | | CD56 (NKH1) (n = 44) | | Augmented NK (IFK25) (n = 33) | |
|---|---|---|---|---|---|---|---|---|
| | r | p | r | p | r | p | r | p |
| Anxiety | −0.32 | 0.013** | −0.24 | 0.066 | −0.08 | 0.618 | −0.37 | 0.035* |
| Depression | −0.32 | 0.012** | −0.12 | 0.355 | −0.24 | 0.124 | −0.33 | 0.059 |
| Anger | −0.39 | 0.002** | −0.17 | 0.180 | −0.18 | 0.246 | −0.45 | 0.008** |
| Confusion | −0.17 | 0.183** | −0.09 | 0.471 | −0.16 | 0.294 | −0.09 | 0.605 |
| Total mood disturbance | −0.28 | 0.030* | −0.11 | 0.403 | −0.17 | 0.271 | −0.15 | 0.407 |

$^*p < .05$, $^{**}p < .01$.

A clear pattern of relationships also emerged between the coping methods and affective state. As effective coping increased, negative affective state decreased. Patients who were coping better felt better psychologically. In turn there were strong relationships between affective state and psychosocial adjustment, quality of life, and some immune parameters. Improvement in psychological state was accompanied by a decreased need for adjustment to illness. When patients felt better psychologically and were requiring less psychosocial adjustment their perception of their overall quality of life improved. Finally, decreases in anxiety, depression, and TMD, and increases in anger were associated with increases in LGLs and augmented NK-cell activity.

The positive psychological effects of this short-term intervention were apparent by the end of the six-week programme. These positive results were either maintained or enhanced over the following six months as the patients practised and improved their newly learned skills.

This study used a structured psychiatric group intervention encompassing various modalities (that is education, problem solving, stress management through relaxation, and psychological support). Since the intervention was structured and time-limited, it can be implemented in research studies and/or clinical care areas to help patients adjust to the diagnosis and treatment of cancer.

While other studies dealt mainly with patients with advanced disease and poor prognosis, our patients had early-stage cancer and good prognoses. These patients are part of a rapidly growing group of individuals who must learn to live with having had cancer, and they are ideal subjects to benefit from early interventions. These interventions should assist patients to overcome the crisis of cancer and return to fully productive, enjoyable lives by replacing initial feelings such as lack of vigour, confusion–bewilderment, helplessness, and hopelessness with a sense of energy, mastery, confidence, and hope.

# 4   Five-year survival

Although our structured, short-term psycho-educational intervention can be useful in enhancing coping and lowering levels of distress for some patients, determining the impact of the intervention on survival was not among the goals of the original study. The study was not specifically designed to investigate such an impact and the number of patients involved is quite small. This severely limits generalizations. Despite the small sample size, especially in the high risk category, the results warrant further research in this area with a larger number of properly stratified subjects.

However, we have studied the intervention effects on survival. This analysis indicates that those subjects who participated in the structured, six-week, psycho-educational intervention had a statistically significant better survival rate than the control subjects (see Table 11). Since our control group was shown to be representative of the norm, and since our control and experimental groups were well-matched groups that had been randomly assigned, these results suggest that the intervention could well have played some role in the differential survival outcomes (71, 72).

A number of explanations are possible. The intervention may have fostered (via increased knowledge and encouragement) improved health habits (for example sunblock use, time of sun exposure, better nutrition, and exercise regimens). Effective coping may have been increased resulting in such things as good doctor–patient partnerships, positive mental attitudes, and greater compliance with treatment and follow-up regimens.

Richardson *et al.* (73) found that special educational and supportive programmes designed to improve patient compliance were associated with significant prolongation of patient survival due to, as well as independent of, their effects on compliance. Subjects in the present study may have learned to better manage their stress by eliminating or altering their personal stressors through problem-solving, changing their attitudes towards stressors (for example perceiving them as less important and, therefore, less stressful), and/or altering their physiological response to stress through relaxation techniques.

Social support has been reported to be related to health outcomes (74–77). Patients in the intervention group received a great deal of social support from their participation in the groups. They were able to express their feelings freely to an understanding and sympathetic audience. They also had the benefit of hearing how others were dealing with the stresses of the same disease. Although the intervention appears to have benefited some patients, we cannot specify which parts of the intervention were most beneficial for particular individuals.

**Table 11**   The effect of intervention on survival

| Outcome | Control | Experimental | Log Rank Test |
|---------|---------|--------------|---------------|
|         | (out of 37) | (out of 37) |              |
| **Survival** |    |              | $p = .008$ |
| Dead    | 12      | 3            |               |
| Alive   | 25      | 34           |               |

# 5   Summary and conclusions

The diagnosis of cancer frequently produces psychological distress. This distress may in turn impact on the immune system although the mechanisms by which this may occur as well as the clinical implications involved are still largely hypothetical. What is clear is that the studies we have reviewed show that early-stage interventions that encourage active-behavioural coping and active-cognitive coping rather than avoidance or passive acceptance of the illness can be helpful psychologically. These active behavioural and cognitive coping behaviors, which can be learned, can attenuate the psychological distress caused by stressful illness, decrease the amount of psychosocial adjustment to the illness needed, improve overall quality of life, and may also be associated with longer survival time (4, 51–52, 75, 78–80).

5.1   ACKNOWLEDGEMENTS

This study was supported by a grant from the UCLA Neuropsychoimmunology Task Force and the authors wish to express their deep appreciation for the Task Force's ongoing support.

# 6   References

1.  Schmale, A. H. (1974). Perspective: The psychosocial interaction of the patient, the cancer and their physicians. In *Clinical Oncology for Medical Students and Physicians, a Multidisciplinary Approach*, (4th edn), (ed. P. Rubin) American Cancer Society, Atlanta, USA.

2.  Holland, J. (1973). Psychological aspects of cancer. In *Cancer Medicine*, (eds J. R. Holland and E. Frei), pp. 991–1021. Lea and Febiger, Philadelphia.

3.  Pfefferbaum, B., Pasnau, R. O., Jamison, K., and Wellisch, D. K. (1977). A comprehensive program of psychosocial care for mastectomy patients. *Int. J. Psychiatry Med.*, 8, 63–71.

4.  Greer, S., Morris, T., and Pettingale, K. W. (1979). Psychological response to breast cancer: Effect on outcome. *Lancet*, 2, 785–787.

5. Parkes, C. M. (1975). The emotional impact of cancer on patients and their families. *J. Laryngol. Otol.*, **89**, 1271–1279.

6. Morris, T., Greer, H. S., and White, P. (1977). Psychological and social adjustment to mastectomy: A two-year follow-up study. *Cancer*, **40**, 2361–2387.

7. Maguire, G. P., Lee, E. G., Bevington, D. J., Kuchemann, C., Crabtree, R. J., and Cornell, C. E. (1978). Psychiatric problems in the first year after mastectomy. *Br. Med. J.*, **1**, 963–965.

8. Fawzy, F. I. and Fawzy, N. W. (1982). Psychosocial aspects of cancer. In *Diagnosis and Management of Cancer*, (ed. D. W. Nixon), pp. 111–123. Addison-Wesley, Menlo Park, CA.

9. Peck, A. (1972). Emotional reactions to having cancer. *Am. J. Roentgenol. Radium Ther. Nucl. Med.*, **114**, 591–599.

10. Bahnson, C. (1975). Psychologic and emotional issues in cancer: The psychotherapeutic care of the cancer patient. *Sem. Oncol.*, **2**, 293–309.

11. Namir, S., Wolcott, D. L., Fawzy, F. I., and Alumbagh, M. J. (1987). Coping with AIDS: Psychological and health implications. *J. Appl. Psychol.*, **17**, 309–328.

12. Bloom, J. R. (1982). Social support, accommodation to stress and adjustment to breast cancer. *Soc. Sci. Med.*, **16**, 1329–1338.

13. Holahan, C. J. and Moos, R. H. (1983). *Life Stress and Health: Personality, Coping and Family Support in Stress Resistance*. Stanford University Social Ecology Laboratory, Palo Alto, CA.

14. Billings, A. G. and Moos, R. H. (1981). The role of coping responses and social resources in attenuating the stress of life events. *J. of Behav. Med.*, **4**, 139–157.

15. Felton, B. J., Revenson, T. A., and Hinrichsen, G. A. (1984). Stress and coping in the explanation of psychological adjustment among chronically ill adults. *Soc. Sci. Med.*, **18**, 889–898.

16. Bartrop, R. W., Luckhurst, E., Lazarus, L., Kiloh, L. G., and Penny, R. (1977). Depressed lymphocyte function after bereavement. *Lancet*, **1**, 834–836.

17. Schleifer, S. J., Keller, S. E., Camerino, M., Thornton, J. C., and Stein, M. (1983). Suppression of lymphocyte stimulation following bereavement. *J. Am. Med. Assoc.*, **250**, 374–377.

18. Irwin, M., Daniels, M., Smith, T. L., Bloom, E., and Weiner, H. (1987). Impaired natural killer cell activity during bereavement. *Brain, Behav. Immun.*, **1**, 98–104.

19. Kiecolt-Glaser, J. K., Fisher, L. D., Ogrocki, P., Stout, J., Speicher, C., and Glaser, R. (1987). Marital quality, marital disruption and immune function. *Psychosom. Med.*, **49**, 13–34.

20. Kiecolt-Glaser, J. K., Kennedy, S., Malkoff, S., Fisher, L., Speicher, C. E., and Glaser, R. (1988). Marital discord and immunity in males. *Psychosom. Med.*, **50**, 213–229.

21. Kiecolt-Glaser, J. K., Garner, W., Speicher, C., Penn, G., Holliday, J., and Glaser, R. (1984). Psychosocial modifiers of immunocompetence in medical students. *Psychosom. Med.*, **46**, 7–14.

22. Dorian, B. J., Garfinkle, P. E., Brown, G., Shore, A., Gladman, D., and Keystone, E. (1982). Aberrations in lymphocyte subpopulations and functions during stress. *Clin. Exper. Immunol.*, **50**, 132–138.

23. Kiecolt-Glaser, J. K., Glaser, R., Dyer, C., Shuttleworth, E., Ogrocki, P., and Speicher, C. E. (1987). Chronic stress and immunity in family caregivers of Alzheimer's Disease victims. *Psychosom. Med.*, **49**, 523–535.

24. Palmblad, J., Cantell, K., Strander, H., Froberg, J., Karlson, C., Levi, L. *et al.* (1976). Stressor exposure and immunological response in man: Interferon-producing capacity and phagocytosis. *J. Psychosom. Res.*, **20**, 193–199.

25. Linn, B. S. and Jensen, J. (1983). Age and immune response to a surgical stress. *Arch. Surg.*, **118**, 405–409.

26. Kronfol, Z., Silva, Jr. J., Greden, J., Dembinski, S., Gardner, R., and Carroll, B. (1983). Impaired lymphocyte function in depressive illness. *Life Sci.*, **33**, 241–247.

27. Kronfol, Z., Turner, R., Nasrallah, H., and Winokur, G. (1984). Leukocyte regulation in depression and schizophrenia. *Psychiatry Res.*, **13**, 13–18.

28. Kronfol, Z. (1987). Depression and the immune system. In *Presentations of Depression: Depressive Symptoms in Medical and Other Psychiatric Disorders*, (ed. O. G. Cameron), pp. 341–353. John Wiley, New York.

29. Krueger, R. B., Levy, E. M., Cathcart, E. S., Fox, B. H., and Black, P. H. (1984). Lymphocyte subsets in patients with major depression: Preliminary findings. *Advances: J. Inst. Advance. Health*, **1**, 5–9.

30. Linn, M. W., Linn, B. S., and Jensen, J. (1984). Stressful events, dysphoric mood, and immune responsiveness. *Psychol. Rep.*, **54**, 219–222.

31. Albrecht, J., Helderman, J. H., Schlesser, M. A., and Rush, A. J. (1985). A controlled study of cellular immune function in affective disorders before and during somatic therapy. *Psychiatry Res.*, **15**, 185–193.

32. Stein, M., Keller, S. E., and Schleifer, S. J. (1985). Stress and immunomodulation: The role of depression and neuroendocrine function. *J. Immunol.*, **135**, 827s–833s.

33. Schleifer, S. J., Keller, S. E., Meyerson A. T., Raskin, M. J., Davis, K. L., and Stein, M. (1984). Lymphocyte function in major depressive order. *Arch. Gen. Psychiatry*, **41**, 484–486.

34. Schleifer, S. J., Keller, S. E., Bond, R. N., Cohen, J., and Stein, M. (1989) Major depressive disorder and immunity: Role of age, sex, severity, and hospitalization. *Archives of General Psychiatry*, **46**, 81–87.

35. Kemeny, M. E., Cohen, F., Zegans, L. S., and Conant, M. A. (1989). Psychological and immunological predictors of genital herpes recurrence. *Psychosom. Med.*, **51**, 195–208.

36. Kiecolt-Glaser, J. K., Ricker, D., George, J., Messick, G., Speicher, C., Garner, W., and Glaser, R. (1984). Urinary cortisol levels, cellular immunocompetence, and loneliness in psychiatric patients. *Psychosom. Med.*, **46**, 15–23.

37. Glaser, G., Kiecolt-Glaser, J. K., George, J. M., Speicher, C. E., and Holliday, J. E. (1985). Stress, loneliness, and changes in herpes virus latency. *J. Behav. Med.*, **8**, 249–260.

38. Laudenslager, M. L., Ryan, S. M., Drugan, R. C., Hyson, R. L., and Maier, S. F. (1983). Coping and immunosuppression: Inescapable but not escapable shock suppresses lymphocyte proliferations. *Science*, **221**, 568–570.

39. Pennebaker, J. W., Kiecolt-Glaser, J. K., and Glaser, R. (1988). Disclosure

of traumas and immune function: Health implications for psychotherapy. *J. Consult. Clin. Psychol.*, **56**, 239–245.

40. Pettingale, K. W., Greer, S., and Tee, D. E. H. (1977). Serum IgA and emotional expression in breast cancer patients. *J. Psychosom. Res.*, **21**, 395–399.

41. Linn, B. S. and Harris, R. (1982). Effects of counseling for late stage cancer patients. *Cancer*, **49**, 1948–1055.

42. Gordon, W. A., Freidenbergs, I., Diller, L., Hibbard, M., Wolf, C., Levine, L. *et al.* (1980). Efficacy of psychosocial intervention with cancer patients. *J. Consult. Clin. Psychol.*, **48**, 743–759.

43. Zimbardo, P. and Ebbeson, E. B. (1970). *Influencing Attitudes and Changing Behavior*. Addision Wesley, Reading, MA.

44. Ali, N. and Khalil, H. (1989). Effects of psychoeducational intervention on anxiety among Egyptian bladder cancer patients. *Cancer Nurs.*, **12**(4), 236–242.

45. Burish, T. G. and Lyles, J. N. (1981). Effectiveness of relaxation training in reducing adverse reactions to cancer chemotherapy. *J. Behav. Med.*, **4**, 65–78.

46. Burish, T. G., Snyder, S. L., and Jenkins, R. A. (1991). Preparing patients for cancer chemotherapy: effect of coping preparation and relaxation interventions. *J. Consult. Clin. Psychol.*, **59**(4), 518–525.

47. Bridge, L. R., Benson, P., Pietroni, P. C., and Priest, R. G. (1988). Relaxation and imagery in the treatment of breast cancer. *Br. Med. J.*, **297**, 1169–1172.

48. Ferlic, M., Goldman, A., and Kennedy, B. J. (1979). Group counseling in adult patients with advanced cancer. *Cancer*, **43**, 760–766.

49. Gordon, W. A., Freidenbergs, I., Diller, L., Hibbard, M., Wolf, C., Levine, L. *et al.* (1980). Efficacy of psychosocial intervention with cancer patients. *J. Consult. Clin. Psychol.*, **48**, 743–759.

50. Vachon, M. L. and Lyall, W. A. (1976). Applying psychiatric techniques to patients with cancer. *Hosp. Commun. Psychiatry*, **27**, 582–584.

51. Parsell, S. and Taglarena, E. M. (1975). Cancer patients help each other. *Am. J. Nurs.*, **74**, 650–651.

52. Spiegel, D., Bloom, J. R., and Yalom, I. D. (1981). Group support for metastatic cancer patients: A randomized prospective outcome study. *Arch. Gen. Psychiatry*, **38**, 527–533.

53. Spiegel, D., Bloom, J. R., Kraemer, H. C., and Gottheil, E. (1989). Effect of psychosocial treatment on survival of patients with metastatic breast cancer. *Lancet*, **2**, 888–891.

54. Greer, S., Moorey, S., Baruch, J. D. R., Watson, M., Robertson, B. M., Mason, A. *et al.* (1992). Adjuvant psychological therapy for patients with cancer: a prospective randomized trial. *Br. Med. J.*, **304**, 675–680.

55. Edgar, L., Rosberger, Z., and Nowlis, D. (1992). Coping with cancer during the first year after diagnosis: assessment and intervention. *Cancer*, **69**, 817–828.

56. Kiecolt-Glaser, J. K., Glaser, R., Williger, D., Stout, J., Messick, G., Sheppard, S. *et al.* (1985). Psychosocial enhancement of immunocompetence in a geriatric population. *Health Psychol.*, **4**, 25–41.

57. Kiecolt-Glaser, J. K., Glaser, R., Strain, E., Stout, J., Tarr, K., Holliday, J.

et al. (1986). Modulation of cellular immunity in medical students. J. Behav. Med., 9, 5-21.

58. Gruber, B. L., Hall, N. R., Hersh, S. P., and Dubois, P. (1988). Immune System and psychological changes in metastatic cancer patients using relaxation and guided imagery: A pilot study. Scand. J. Behav. Ther., 17, 25-35.

59. Thestrup-Pedersen, K. (1975). Suppression of tuberculin skin reactivity by prior tuberculin skin testing. Immunology, 28, 342-348.

60. Black, S., Humphrey, J. H., and Niven, J. S. (1963). Inhibition of Mantoux reaction by direct suggestion under hypnosis. Br. Med. J., 6, 1649-1652.

61. Smith, G. R. and McDaniel, S. M. (1983). Psychologically mediated effect on the delayed hypersensitivity reaction to tuberculin in humans. Psychosom. Med., 45, 65-70.

62. Zachariae, R., Bjerring, P., and Arendt-Nielsen, L. (1989). Modulation of Type I immediate and Type IV delayed immunoreactivity using direct suggestion and guided imagery during hypnosis. Allergy, 44, 537-542.

63. Fawzy, F. I., Cousins, N., Fawzy, N. W., Kemeny, M. E., Elashoff, R., and Morton, D. (1990). A structured psychiatric intervention for cancer patients, I: Changes over time in methods of coping and affective disturbances. Arch. Gen. Psychiatry, 47, 720-725.

64. Fawzy, F. I., Cousins, N., Kemeny, M. E., Fawzy, N. W., Elashoff, R., Morton, D. et al. (1990). A structured psychiatric intervention for cancer patients, II: Changes over time in immunological parameters. Arch. Gen. Psychiatry, 47, 729-735.

65. McNair, D. M., Lorr, M., and Doppelman, L. F. (1971). Profile of Mood States Instrument. In Manual for the Profile of Mood States (eds D. M. McNair, M. Lorr, and L. F. Doppelman). Educational and Industrial Testing Service, San Diego, CA.

66. Derogatis, L. R. (1983). Administration Manual for the Psychosocial Adjustment to Illness Scale (PAIS). Clinical Psychometric Research, Maryland.

67. Padilla, G. V., Presant, C. A., Grant, M., Baer, C., and Metter, G. (1981). Assessment of quality of life in cancer patients. Proceedings of the American Association for Cancer Research (72nd Annual Meeting) and the American Society of Clinical Oncology (17th Annual Meeting), 22, 397.

68. Barlozzari, T., Leonhardt, J., Wiltrout, R. H., Herberman, R. B., and Reynolds, C. W. (1985). Direct evidence for the role of LGL in the inhibition of experimental tumor metastases. J. Immunol., 134, 2783-2789.

69. Sobel, H. J. and Worden, J. W. (1982). Helping Cancer Patients Cope: Practitioner's Manual. Guilford Publications, New York.

70. Weisman, A. D., Worden J. W., and Sobel, H. J. (1980). Psychosocial screening intervention with cancer patients. Project Omega, Boston.

71. Fawzy, F. I. and Fawzy, N. W. (1994). Psychoeducational interventions and health outcomes. Handbook on Stress and Immunity. (In press.)

72. Fawzy, F. I., Fawzy, N. W., Hyun, C., Elashoff, R., Guthrie, D., Fahey, J. et al. (1994). Malignant melanoma: Effects of an early structured psychiatric intervention, coping, and affective state on recurrence and survival six years later. Arch. Psychiatry. (In press.)

73. Richardson, J. L., Shelton, D. R., Krailo, M., and Levine, A. M. (1990). The effect of compliance with treatment on survival among patients with hematologic malignancies. *J. Clin. Oncol.*, **8**, 356–364.

74. Rabkin, J. and Streuning, E. (1976). Life events, stress, and illness. *Science*, **194**, 1013–1020.

75. Rogentine, Jr. G. N., Van Kammen, D. P., Fox, B. H., Docherty, J. P., Rosenblatt, J. E., Boyd, S. C. *et al.* (1979). Psychological factors in the prognosis of malignant melanoma: A prospective study. *Psychosom. Med.*, **41**, 647–655.

76. Sklar, L. and Anisman, H. (1981). Stress and cancer. *Psychol. Bull.*, **89**, 369–406.

77. Soloman, G. S. and Amkrant, A. A. (1981). Psychoneuroendocrinological effects on the immune response. *Ann. Rev. Microbiol.*, **35**, 155–184.

78. Derogatis, L. R., Abeloff, M. D., and Melisaratos, N. (1979). Psychological coping mechanisms and survival time in metastatic breast cancer. *J. Am. Med. Assoc.*, **242**, 1504–1508.

79. Greer, S. (1991). Psychological response to cancer and survival. *Psychol. Med.*, **21**(1), 43–49.

80. Ornish, D., Brown, S. E., Scherwitz, L. W., Billings, J. H., Armstrong, W. T., Ports, T. A. *et al.* (1992). Can lifestyle changes reverse coronary heart disease? *Lancet*, **336**(8708), 129–133.

# 12

# Correlation of psychological, endocrine, and immune parameters in cancer patients: the WITTEN study

## K. S. ZANKER

## 1  Introduction

### 1.1 THE IMPACT OF EMOTIONAL STATUS ON DISEASE: HISTORICAL PERSPECTIVES

As our understanding of the molecular pathogenesis of infectious diseases and cancer has increased, it has become increasingly apparent that patients do not develop illnesses simply because of the presence of a pathogenic micro-organism or a carcinogen. An array of factors associated both with the host and the pathogen/carcinogen interact to influence disease outcome. Both clinicians and laypersons here noted that the emotional or psychological stresses of life have an effect on general physical well-being and health.

Based on numerous historical reports that emotional stress appeared to influence susceptibility to, and rate of recovery from, infectious diseases, several groups of investigators have attempted to develop experimental animal systems to study these phenomena under controlled laboratory conditions. Most of these were conducted during the late 1950s and 1960s at the Universities of Los Angeles, Rochester, and Stanford, USA.

The UCLA (1) studies were carried out using Swiss mice as the experimental host with the main stressor being an avoidance-learning shuttle box apparatus. The results of these experiments showed that avoidance-learning and confinement stress induced such changes as hypotrophy of the adrenal gland, spleen, and thymus, as well as leukopaenia. They also showed that young mice, when inoculated with polyoma virus and subjected to a combination of sound and avoidance-learning stress, developed a higher incidence of tumours than non-stressed control mice. The Rochester group (2) attempted to develop an animal model to help elucidate the physiological and social factors which influence host resistance to disease processes. Other studies were conducted by these workers on the influence of stress on tumour growth in rats.

The Stanford group (3) explored the possible interrelationship between emotional stress and immunological functions. While much of this work was concerned with the possible influence of stress on cancer and autoimmune diseases, many of these studies dealt with basic immune responses. What at that time began to emerge from these results was the concept that the effects of emotional stress on the host–parasite/tumour relationships are often subtle. The original concepts that the influence of stress are cumulative and always in the direction of increased susceptibility were not always supported by experimental findings.

Human studies were also undertaken in parallel with these animal experiments. A number of these indicated an increase in the numbers of infectious diseases in individuals of a group or culture undergoing major social adjustment. Other forms of emotional stress have been clearly correlated with increased recurrence of herpes simplex virus lesions. However, it should be noted that some studies failed to show this association. Employees who were burdened with extra responsibilities, frustrations, and worries were seen to be more likely to be absent from work as a result of common illness than were their more contented, well-adjusted co-workers. Moreover, students who had good psychological health had a more rapid rate of recovery from infectious mononucleosis than students who had a low ego-strength.

During the 1970s, there was a marked increase in the number of valid studies measuring emotional entities and employing newly improved techniques to determine the neurochemical messengers involved. At the same time, knowledge of the factors regulating the function of immune cells system grew exponentially. As neuroendocrine and immune parameters were not directly measured in early studies of the psychological aspects of health/disease, results published during the decade of the 1980s could only be interpreted as indicating that stress, in some undefined way, altered the incidence and development of infectious and malignant diseases in animals. Although preliminary data indicated that some stressful procedures might suppress immune functions by altering brain and plasma levels of certain neuropeptides and hormones, the lack of solid information correlating psychological, endocrine, and immune parameters seems to have been a hallmark in early studies in psychoneuroimmunology. There have been few prospective studies in which psychosocial factors have been correlated with neuroendocrine and immunological parameters for the same patients.

Greer and colleagues performed a seminal study (the longest prospective study of its kind, to date) on the relationship between the psychological response to cancer and disease outcome. It suggested that patients who responded with fighting spirit or with denial were significantly more likely to be alive and free of recurrence than were patients with a fatalistic or help-less response (4, 5). A second prospective study on the effect on survival of psychological support for cancer patients was published by Spiegel and colleagues (6). They reported that psychosocial intervention can enhance survival of patients with metastatic breast cancer.

One major shortcoming of both studies was that the relevant neuro-endocrine or immunological variables which might have influenced survival were not examined. The challenging clinical implications of these prospective studies now need to be extended both to other types of malignancy and to include measurement of the endocrine and immune parameters in the same patient population.

Before outlining our own prospective study (the WITTEN study) in this area, a brief outline of some of the possible physiological links in the brain–endocrine–immune axis is provided (the reader is also referred to Chapters 1–3 of this volume for more detailed accounts).

## 1.2 LINKING THE BRAIN WITH ENDOCRINE FUNCTIONS

The brain is arguably the most exciting area of the human body to study. The immense cytoarchitecture and functional complexity of this tissue provides an outstanding facility for a network of intercommunication with other systems. The communication between representative cells of such different complex biochemical systems as different compartments in the body (fluid or tissue) is largely mediated by multifunctional peptide/protein signals. These comprise a series of newly characterized substances found throughout the central and autonomic nervous (neuropeptides), endocrine (hormones), and immune (cytokines) systems (7, 8).

Two classical pathways of communication are used by the brain to modulate other bodily systems; humoral connections through the endocrine system and direct neuronal connections via the autonomic nervous system as studies of sympathetic innervation of lymphoid organs have recently suggested (see Chapter 2). Signals travel down two major axes, the hypothal-amic–pituitary–adrenocortical system and the sympathetic–adreno–medullary system. The release and co-release of chemical messengers to which cells respond is the mode of intercellular communication used, which is established by binding of these chemical messengers to the receptors on the surface of target cells. As indicated in Chapter 2, immune cells have been shown to bear receptors for a wide variety of hormones, neuropeptides, and neurotransmitters. Furthermore, recent data have suggested that immune cells may contribute such extracellular signals as cytokines and hormones to an afferent feedback of adaptive control for CNS activity (see Section 1.4) (9).

The stimulation by a significant challenge of a cascade of neuroendocrine events, mainly along the aforementioned axes, mobilizes an array of responses that involve both the metabolic and functional processes of a number of tissues and organ systems. Thus, the response of an organism to mental or emotional stimuli usually involves common sympatho- and pituitary–adrenal components. However, it should be noted that the exact combination of ancillary autonomic, endocrine, and immune adjustments evoked by a particular stimulus is unique to each person.

Taking into account the similar phylo- and ontogenetic development of the nervous and immune systems, and the similarity in some of their properties (Table 1) it is feasible to suggest that a set of integrated neurohumoral mechanisms may form the basis for the development of both immunological and some kinds of psychological memory where the endocrine system functions as a buffer between the brain and the immune system.

## 1.3 LINKING THE ENDOCRINE AND IMMUNE SYSTEMS OF THE BODY

In the last decade, many neuropeptides and hypophyseal hormones have been shown to modulate immune function (see Chapter 2). Arginine vasopressin (AVP) potentiates the release of adrenocorticotrophic hormone (ACTH) by corticotrophin-releasing factor (CRF), and is thus involved in modulating the activation of the hypothalamic–pituitary–adrenal axis (10). AVP has been found to promote the production of gamma-interferon in mitogen-stimulated lymphocytes and AVP receptors have been identified on T-lymphocytes.

Almost any aspect of the immune system can be modulated to some degree by glucocorticoids. Although most of the effects of CFR and ACTH on immunity are mediated by the release of glucocorticoids, both peptides may act directly on the immune system. High- and low-affinity ACTH receptors have been described on lymphocytes, furthermore, an ACTH receptor expressed on the surface of mouse and human mononuclear cells was found to be similar to that present on the cortical cells of the adrenal gland (11). CRF receptors have been characterized on mouse splenic cells, and intraventricular administration of CRF suppresses natural killer (NK) cell activity and increases plasma noradrenaline levels. Similar changes also occur, when brain concentrations of acetylcholine and/or serotonin are increased. Certain lymphoid cells lines and normal mouse thymocytes have been shown to

**Table 1**   Comparisons between the brain and the immune system

| Category | Brain | Immune system |
|---|---|---|
| Smallest functional unit | Neuron | Lymphocyte |
| Accessory units | Glial cells, macrophages, epithelial cells | Dendritic cells |
| Communication structures | Synapsis | Cell-surface receptors |
| Communication molecules neurotransmitters | Neuropeptides, cytokines | Cytokines |
| Mode of action | Endo/paracrine, neurocrine | Para-/endocrine, juxtacrine |
| Diversity | Map of neural representation | Phenotypes of lymphocytes |
| Perceptual function | Identifying objects | Recognition |
| Learning and educating | Changes in synaptic connections | Thymus and antigens-derived education |
| Memory | Engram | Memory cells |
| Information processing | Actively seeking out | Self/non-self discrimination |
| Meaning | Language and semantic | Molecular, linguistic |
| Computation | Artificial intelligence | Network of algorithms |
| Creating new entities | Knowledge and analysis of ambiguity | Mutation and recombination of genes |
| Ontology of cross-talk between body and mind | Consciousness and self-consciousness | Self-regulatory and intercommunicative |

express specific and high-affinity receptors for growth hormone (GH) (12). GH is a pituitary hormone which appears to be modulated by CRF. In humans, nanogram concentrations of GH potentiate colony formation by normal T-cells and induce lymphoproliferation, and NK-cell activity in GH-deficient children is significantly reduced (13). However, the interdependent role of GH and CRF in modulating immune responses remains to be fully elucidated. The release of another pituitary hormone, Prolactin (PRL), is also stimulated by many types of physical and emotional stress. The expression of PRL receptors on both lymphocytes and monocytes has been reported, and PRL restores some impaired immune functions in hypophysectomized animals, such as an antibody response to sheep red blood cells. PRL release is tonically inhibited by dopamine and stimulated by serotonin and histamine (14).

The classical response to stress, as conceived by Hans Selye (15), is thought to be the activation of the hypothalamic–pituitary–adrenal axis, with a rise in corticosteroids being the ultimate event. This tends to lead to the suppression of various immune functions. Activation of CRF leads to the release of both ACTH and β-endorphin. ACTH stimulates the adrenal cortex to release cortisol into the bloodstream and β-endorphin may act on a number of target organ(s) in an endocrine manner. Whether the immune system may represent an important target organ for β-endorphin remains to be determined, although evidence exists for opiate receptors on monocytes, granulocytes, lymphocytes, and mast cells. Furthermore, structural similarities between interferon, ACTH, and the endorphins have been described (16).

In our laboratory, we were not able to show in *in vitro* experiments, using ConA pre-stimulated human peripheral blood lymphocytes, that β-endorphin has any influence on the proliferation rate and the regulation of IL-2 receptors, when used at physiological concentrations (K. Zanker, unpublished observations). Other studies, however, have reported a two- to four-fold increase in T-cell proliferation in the presence of ConA and β-endorphin (17) (see Chapter 16).

ACTH, melanocyte-stimulating hormone, met-enkephalin, and the inactive prohormone of the endorphins, beta-lipotropin, have all been found to be derived from pro-opiomelanocortin (POMC), a macromolecular glycoprotein found in anterior pituitary cells and in nerve cell bodies in the arcuate nucleus of the hypothalamus. It is noteworthy that high molarities of met-enkephalin and low leu-enkephalin concentrations enhance lymphocyte blastogenesis in the presence of the mitogen, phytohaemagglutinin (see Chapter 17). This network of putative endocrine influences on the immune system takes on added significance in the light of recent research showing that cells of the immune system produce factors themselves which perform endocrine functions in regulating the activity of various brain structures.

## 1.4 LINKING IMMUNE FUNCTIONS WITH BRAIN ACTIVITY: COMPLETING THE LOOP

Cytokines are a well characterized group of intracellular messengers used extensively within the immune system. These signals co-ordinate the various activities of immune cell types in the body. Many neurons resemble T-cells inasmuch as they have CD4 receptors on their surface (as do helper-T cells). Stimulated helper-T cells secrete the cytokine, interleukin-2 (IL-2), which interacts with specific IL-2 receptors to induce the proliferation of the T-cells. By contrast, exposure of neonatal rat oligodendrocyte progenitor cells to IL-2 at physiological concentrations blocks their rate of proliferation. Activated lymphocytes have been shown to secrete a number of other cytokines *in vitro*, several of which have antiproliferative activity. Concanavalin A (ConA)-stimulated human peripheral blood mononuclear cells release a factor which slows the rate of growth of both a human glioblastoma cell line and a human B-cell lymphoma line *in vitro* (18).

A central part of the immune system, the bone marrow, synthesizes peptides called myelopeptides which appear to influence the nervous system. These have both immunoregulatory and opiate-like, analgesic activities, and can also be produced by monocytes. The potential amplitude evoked following electric nociceptive stimulation was markedly reduced when healthy humans were injected subcutaneously with myelopeptides (19).

Other, so-called, immunomodulatory proteins also transmit information from the immune system to the nervous system. These include thymic peptides (20), interferons (21), and certain interleukins (22, 23). Alpha-thymosin was shown to bind to neurons of various subcortical structures. Thymosin-like peptides displace labelled opiates from specific binding sites on human lymphocytes and rat brain cells.

Interleukin-1 (IL-1) influences the reactivity of neurons of the central nervous system to cause fever and to prolong sleep. Once thought to be primarily produced by monocytes and macrophages, this cytokine is now known to be generated by a variety of other cell types including epithelial cells, mesangial cells, astrocytes, and microglial cells of the brain. Of particular interest is the observation that IL-1 can both up and down regulate the release of multiple hormones by the pituitary. It has been reported that IL-1 can stimulate release of ACTH by a direct action on pituitary cells. IL-1 can also exert an effect on the pituitary by stimulating the release of CRF from the hypothalamus.

Lymphocytes are themselves a source of ACTH, $\beta$-endorphin, and the $\beta$-endorphin fragment, gamma-endorphin (24). Murine and human peripheral blood mononuclear cells can produce ACTH *in vitro*. Newcastle disease virus infection causes mouse splenic cells to exhibit ACTH-like immunoreactivity and induces physiological levels of corticosterone. The demonstration of CRF receptors on mouse splenic macrophages further indicates that the interaction of monocytes/macrophages with the hypothalamic–pituitary–adrenocortical axis may represent a significant component of the regulatory circuit interconnecting the immune system with the hypothalamic–pituitary–adrenocortical axis.

A recent study has suggested that mouse helper-T cells produce pre-pro-enkephalin A in the presence of ConA and release measureable amounts of met-enkephalin. Met-enkephalin activates the expression of IL-2 receptors as well as the production of IL-2 blood levels. Human IL-2, formerly termed T-cell growth factor, represents the central mediator in a regulatory network of cell-mediated immunity. It is noteworthy that in schizophrenic patients, and in those with paranoid-type schizophrenia and affective disorders, the production of IL-2, measured in the supernatant from E-rosetting T-cell cultures is lower than in normal controls (see Chapter 1) (25).

After administration of murine interferon to C3H and A2G strains of mice, they became carriers of the mouse hepatitis virus and developed progressive neurological disorders lasting from weeks to months. Similar observations have been made by clinicians using high-dose interferon therapy in cancer patients. Without showing any signs of fever, apathy, and somnolence, aggressiveness was a common side-effect of the therapy, suggesting a direct or indirect effect of this cytokine administered on CNS structures.

Thus, a plethora of soluble mediators can be released by immunocompetent cells and may through multiple amplification loops, perpetuate or inhibit the cascade of neuroendocrine responses to a given stimulus or condition.

Considering immunopeptides and related signals have largely to reach the central nervous system to influence neuronal activity, the blood–brain barrier should be mentioned. As its name suggests, the blood–brain barrier affords the separation of the brain and the systemic circulation. This prevents mingling of cells and macromolecules from the two compartments and results from the formation of tight junctions between the endothelial cells of the blood vessels of the brain. This phenomenon may contribute to the 'immunologically privileged' status of the brain and when an immune reaction is necessary, astrocytes could, in theory, regulate the infiltration and activity of T-lymphocytes. Another explanation could be based on the fact that similar and even identical molecules (neuromediators, cytokines) are used for very different functions in the nervous and the immune systems. In the absence of a blood–brain barrier a complete confusion of signals would be created. Therefore, the blood–brain barrier separates these two cellular systems (that is neurons and leucocytes) of comparable complexity and allows them to communicate in two different languages using identical or closely related molecules.

## 2 The WITTEN study

There is increasing evidence that personality and psychosocial/emotional factors contribute to the progression of cancer, and subsequently to survival time. Research in this area, however, is dogged by inconsistent and contradictory results and methodological problems (26).

Grossarth-Maticek investigated the relationship between a number of psychosocial factors and cancer outcome. This was a prospective epidemiological study carried out in Yugoslavia and subsequently confirmed in a German study (27). Spectacular findings from these studies purported to demonstrate that psychosocial variables could be strong and specific predictors of cancer. Whilst this result is generally consistent with those of other investigators, some critics have questioned the credibility of his data.

Generally, studies that have attempted to assess the relationship between psychological variables and cancer in humans have typically been retrospective, prospective, or prognostic in orientation. The majority of retrospective studies have revealed a relationship between life-events, coping style, and neoplastic disease. For example, the incidence and progression of cancer has been found to be particularly high among individuals who recently suffered the loss of an important emotional relationship (28). Indeed, inability to cope with stressful life events has been linked to the development of cervical cancer. In addition, other psychological variables such as poor emotional expression, reduced aggressive expression, and a masochistic personality have all been associated with cancer development. Retrospective research indicates that the experience of stressful life events and inability to cope with stress may play a part in the onset of cancer, but that may actually be more influential in the progression and rate of formation of metastasic deposits by the tumour (29).

However, a number of considerations render these conclusions somewhat provisional. Cancer patients may recall more traumatic life-events than 'control' individuals, simply because the knowledge of having cancer may influence the individual's perception or interpretation of previous experiences. Furthermore, cancer may have physiological consequences which also influence psychological and behavioural functions. After all, the central nervous system may have been altered by undetected metastases or by neurological and endocrine metabolic changes due to the disease processes.

When Spiegel and colleagues (6) published their data, we had just examined prospectively immunological, neuroendocrine, and psychological variables in breast and colon cancer patients. The WITTEN study was designed as a prospective (that is over 18 months), controlled study. Thirty-seven breast cancer patients, 13 colon cancer patients, and 25 female, aged-matched healthy subjects were enrolled. The conceptual framework for the psychological aspects of this research was provided by Dr Charles Spielberger (Tampa, FL, USA), a leading expert in this field, who guided the construction and development of the psychometric measures. These scores differentiated between transient emotional 'states' and differences in relatively stable personality 'traits' (The State/Trait Concept) (30). This entailed Trait-anxiety/State-anxiety, Trait-Anger/State-Anger, Anger-in/Anger-out, and Anger-control inventories together with Trait-Curiosity and the Rationality/Emotional Defensiveness Scales. The results obtained by the WITTEN study demonstrated the feasibility of studies attempting to correlate prospectively trait and state characteristics with neurochemical and immunological data for the same patients.

After informed (written) consent was obtained, 50 cancer patients (breast: $n = 37$; colon: $n = 13$) with the initial clinical staging TO (tumour invasive); 1; NO (local nodal involvement); 1; MO (disseminated tumour); O; entered the study for 18 months. The battery of psychometric scores were recorded and every four months for a year, peripheral blood was drawn to measure percentages of lymphocyte subpopulations, IL-2 receptor expression as well

**Table 2** Spearman's correlation between various personality traits and endocrine or immune variables in breast and colon cancer patients

| Trait-personality | Endocrine immunological parameters | Correlation coefficient ($r$) | Significance level ($p$) |
|---|---|---|---|
| Anger-in | ACTH | 0.29 | 0.08 |
| Anger-out | ACTH | −0.43 | 0.007* |
| Anger-control | $\beta$-endorphin | −0.35 | 0.018* |
| Rationality/Emotional Defensiveness | $\beta$-endorphin | −0.36 | 0.01* |
| Curiosity | ACTH | 0.44 | 0.009* |
|  | NK cells | −0.28 | 0.09 |
|  | CD4 cells | −0.34 | 0.016* |

* Achieved statistical significance (that is $p < 0.05$).

as $\beta$-endorphin and ACTH (two of the main fragments of POMC). Table 2 and Table 3 show the final results after 18 months follow-up.

In general, it is thought that episodes of distress lead to immunosuppression. However, the data in Table 2 suggest that the expression of anger may correlate with decreased ACTH secretion. Furthermore, anger control— inability to express anger—was significantly correlated with decreased blood $\beta$-endorphin levels in breast cancer (Table 2 and Figure 1) and colon cancer patients (Table 2). In this context, it is important to remember that ACTH secretion suppresses antibody production, NK-cell activity, and cytokine production by means of glucocorticoid release, and that $\beta$-endorphin can increase antibody synthesis, macrophage activation, and T-lymphocyte response. Thus, alterations in the systemic levels of ACTH and $\beta$-endorphin may have widespread effects on a number of immune parameters of possible clinical significance to cancer patients.

Our findings of a correlation between anger control and plasma $\beta$-endorphin levels in breast cancer patients also accords well with the data presented in Figure 2 and Table 2, which also significantly correlate $\beta$-endorphin levels in breast and colon cancer patients with rationality/ emotional defensiveness.

Further studies of the impact of emotional status on the immune system might benefit from a more extensive examination of different types of activity of immunocompetent cells in the peripheral blood. Furthermore, the differential activity of lymphocytes trafficking between the peripheral blood, various tissues, and the lymph vessels/organs may also be important in the anti-tumour defense mechanism of the body. It could be argued that the peripheral blood is not the most appropriate compartment in which to measure the activity of immunocompetent cells in cancer patients. Perhaps it is hardly

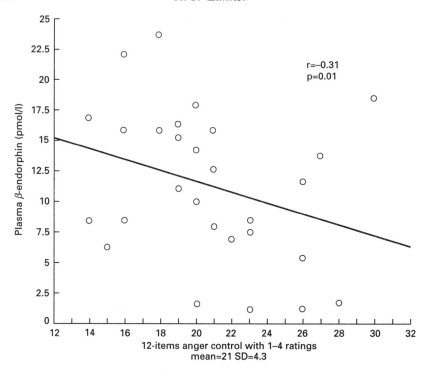

**Figure 1** Correlation of plasma β-endorphin levels (pmol/ℓ) and the results of a 12-item anger-control inventory for eligible breast cancer patients in the WITTEN study: $r$ = correlation coefficient; $p$ = significant level.

surprising, therefore, that trait/curiosity (a so-called, 'positive' emotion) did not improve immune function in the peripheral blood (Table 2). This finding suggests that (i) the control of immune status may depend on the net change of many psychoneuroimmunological variables in the body, many of which remain to be fully elucidated, and (ii) where feasible to do so, immune cell activity in other compartments of the body (for example blood, vs. tumour vs. lymphoid tissue) should also be investigated where possible.

The rationale applied to persevering further with the correlation of the Trait/state concept with neuroendocrine and immunological parameters in such a study as this is demonstrated in Table 3 and Figure 3.

IL-2 receptors were down regulated when a patient experienced situation-dependent high anxiety and she/he was unable to cope (Table 3). State-curiosity and β-endorphin were positively correlated; the more curious a given patient was about her/his situation, the more the β-endorphin levels rose in the plasma (Table 3). The validity of applying the Trait/State concept in

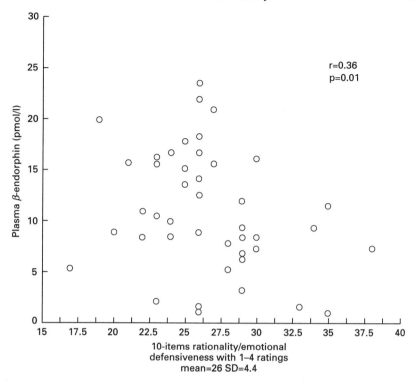

**Figure 2** Correlation of plasma β-endorphin levels (pmol/ℓ) and the scoring of eligible breast and colon cancer patients on a 10-item rationality/emotional defensiveness scale: *r* = correlation coefficient; *p* = significant level.

psycho-oncology is enhanced by these results, as even transitory emotional states could be correlated with altered β-endorphin release (minutes) and mutable (few hours) IL-2 receptor expression on the surface of peripheral blood lymphocytes. Traits (stable personality characteristics) concerning anxiety and curiosity failed to show any correlation with such rapidly changing immune parameters (data not shown).

The three-dimensional and centroid-structured data base related to the enumeration of CD4- and CD8-positive human peripheral lymphocytes and β-endorphin plasma levels (Figure 3), showed two clusters; one cluster, in which the computed values for these three parameters are *narrowly centred* around the centroid (healthy subjects) and a second cluster, where the computed values for the same parameters were *widely distributed* around the centroid (breast cancer patients). Apart from the absolute numerical separation of these two custers, the 3-D graphic suggests that different mechanisms might exist to regulate the presence of different subgroups of T-cells in

**Table 3**   Spearman's correlation between anxiety or curiosity (that is 'State' characteristics) and certain immune or endocrine parameters in breast and colon cancer
patients

| State-personality | Immunological/endocrine parameters | Correlation coefficient ($r$) | Significance level ($p$) |
|---|---|---|---|
| Anxiety | IL-2 receptor | −0.45 | 0.012* |
| Curiosity | β-endorphin | +0.42 | 0.025* |

*Achieved statistical significance (that is $p < 0.05$).

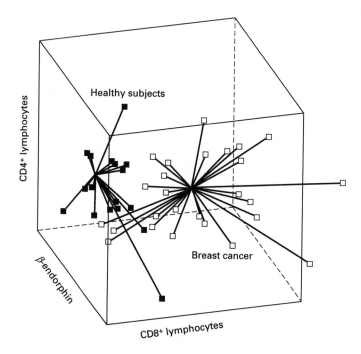

**Figure 3**   Three-dimensional and centroid-structured data base for eligible breast
cancer patients and age-matched controls. The data are taken from the second set of
measurements after enrollment into the WITTEN study.

peripheral blood and β-endorphin levels in the plasma in healthy subjects vs.
breast cancer patients. This graph could be (cautiously) interpreted as indicating that the interdependence of immunological and neuroendocrine parameters is less regulated in cancer patients that in healthy subjects; possibly
leading to—or caused by—disrupted molecular interactions and/or signalling
in the psychoimmune pathways of the former group.

# 3   Summary and conclusions

There is general agreement amongst researchers in psychoneuroimmunology that the response of the immune system to various antigens is modulated by the central nervous and neuroendocrine systems of the body. Moreover, that the functions of these systems may be reciprocally influenced by proteins produced by immune cells under certain conditions. The brain and the immune system share an array of common molecules by which they communicate. In order to perform this cross-talk, two classical neuro/endocrine axes are used; the hypothalamic–piuitary–adrenal axis and the sympathetic-adreno–medullary axis. We are far from understanding the semantic behind the human behaviour and psychological responses to exogenous and endogenous stimuli at a molecular level, but we are gradually unearthing something of the vocabulary used in the triadic communication between the neuron, the endocrine cell, and the immune cell.

Modern laboratory techniques have opened the door to measuring subtle changes in endocrine and immune functions in humans, and ever-increasing numbers of valid inventories are developed each year to measure changes in psychological parameters. These scientific and clinical advances offer the possibility of taking a more complete and logistic approach to the study of the psycho–neuro–immune axis, and with it, the treatment of cancer patients.

# 4   References

1.  Marsh, J. T. and Rasmussen, A. F. (1960). Response of adrenals, thymus, spleen and leucocytes to shuttle box and confinement stress. *Proc. Soc. Exp. Biol. Med.*, **104**, 180.
2.  Ader, R. and Friedman, S. B. (1965). Social factors affecting emotionality and resistance to disease in animals. *Psychosom. Med.*, **17**(2), 119–124.
3.  Solomon, G. F. (1969). Emotions, stress, the central nervous system and immunity. *Ann. N.Y. Acad. Sci.*, **164**, 335–340.
4.  Pettingale, K. W., Morris, T., and Greer, S. (1985). Mental attitudes to cancer: an additional prognostic factor. *Lancet*, **i**, 750.
5.  Greer, S., Morris, T., Pettingale, K. W., and Haybittle, J. L. (1990). Psychosocial response to breast cancer and 15-year outcome. *Lancet*, **i**, 49–50.
6.  Spiegel, D., Bloom, H. R., Kraemer, H. C., and Gottheil, E. (1989). Effect of psychosocial treatment on survival of patients with metastatic breast cancer. *Lancet*, **ii**, 888–891.
7.  Brown, M. R. (1989). Neuropeptide regulation of the autonomic nervous system. In *Neuropeptides and Stress* (eds T. Tache, J. E. Morley, and M. R. Brown), pp. 107–120. Springer, New York.

8. Blalock, J. E., Bost, K. E., and Smith, E. M. (1985). Neuroendocrine peptide hormones and their receptors in the immune system. *J. Neuro-immun.*, **10**, 31–40.

9. Wekerle, H., Linington, C., Lassmann, H., and Meyermann, R. (1986). Cellular immune reactivity within the CNS. *TINS*, **9**, 271–277.

10. Sawchenko, P. E., Swanson, L. W., and Vale, W. W. (1984*b*). Corticotropin-releasing factor: Co-expression within distinct subsets of oxytocin-, vasopressin-, and neurotensin-immunoreactive neurons in the hypothalamus of the male rat. *J. Neurosci.*, **4**, 1118–1129.

11. Blalock, J. E., Bosi, K.L., and Smith, E. M. (1985). Neuroendocrine peptide hormones and their receptors in the immune system. *J. Neuro-immunol.*, **10**, 31–40.

12. Brown, G. M. and Martin, J. B. (1974). Patterns of growth hormone and cortisol responses to handling and new environment in the rat. *Psychosom. Med.*, **36**, 241–247.

13. Kies, W., Holtmann, H., Butenanch, O., and Eife, R. (1983). Modulation of lymphoproliferation by human growth hormone. *Eur. J. Pediatr.*, **150**, 47–50.

14. Kant, G. J., Len, J. R., Anderson, S. M., and Mongey, E. (1987). Effect of chronic stress on plasma corticosterone, ACTH and prolactin. *Physiol. Behav.*, **40**, 775–779.

15. Selye, H. (1970). The evolution of the stress concept. *Am. Sci.*, **61**, 692–699.

16. Blalock, J. E. and Smith, E. M. (1980). Human leukocyte interferon: Structural and biological relatedness to adreno-corticotropic hormone and endorphins. *Proc. Natl. Acad. Sci. USA*, **77**, 5972–5974.

17. Gilman, S. C., Schwartz, J. M., Milner, R. J., Bloom, F. E., and Feldman, J. D. (1981). Enhancement of lymphocyte proliferative response by β-endorphin. *Soc. Neurosci.*, **7**, 880.

18. Kuppner, M. C., Hammon, M. F., and DeTribolet, N. (1988). Cytotoxic response of cultured tumor infiltrating lymphocytes to autologous human glioblastoma cells. *Ann. N.Y. Acad. Sci.*, **540**, 401–402.

19. Petrov, R. V., Mikhailova, A. A., and Zakharova, L. A. (1987). Myelopeptides: Mediators of interaction between the immune and the nervous system. *Ann. N.Y. Acad. Sci.*, **496**, 271–277.

20. Goldstein, A. L., Low, T. L., Thurman, G. B., Zata, M. M., Hall, N. R., Chen, J. *et al.* (1981). Current status of thymosin and other hormones of the thymus gland. *Recent Progr. Horm. Res.*, **37**, 369–415.

21. Blalock, J. E. and Smith, E. M. (1981). Human leukocyte interferon (HuIFN-alpha): Potent endorphin-like opioid activity. *Biochem. Biophys. Res. Commun.*, **101**, 472–478.

22. Besedovsky, H. O., DelRey, A., and Sorkin, E. (1981). Lymphokine-containing supernatants from ConA-stimulated cells increase corticosterone blood levels. *J. Immunol.*, **126**, 385–387.

23. Besedovsky, H. O., Sorkin, E., Felix, D., and Haas, H. (1977). Hypothalamic changes during immune response. *Eur. J. Immunol.*, **7**, 325–328.

24. Bernton, E. W., Beach, J. E., Holaday, J. W., Smallbridge, R. C., and Fein, H. G. (1987). Release of multiple hormones by a direct action of interleukin-1 on pituitary cells. *Science*, **238**, 519–521.

25. Morley, J. E., Kay, N. E., Solomon, G. F., and Plotnikoff, N. P. (1987). Neuropeptides: Conductors of the immune orchestra. *Life Sci.*, **41**, 527–544.

26. Riley, V. (1979). Cancer and stress: Overview and critique. *Cancer Detect. Prevent.*, **2**, 163–165.

27. Grossarth-Maticek, R., Bastiaans, J., and Kanazir, D. T. (1985). Psychosocial factors as strong predictors of mortality from cancer, ischemic heart disease and stroke: The Yugoslav prospective study. *J. Psychosom. Res.*, **29**, 167–176.

28. Zänker, K. S. and Kroczek, R. (1988). Immunophenotyping, immunointervention and depression in cancer patients. A follow up study in five bereaved patients. *Int. J. Immunotherapie*, **IV** (4), 235–241.

29. Bahnson, C. B. and Bahnson, M. B. (1966). Role of ego defenses: Denial and repression in the etiology of malignant neoplasm. *Ann. N. Y. Acad. Sci.*, **125**, 828–845.

30. Sharma, S., Dang, R., and Spielberger, C. D. (1986). Effects of trait anxiety and intelligence on academic performance in different school courses. In *Cross-Cultural Auxiety* (eds C. D. Spielberger and R. Diaz-Guerrero), Vol. 3, pp. 1–9. Hemisphere Publishing Corporation, Washington.

# 13

# The effects of psychological intervention on cortisol levels and leukocyte numbers in the peripheral blood of breast cancer patients

M. SCHEDLOWSKI, U. TEWES, AND H.-J. SCHMOLL

## 1 Introduction

Research in psychoneuroimmunology has provided growing evidence for the integration of nervous, endocrine, and immune systems in the body. Different stressful situations such as bereavement or examinations can alter a variety of immunological functions (1–4), and psychological factors such as inadequate social support, loneliness, and depression were reported to be negatively correlated with humoral and cellular immune functions in healthy individuals (5, 6). Similar results were found with breast cancer patients (7, 8).

The potential clinical relevance of stress-induced changes in immune functions have been shown in a plethora of animal experiments where exposure to stress was associated with increased growth of transplanted tumours and decreased survival time (9–13). These effects seemed to be mediated via a stress-induced suppression of immune functions. In a tumour model in which lung metastasis are controlled by natural killer (NK) cells, the stress induced by forced swimming decreased NK-cell activity and resulted in a two-fold increase in lung metastases (14).

It is postulated that immunological changes after stress exposure are mediated by the endocrine system since lymphocytes have been shown to express receptors for a variety of hormones (15). However, the question of whether psychological stress influences the number and function of human peripheral blood lymphocytes, and which hormones are involved have yet to be fully established (see Chapter 2).

## 1.1 STRESS-INDUCED ALTERATIONS IN CELL-MEDIATED IMMUNE FUNCTIONS

A human stress model of high experimental control was chosen (16) to establish if and how acute psychological stress might influence the function of immune cells (particularly NK cells) and to elucidate the role of endocrine factors in these stress-induced alterations.

Forty-five first-time tandem parachutists were continuously monitored for plasma concentrations of cortisol and catecholamines before, during, and after jumping (17). Lymphocyte subsets and NK-cell activity were determined before, immediately after, and one hour following jumping. There was a significant increase in sympathetic-adrenal hormones during (adrenaline, noradrenaline) and shortly after jumping (cortisol). There was also 100 per cent increase in NK-cell numbers (that is CD56$^+$ cells) immediately after jumping followed by a significant decrease below baseline values one hour later. These changes were paralleled by changes in NK-cell cytotoxicity or NK-cell activity (Table 1). Additional calculation of lytic units suggested that the functional changes observed not only reflected alterations in NK-cell numbers, but also in the activity of individual NK cells. Such an alteration in NK-cell number and cytotoxic activity was significantly correlated with plasma concentrations of noradrenaline.

These changes in cellular immune functions, in particular the quick mobilization and subsequent decrease in NK-cell number and function may be interpreted as one major mechanism for an effective and rapid adaptation of the immune system to environmental stimuli. In this model, the adaptation process of cellular immune functions seemed to be mediated by the catecholamine, noradrenaline. Since there is evidence for diminished NK-cell numbers after psychological stress, it is of further interest whether this is a transient or long-lasting effect which might enhance susceptibility to infections.

**Table 1** Numbers of peripheral blood lymphocytes, T-lymphocyte subsets (CD4$^+$, CD8$^+$) and NK cells (CD56$^+$), and NK activity (specific lysis/%) two hours before (baseline), immediately, and one hour after a parachute jump. (Data presented are means ± S.E.M.)

| Cell number/$\mu$l | Baseline | Immediately after jumping | One hour after jumping |
|---|---|---|---|
| Total lymphocytes | 2718 ± 124 | 3484 ± 214* | 2043 ± 102 |
| CD4$^+$ cells | 1205 ± 70 | 1280 ± 100 | 1024 ± 65 |
| CD8$^+$ cell | 771 ± 49 | 1172 ± 85* | 574 ± 36* |
| CD56$^+$ NK cells | 543 ± 62 | 1081 ± 100* | 292 ± 27* |
| NK activity | 34 ± 1.9 | 48.6 ± 2* | 28 ± 1.9* |

* $p < 0.01$, significantly different from respective baseline value.

## 1.2 INTERACTION OF THE NEUROENDOCRINE AND IMMUNE SYSTEMS OF THE BODY

Although increases in NK-cell number and cytotoxicity have been demonstrated after administration of adrenaline, the *in vivo* effects of noradrenaline on human peripheral blood lymphocyte subsets and other NK-cell functions have not been established. In order to prove a causal relationship between noradrenaline and cellular immune functions, a study was designed to compare the effects of noradrenaline and adrenaline on the function of lymphocyte subsets, and then to analyse the time kinetics of catecholamine-induced alterations of cellular immune functions. Healthy male subjects were given a subcutaneous injection of either physiological saline (NaCl), adrenaline, or noradrenaline. Catecholamine concentrations, subsets of peripheral blood lymphocytes, and NK-cell activity were analysed before (baseline) and 5, 15, 30, 60, and 120 minutes after injection. NK-cell number and cytotoxicity increased significantly after injection of adrenaline and noradrenaline, reaching highest values 15 to 30 minutes postinjection, and subsequently declining to baseline values 60 (noradrenaline) and 120 (adrenaline) minutes after injection (Table 2) (18).

These data suggest that some cellular immune functions, such as NK-cell number and function, can be modulated within minutes via catecholamines. This is in accordance with other studies dealing with acute emotional stress where alterations in immune functions have been observed immediately after exposure to stress, and where catecholamines or neuropeptides were thought to be responsible for the observed effects (19, 20). Taken together, these studies provide further evidence for a close and sensitive interaction between the CNS and parts of the immune system.

**Table 2** NK cells (CD56$^+$) and NK activity (specific lysis/%) before (baseline) and 5, 15, 30, 60 and 120 minutes after injection of NaCl, adrenaline, or noradrenaline. (Data presented are means ± S.E.M.)

| | Baseline | 5 | 15 | 30 | 60 | 120 | P |
|---|---|---|---|---|---|---|---|
| **Percentage of CD56$^+$ NK cells** | | | | | | | |
| NaCl | 14.1 ± 2.1 | 14.3 ± 0.9 | 13 ± 0.5 | 14.2 ± 1 | 15 ± 1.7 | 16.9 ± 2.2 | |
| Adrenaline | 10.3 ± 2.2 | 25.7 ± 3.5 | 26.8 ± 3.7 | 29 ± 3.9 | 25.5 ± 3.3 | 9.9 ± 1 | * |
| Noradrenaline | 13.7 ± 2 | 20.9 ± 2.7 | 26.6 ± 2.9 | 20.4 ± 2.7 | 11.1 ± 1.3 | 14.8 ± 2.6 | * |
| **NK Acticity** | | | | | | | |
| NaCl | 18.3 ± 0.9 | 18.9 ± 0.5 | 19.3 ± 0.8 | 20.5 0.7 | 19.5 ± 0.9 | 19.7 ± 0.9 | |
| Adrenaline | 18.9 ± 1.9 | 30.6 ± 2.4 | 35.1 ± 2.3 | 39.7 ± 1.5 | 40.2 ± 1.3 | 23.5 ± 2.82 | * |
| Noradrenaline | 23.4 ± 2.9 | 35.6 ± 4.2 | 43.1 ± 4.7 | 32.2 ± 4.5 | 18.6 ± 1 | 24.6 ± 1.4 | * |

* $p < 0.001$ significantly different from respective NaCl group ANOVA.

## 2 Intervention-induced changes in endocrine and immune functions

Studies assessing the effects of various short-term psychological stressors reported an immediate enhancement of NK-cell number and activity after exposure to stress. It has also been documented that short-term physical stress induced by exercise results in a transient increase in NK cells and their cytotoxicity (21, 22).

These observations, together with data indicating a close interaction between the nervous, endocrine, and immune systems (23) (see Chapter 2), provide a biochemical basis for possible improvement of immune functions by behavioural strategies such as psychological intervention. This hypothesis is supported by observations that interventions such as relaxation, self-disclosure, and social support increased cell-mediated immune functions in students and older adults (4, 24–26). Moreover, patients with malignant melanoma showed increased NK-cell numbers and function six months after a psychiatric group intervention (27) (see also Chapters 00 and 00 of this volume).

However, there are very limited data of the impact of behavioural intervention on immune functions in cancer patients (28). In order to extend the previous reported data we designed a study to investigate the effects of short- (pre- vs. post intervention session) and longer-term (nine weeks) behavioural group intervention on illness-related coping, plasma levels of cortisol, and white blood cell counts (WBC) in breast cancer patients. This study is outlined below.

## 2.1  METHODOLOGICAL APPROACH

### 2.1.1  *Patients*

Twenty-four Stage I and II breast cancer patients (aged 40–62 years) participated in this study after giving their informed consent. All patients had undergone standard surgical treatment of their tumours and were not undergoing adjuvant (chemo/radiation) therapy. Subjects with drug or alcohol abuse or medication were excluded. A voluntary allocation procedure was used in which patients were given the option of participating in the first intervention group or acting as controls during this time, and then participating in the next intervention group starting three months later. Fourteen patients (average age, 51 years) remained in the intervention group while 10 patients (average age, 50.6 years) served as controls. There was no significant difference concerning the period of time between surgical tumour treatment and entry in the study between the intervention ($21.1 \pm 7$ months) and the control ($25.2 \pm 10$ months) group.

### 2.1.2  *Intervention procedure*

Intervention took place once a week for two hours from 6:00 to 8:00 p.m. over a period of 10 weeks. Blood samples were taken before and immediately after the second and tenth session to determine plasma concentration of cortisol and WBC. Illness-related coping was assessed twice; before and after the completion of intervention period. Personality factors were assessed once at the beginning of the study.

Control patients were assessed twice; two days after the second and tenth session of the intervention group. They received the same psychological, endocrine, and immunological assessments. During the two-hour periods between blood collections (6:00–8:00 p.m.), control patients were waiting in the same room where the intervention took place. However, only six out of ten patients of the control group participated in the first and second control session as well. Therefore, only data from these six patients were used as controls for blood analysis.

The intervention consisted of relaxation techniques, information about the 'body-network', health education, and development and enhancement of stress- and illness-related coping skills. The relaxation technique is a modification of the autogenic training (29), including guided imagery. The relaxation technique was done twice; at the beginning and the end of each session. Patients were encouraged to practice these techniques at least twice a day. The information about the 'body-network' consisted of information about cancer and the immune system, the psychobiology of stress, and the biochemical

**Table 3** Means (± S.E.M) and standard deviations of FEKB subscales for intervention ($n = 14$) and control group ($n = 10$) before (Pre) and after (Post) the intervention period.

| | | FEKB subscales | | | | |
|---|---|---|---|---|---|---|
| | | RU | SA | TM | SI | SR |
| Intervention group | Pre | 29.3 ± 6.6 | 38.2 ± 4.8 | 42.1 ± 2.6 | 32 ± 3.6 | 9.7 ± 4.1 |
| | Post | 28.6 ± 8.6 | 40.2 ± 5.3 | 40.7 ± 3.6 | 31.7 ± 6.5 | 9.5 ± 3.7 |
| Control group | Pre | 29.9 ± 9.4 | 37.7 ± 7.9 | 38.6 ± 7.3 | 26.2 ± 10.5 | 9.9 ± 4.5 |
| | Post | 32.1 ± 7.5 | 38.3 ± 7 | 39.9 ± 4.9 | 29.3 ± 11.1 | 9.8 ± 5.1 |

links between the nervous, endocrine, and immune systems. In this context, the possibility of improving immune functions by behavioural techniques was carefully emphasized. The content of the health education component was mainly structured by the patients' needs and included information about nutrition, diet, exercise, etc. Behavioural and cognitive techniques were used to develop and improve stress- and illness-related coping skills (30). Problems were discussed in the group, strategies to resolve the problems were developed and, if possible, incorporated into the work of the group.

### 2.1.3 Measurement of psychological parameters

Coping with chronic disease was assessed using the questionnaire for the assessment of modes of coping with severe bodily disease (FEKB) (31). This 64-item inventory assesses five coping strategies: (1) rumination (RU/9 items) which describes intrapsychic processes focusing on the disease and leading to social withdrawal; (2) search for affiliation (SA/9 items); a highly sociable coping behaviour leading to intentional diversion and distraction from disease; (3) threat minimization (TM/8 items), which covers items that describe intrapsychic, emotion-focused coping reactions like self-instruction towards positive thinking and maintaining trust in the medical treatment; (4) search for information (SI/8 items), which reflects overt reactions aimed at gaining knowledge about the disease and its medical treatment particularly from the interaction with other patients; (5) search for meaning in religion (SR/3 items); this attempts to find meaning in the illness experience with special reference to religious issues. The higher the score on these subscales, the greater the use of a particular coping strategy. Previous study with cancer patients ($n = 333$) has shown the questionnaire to be sufficient, reliable, and consistent (31).

To control for *a priori* differences in personality factors between intervention and control groups the 'Freiburger Personality-Inventory' (FPI-R)

(32) was administered before the intervention period. The 138 items of the FPI-R assesses relatively stable dimensions of personality on 12 subscales (for example social orientation, aggressiveness, psychosomatic complaints, and extraversion). In addition, information about daily coffee and alcohol intake, smoking, physical exercise, and average number of sleeping hours per night were obtained before and after the intervention period (33).

All blood samples were collected in heparinized tubes. White blood cell counts (WBC) were assessed the same evening immediately after the last blood sample was collected using standard techniques (Coulter Electronics, Krefeld, Germany). Samples for the endocrine analyses were centrifuged at 4 °C, and stored frozen at 70 °C until assayed. The concentration of cortisol in the plasma was determined by radioimmunoassay (Biermann GmbH, Bad Nauheim, Germany).

To determine intervention effects on coping strategies and on short- (pre- vs. post-second and tenth session) and longer- (pre-second vs. pre-tenth session) term alterations in plasma cortisol concentrations and WBC, an analysis of variance (ANOVA) of repeated measurements (Group × Time) were performed. Student t-tests were used to test for differences between intervention and control groups with respect to personality factors and control variables. Pearson correlations were performed to determine correlations between cortisol and WBC.

## 2.2 RESULTS

There were no significant differences in personality, coffee/alcohol consumption, smoking, physical exercise, or sleep between intervention and control groups, pre- and post-treatment for either group. Coping strategies measured by FEKB before and after the treatment showed no initial differences between groups. Furthermore, these remained unaffected by the intervention (Table 1). However, there was a significant reduction in plasma concentration of cortisol in the intervention group after the second session (Figure 1) which was confirmed by a marked Time × Group interaction effect ($F = 8.47$; $p < 0.01$). Cortisol concentrations remained reduced in the intervention group in comparison with the control group when plasma levels were determined before the tenth session, and further decreased after the tenth session. However, the short-term (pre- vs. past-tenth session) (Group × Time) effect ($F = 0.64$; $p < 0.43$) and the decrease in plasma cortisol levels over the nine-week period (pre-second vs. pre-tenth session) ($F = 3.79$; $P < 0.07$) failed to reach statistical significance. Separate analysis for both groups with respect to changes over time revealed significant short-term effects for the second ($F = 25.82$; $p < 0.001$) and tenth session ($F = 11.70$; $p < 0.01$) for the intervention group alone, as well as a significant decrease in plasma cortisol levels in this

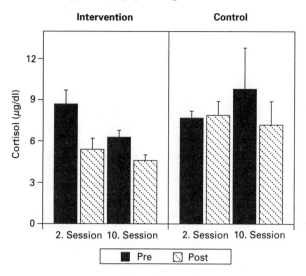

**Figure 1**   Plasma concentrations before and after the second and tenth intervention session ($n = 14$) and equivalent time points for the control group ($n = 6$). (Data presented are means ± S.E.M.)

group over the 9-week period (pre-second vs. pre-tenth session) ($F = 7.10$; $p < 0.05$).

Analyses of WBC revealed no significant differences in the absolute numbers of leukocytes and monocytes either between the different groups and/ or the different time points. However, an increase in lymphocyte numbers was observed in the intervention group after the second session (Figure 2). ANOVA revealed a significant Group × Time interaction (pre- vs. second session) ($F = 5.32$; $p < 0.05$). Elevated lymphocyte numbers were observed in the intervention group after a period of nine weeks (pre-second vs. pre-tenth session) ($F = 3.43$; $p < 0.09$) with a further, but not significant increase after the tenth session (pre- vs. tenth session) ($F = 0.32$; $p < 0.58$). However, separate analysis for both groups showed significant increases in lymphocyte numbers only for the intervention group after the second ($F = 18.88$, $p < 0.001$) and tenth session ($F = 5.28$; $p < 0.05$) and a significant longer-term increase of peripheral blood lymphocytes over a period of the nine weeks (pre-second vs. pre-tenth session) ($F = 10.88$; $p < 0.01$).

Pearson correlation analyses were performed between cortisol levels and WBC counts at different points in time for each group in order to analyse the association between the observed decreases in cortisol plasma concentrations and increases in peripheral blood lymphocytes. There were no significant

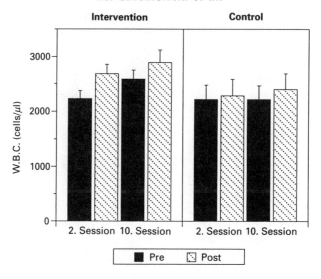

**Figure 2** Numbers of white blood cells (WBC) before and after the second and tenth intervention session ($n = 14$) and equivalent time point for the control group ($n = 6$). (Data are presented as means ± S.E.M.)

correlations between cortisol levels and numbers of leukocytes, monocytes, or lymphocytes for either group at any time (data not shown).

## 2.3 SUMMARY AND CONCLUSIONS

The results of the present study support the hypothesis that behavioural group intervention could have immediate and longer-term positive effects on immune functions in breast cancer patients. The treatment had no effects on illness-related coping skills measured before and after intervention. However, patients in the intervention group displayed a short- and longer-term increase in the absolute numbers of WBC, which was paralleled by a reduction in plasma concentrations of cortisol. These data accord with those of other studies reporting relaxation/intervention-induced increases in certain lymphocyte subsets and functions in healthy populations and cancer patients (24–27).

In this study, there were no differences between intervention and control group with respect to age, tumour stage, surgical cancer treatment, time of entry into the study, or measurable personality factors. In addition, health-influencing behaviour, such as coffee and alcohol intake, smoking, exercise, and sleep were found to be similar and stable with time (pre- vs. post-intervention period) for both groups. Therefore, it is conceivable that the observed short- and longer-term alterations in plasma cortisol concentrations and WBC numbers recorded for the intervention group may have been due to the treatment itself.

Cortisol is largely responsible for impaired immune function following stress (34). Although in the present study the increases in WBC numbers were paralleled by decreases in plasma levels of cortisol, there was no significant correlation between these endocrine and immune variables. Besides glucocorticoids, neuroendocrine factors such as catecholamines and/or $\beta$-endorphin have been shown to be potent modulators of cell-mediated immune functions (18, 35, 36) and these might induce lymphocyte mobilization from their respective reservoirs, such as the spleen.

Alterations in immune cell functions have been reported after acute psychological stress (17, 37), where the observed changes seemed to occur within minutes of stress exposure. The data of this study, in particular the increases in lymphocyte numbers evident immediately following both intervention sessions suggest that rapid changes in lymphocyte distribution can be achieved by such intervention techniques as well.

NK-cell number and cytotoxity have been reported to be affected by acute emotional stress, physical exercise, or psychological intervention. NK cells are thought to act as a first-line of defence in the immune system without MHC restriction, and to play a significant role in immunosurveillance against tumours. Although immunophenotypic analysis of lymphocyte subpopulations was not performed in this study, it is tempting to speculate that the increases in lymphocyte numbers in the intervention group may have involved an increase in NK-cell numbers. However, because of the relatively preliminary nature of this study (low total subject number, loss of some subjects in the control group resulting in blood data for only 6 individuals, lack of functional data on immune status, isolated measurements of cortisol concentrations) caution must be exerted in the interpretation of the results obtained.

It is not known whether the intervention-induced increase in WBC numbers was long-lasting. This might have been a transient effect which was curtailed shortly after the intervention period ended and without substantial health benefits for the patients concerned.

Furthermore, the potential clinical consequences, if any, of such psycho-neuroimmunological data remains a contentious issue. In this context, it has been suggested that, for example, stress- or intervention-induced changes in immune functions, whilst achieving statistical significance, may not have any clinical impact (for example actually affect cancer progression). However, a ten-year follow-up study has demonstrated a significantly extended survival time for breast cancer patients undergoing such behavioural intervention regimens compared with untreated control groups (36, 38). Unfortunately, no immunological data were collected in these studies so that the causal relationship between behavioural intervention, immune functions, and disease progression in cancer has yet to be unequivocally established. There is clearly a need for carefully controlled, prospective studies to address the links in this axis.

Although the prognostic implications of intervention-induced changes in lymphocyte numbers, subsets, and functions remain unclear, the results of this study, together with the data of other intervention studies, point to the possibility that behavioural intervention following surgery could have considerable impact on treatment strategies for breast cancer patients.

# 3 References

1. Bartrop, R., Luckhorst, Lg., Lazarus, E., Kiloh, L. G., and Penny, R. (1977). Depressed lymphocyte function after bereavement. *Lancet*, 1, 834–836.

2. Schleifer, S. J., Keller, S. E., Camerino, M., Thornton, J. C., and Stein, M. (1983). Suppression of lymphocyte stimulation following bereavement. *J. Am. Med. Assoc.*, **250**, 374–377.

3. Glaser, R., Kiecolt-Glaser, J. K., Bonneau, R. H., Malarkey, W., Kennedy, S., and Hughes, J. (1992). Stress-induced modulation of the immune response to recombinant hepatitis B vaccine. *Psychosom. Med.*, **54**, 22–29.

4. Glaser, R., Rice, J., Speicher, C. E., Stout, J. C., and Kiecolt-Glaser, J. K. (1986). Stress depresses interferon production by leukocytes concomitant with a decrease in natural killer cell activity. *Behav. Neurosci.*, **100**, 675–678.

5. Kiecolt-Glaser, J. K., Ricker, D., George, J., Messick, G., Speicher, C. E., Garner, W. *et al.* (1984). Urinary cortisol levels, cellular immunocompetency and loneliness in psychiatric impatients. *Psychosom. Med.*, **46**, 15–24.

6. Glaser, R., Kennedy, S., Lafuse, W. P., Bonneau, R. H., Speicher, C., Hillhouse, J. *et al.* (1990). Psychological stress-induced modulation of interleukin 2 receptor gene expression and interleukin 2 production in peripheral blood leukocytes. *Arch. Gen. Psychiatry*, **47**, 707–712.

7. Levy, S., Herberman, R., Lippman, M., and d'Angelo, T. (1987). Correlation of stress factors with sustained depression of natural killer cell activity and predicted prognosis in patients with breast cancer. *J. Clin. Oncol.*, **5**, 348–353.

8. Levy, S. M., Herberman, R. B., Whiteside, T., Sanzo, K., Lee, J., and Kirkwood, J. (1990). Perceived social support and tumor estrogen/progesterone receptor status as predictors of natural killer cell activity in breast cancer patients. *Psychosom. Med.*, **52**, 73–85.

9. Riley, V. (1975). Mouse mammary tumors: Alteration of incidence as appartent function of stress. *Science*, **189**, 465–467.

10. Sklar, L. S., and Anisman, H. (1979). Stress and coping factors influence tumor growth. *Science*, **205**, 513–515.

11. Visintainer, M. A., Volpicelli, J. R., and Seligman, M. E. P. (1982). Tumor rejection in rats after inescapable or escapable shock. *Science*, **216**, 437–439.

12. Weinberg, J. and Emerman, J. T. (1989). Effects of psychosocial stressors on mouse mammary tumor growth. *Brain Behav. Immune.*, 3, 234–246.
13. Basso, A. M., Depiante-Depaoli, M., and Molina, V. A. (1992). Chronic variable stress facilitates tumoral growth: Reversal by imipramine administration. *Life Sci*, 50, 1789–1769.
14. Ben-Eliyahu, S., Yirmiya, R., Liebeskind, J. C., Taylor, A. N., and Gale, R. P. (1991). Stress increases metastatic spread of a mammary tumor in rats: Evidence for mediation by the immune system. *Brain Behav. Immun.*, 5, 193–205.
15. Plant, M. (1987). Lymphocyte hormone receptors. *Ann. Rev. Immunol.*, 5, 621–669.
16. Schedlowski, M. and Tewes, U. (1992). Physiological arousal and perception of bodily state during parachute jumping. *Psychophysiology*, 29, 95–103.
17. Schedlowski, M., Jacobs, R., Stratmann, G., Richter, S., Hadicke, A., Tewes, U. *et al.* (1993a). Changes of natural killer cells during acute psychological stress. *J. Clin. Immunol.*, 13, 119–126.
18. Schedlowski, M., Falk, A., Rohne, A., Wagner, T. O. F., Jacobs, R., Tewes, U. *et al.* (1993b). Catecholamines induce alterations of distribution and activity of human natural (NK) cells. *J. Clin. Immunol.*, 13, 344–351.
19. Naliboff, B. D., Benton, D., Solomon, G. F., Morley, J. E., Fahey, J. L., Bloom, E. T. *et al.* (1991). Immunological changes in young and old adults during brief laboratory stress. *Psychosom. Med.*, 53, 121–132.
20. Brosschot, J. F., Benschop, R. J., Godaert, G. L. R., De Smet, M. B. M., Olff, M., Heijnen, C. J. *et al.* (1992). Effects of experimental psychological stress on distribution and function of peripheral blood cells. *Psychosom. Med.*, 54, 394–406.
21. Kendall, A., Hoffman-Goetz, L., Houston, M., MacNeil, B., and Arumugam, Y. (1990). Exercise and blood lymphocyte subset responses: Intensity, duration and subject fitness effects. *J. Appl. Physiol.*, 69, 251–260.
22. Murray, D. R., Irwin, M., Rearden, C. A., Ziegler, M., Motulsky, H., and Maisel, A. S. (1992). Sympathetic and immune interactions during dynamic exercise. *Circulation*, 86, 203–213.
23. Ader, R., Felten, D. L., and Cohen, N. (1991). *Psychoneuroimmunology*. Academic Press, San Diego.
24. Kiecolt-Glaser, J. K., Glaser, R., Strain, E. C., Stout, J., Tarr, K. L., Holliday, J. F. *et al.* (1986). Modulation of cellular immunity in medical students. *J. Behav. Med.*, 9, 5–21.
25. Kiecolt-Glaser, J. R., Ricker, D., George, J., Messick, G., Speicher, C. E., Garner, W. *et al.* (1984). Urinary cortisol levels, cellular immunocompetency and loneliness in psychiatric impatients. *Psychosom. Med.*, 46, 15–24.
26. Pennebaker, J. W., Kiecolt-Glaser, J. K., Glaser, R. (1988). Disclosure of traumas and immune function: Health implications for psychotherapy. *J. Consult. Clin. Psychol*, 56, 239–245.
27. Fawzy, F. I., Kemeny, M. E., Fawzy, N. W., Elashoff, R., Morton, D., Cousins, N. *et al.* (1990). A structured psychiatric intervention for cancer patients. II. changes over time in immunological measures. *Arch. Gen. Psychiatry*, 47, 729–735.

28. Kiecolt-Glaser, J. K., Cacioppo, J. T., Malarkey, W. B., and Glaser, R. (1992). Acute psychological stressors and short-term immune changes: What, why, for whom, and to what extent? *Psychosom. Med., 54,* 680–685.
29. Lindemann, H. (1975). *Uberleben im Stress. Autogenes Training.* Mosaik, Munchen.
30. Moorey, S. and Greer, S. (1989). *Psychological Therapy for Patients with Cancer: A New Approach.* Heinemann Medical Books, Oxford.
31. Klauer, T., Filipp, S. H., and Ferring, D. (1989). Der 'Fragebogen zur Erfassung von Formen der Karankheitsbewaltigung' (FEKB): Skalenkonstruktion und erste Befunde zu Reliabilitat, Validitat und Stabilitat. *Diagnostica, 35,* 316–335.
32. Fahrenberg, J., Hampel, R., and Selg, H. (1984). *Das Freiburger Personlichkeitsinventar FPI. Revidierte Fassung FPI-R und teilweise geanderte Fassung FPI-A1.* Hogrefe, Gottingen.
33. Kiecolt-Glaser, J. K. and Glaser, R. (1988). Methodological issues in behavioural immunology research with humans. *Brain Behav. Immun., 2,* 67–78.
34. Berczi, I. and Kovacs, K. (1987). *Hormones and Immunity.* MTP Press, Lancaster.
35. Heijnen, C. J., Kavelaars, A., and Ballieux, R. (1991). β-endorphin: Cytokine and neuropeptide. *Immunol. Rev., 119,* 41–63.
36. Crary, B., Hauser, S. L., Borysenko, M., Kutz, I., Hoban, C., Ault, K. A. *et al.* (1983). Epinephrine-induced changes in the distribution of lymphocyte subsets in peripheral blood of humans. *J. Immunol., 131,* 1178–1181.
37. Kiecolt-Glaser, J. K. and Glaser, R. (1992). Psychoneuroimmunology: Can psychological interventions modulate immunity? *J. Consul. Clin. Psychol., 60,* 569–575.
38. Spiegel, D., Bloom, J. R., Kraemer, H. C., and Gottheil, E. (1989). Effect of psychosocial treatment on survival of patients with metastatic breast cancer. *Lancet, 2,* 888–891.

# 14

# Immunological responses to self-regulation training in stage 1 breast cancer patients

S. P. HERSH AND J. F. KUNZ

# 1   Overview and commentary

One view of the human biological system recognizes that we are built of a number of highly differentiated and complex cellular systems interacting chemically and electrically to form a dynamic whole. Our uniqueness as a species seems to reside in our level of self-awareness combined with our adaptability. Insects, of course, far outstrip us in adaptability. Examining some dimensions of the influence of 'self-awareness' on physiological function is the subject of the study presented in this chapter. It was originally entitled, 'Immunological responses of breast cancer patients to behavioural interventions' and published in *Biofeedback and Self-Regulation*, and was written by Barry L. Gruber, Stephen P. Hersh, Nicholas R. S. Hall, Lucy R. Waletzky, John F. Kunz, Joann C. Carpenter, Karan S. Kverno, and Sharlene M. Weiss (1a). It is re-published here in an extended form with permission of the Plenum Publishing Corporation.

Thirteen lymph-node-negative breast cancer patients who had recovered from a modified radical mastectomy were randomly assigned to either an immediate self-regulation training group or a control group (delayed self-regulation training). Multiple pre- and post-training psychological measures were performed. Significant effects were found on natural killer cell activity, mixed lymphocyte responsiveness, concanavalin A responsiveness, and the number of peripheral blood lymphocytes.

In describing this study, we would like to highlight three issues: (1) study design; (2) poststudy five-year follow-up; and (3) our understanding of the mind–body interactions in human beings and other higher animals.

## 1.1   STUDY DESIGN

We wished in our study to examine whether changes in the state of 'self-awareness' (which, of course, resides in the central nervous system) could produce measurable changes in some aspects of the functioning of the immune system. The difficulties of controlling the experimental circumstances and the number of variables that one is examining makes studies of such interactions extraordinarily challenging. Further complicating 'mind/body' studies is the lack of universal agreement concerning the variables that are meaningful expressions of activity of the immune system. The immune system variables we selected were: natural killer (NK) cells, concanavalin A (Con-A) responsiveness, mixed lymphocyte response (MLR); interleukin-2 (IL-2), plasma IgG, IgA, and IgM, peripheral blood lymphocytes (PBL), cortisol, and total white cell count. This selection was based on our review of the literature concerning measurement of immune system functioning in humans and other mammals.

The psychological inventories we chose to use included: the Minnesota Multiphasic Personality Inventory (MMPI), the Millon Behavioural Health Inventory (MBHI), the Sarason Social Support Scale, the Rotter Locus of Control, and two quality of life instruments: the Affects Balance Scale and Greer's Mental Adjustment to Cancer (MAC) scale. These instruments were selected because of their conceptual relevance, their reliability and validity, their extensive use in clinical research, and their demonstrated relevance to cancer patients in general (and breast cancer patients specifically).

Finally, we selected self-regulation training as a replicable and well-established (in western science) approach to influencing states of mind and physiological arousal. The latter is represented by the multitude of studies describing the associations of quieting response training to changes in electromyographic levels, skin conductance response, and peripheral skin temperature.

A sketch of our experimental design follows in Table 1. Our finding that some immune system changes developed some weeks or more after training suggests the need for long-term, preferably longitudinal, experiments in the area of psychoneuroimmunology. Carrying out studies with this type of experimental design is expensive but necessary to investigate the complex interaction of variables. Larger sample sizes are also needed. Finally, our interest in undertaking this study was to explore whether immune system changes would be associated with training in specific relaxation and imagery techniques. Our decision to select cancer patients to examine this question was based on a belief that this group would be more motivated to learn and practice our exercises than adults who had no encounter with a potentially life-threatening illness.

For readers who are specifically interested in the issue of recovery from cancer and in cancer survival, we would like to point out that a prognostic outcome cannot be determined from our study. First, our control group participated in a 6-month waiting-list design, which by definition, exposed all subjects to our experimental (behavioural) intervention. Second, our subjects consisted of women diagnosed and treated for stage 1, node-negative breast cancer. One would expect 95 per cent of these women to be alive at five years—the time of our follow-up. Thus, our subject selection and experimental design obviates any real interpretation about survival. For readers and investigators who are interested in survival outcomes we suggest future studies

EXPERIMENTAL DESIGN

*Cohort 1*
(Experimental)

*Cohort 2*
(Waiting list control)

*Weeks 1–3*
Baseline
3 weekly blood samples

*Weeks 1–3*
Baseline
3 weekly blood samples

*Weeks 4–12*

9 weekly
blood
samples

| Jacobsonian relaxation
| Lazarus's relaxation
| Cancer imagery
| Biofeedback to criterion

*Weeks 4–12*

9 weekly
control
blood
samples

*Weeks 13–52*
Monthly brush-up
and blood samples

*Weeks 13–25*
3 monthly blood samples

*Weeks 26–33*
Begin behavioural
intervention as
with Cohort 1

*Weeks 34–65*
Monthly brush up
and blood samples

employ a design using a true control group (that is in this case, subjects who are not involved in formal self-regulation training) with extensive follow-up of patients over at least ten years.

### 1.2 FIVE-YEAR POST STUDY FOLLOW-UP

With the encouragement of the editors of this volume, we contacted our research volunteers five years after their participation in the Immunologic Response study was completed. One of the 13 patients was lost to follow-up. (She moved out of the area and her oncologist is deceased.)

The 12 contacted patients are all alive and well. They average 6.5 years post-cancer-diagnosis without recurrence of the primary tumour. One patient who entered our study following surgery for a node-negative, intraductal tumour in the left breast developed an unrelated (lobular) tumour in the right breast two years ago. The new tumour was node-negative, treated by surgery alone, with no evidence of recurrence. All participants were pleased with the self-regulation techniques they had learnt in the study and all felt they had incorporated in some fashion the skills they learnt into their lives. Four of our subjects are actively using relaxation skills on a daily basis five years later.

It is important to note that six of our 13 patients were assigned to a waiting list control group. Being 'wait-listed' as a cancer patient adds significantly to one's existential discomfort, producing additional stress. One-third of these patients did not complete their behavioural training. We wonder whether this may have indeed influenced the responses of some of these patients both short-term and long-term.

## 1.3 MIND–BODY INTERACTIONS

Any approach to mind–body studies is usually grounded in the belief that psychological factors are an expression of neocortical activity, indeed possibly even a summation of such activity. Psychological responses function in a bidirectional cascade of chemical, electrical events throughout the complex cellular system of the body. The neuro–endocrine–lymphoid systems have functioned in an autonomous, interactive, stimulus–response fashion through-out evolution in the higher animals. Only recently in evolutionary history have they been influenced by, and modulated through, activity of the neocortex. Current studies show that the neocortex communicates with the limbic system directly via the stria terminalis, through the paraventricular nucleus of the hypothalamus. This communication extends to the medulla oblongata, the pituitary, the spinal cord, and the paravertebral sympathetic chains. Nerve fibres from the medulla oblongata are known to synapse with the lymphoid organs (nodes, spleen, and thymus), and probably into the bone marrow itself. Information of neocortical 'commands/states' could thus be passed directly to the lymphoid organs through direct neurochemical/electrical stimulation, and mobilize B- and T-cells and the non-B/non-T natural killer (NK) cells, as well as modulate the activity of peripheral blood lymphocytes. Furthermore, such 'commands' or 'states' could act through the hypothalamic–pituitary–adrenal axis to stimulate NK-cell activity via increased ACTH and increased beta-endorphins. Any *decrease* in the release of glucocorticoids in this endocrine axis would result in improved peripheral leukocyte migration and enhanced secretion of IL-1, IL-2, and interferon. Increased levels of such cytokines as IL-2 induces the development of cytotoxic T-cells and of B-cell differentiating factor(s). This symphony of events linking the brain with immunity is present at all times in the healthy individual. The question for us as investigators was whether we could measure and document this activity. The study that follows represents a very modest early step in that process.

## 2   Introduction to immunological responses study

Laboratory studies utilizing both whole animals and *in vitro* protocols have clearly demonstrated the existence of bidirectional links between the brain and the immune system. Signals in the form of neurotransmitters and peptide hormones can have profound effects upon the behaviour of lymphocytes and other cellular components of the immune system. In addition, peptides and proteins produced by cells of the immune system can alter the behaviour of the whole organism (2). Tangentially related to these studies are observations using human subjects suggesting that a variety of behavioural interventions can have an impact on the health of the individual. These include the use of social support (3), animal–human bonding (4), guided imagery and relaxation (1b), self-disclosure (5), as well as exercise (6). It is assumed, although not proven, that the beneficial effects of behavioural interventions in human subjects are mediated by pathways similar to those that have been demonstrated to exist using traditional laboratory models.

Guided imagery in conjunction with relaxation was popularized beginning in the late 1970s (7). While widely reported that imagery could be correlated with an improved prognosis in individuals who had tumours, these studies were subject to the valid criticism that little, if any, attempt was made to correlate the improved prognosis with specific changes in the immune system. Thus, few data exist to support the popular claim that imagery boosted the immune system.

Since these early studies, a number of investigations have employed similar techniques in an attempt to either manipulate the immune system/or improve the health status of patients with chronic disease. Relaxation training, especially when augmented with biofeedback, has been found to have efficacy in reducing both the psychological and physical symptoms associated with various disease states (8, 9). It is not clear whether the beneficial effects of relaxation are due to reduced arousal level (10) and/or to a decrease in sympathetic activity within the autonomic nervous system (11). Several studies have, nonetheless, correlated relaxation with specific changes in immune system parameters. In one such study (12) male and female subjects were divided on the basis of their scores on a stress scale. Under baseline conditions, it was found that phagocytic cells from those who reported a high degree of stress had reduced activity in contrast to those with low stress. In a subsequent component of that study it was found that those individuals who measured high on the stress scale benefited more than those in the low stress group following biofeedback training as expressed by increased measures of phagocytic activity. These high stress individuals were also found to have reduced anxiety and improved coping ability following the biofeedback training. Jasnoski and Kugler (13) correlated salivary IgA responses with relaxation either alone or in concert with guided imagery. While no differences in IgA were found between the relaxation and the relaxation plus imagery group, the presence of the relaxation component did correlate with elevated levels of IgA compared with control subjects who were included to control for alertness or mild arousal.

In our pilot study (1b) male and female subjects with a variety of metastatic tumors were studied over the course of one year. Correlated with the behavioural intervention were significant increases in T-lymphocyte function as well as total levels of immunoglobulins G and M. There were also significant increases in mixed lymphocyte responsiveness, the ability of NK cells to lyse tumor cells, and the production of interleukin-2 by stimulated lymphocytes.

The present study was designed to replicate and extend our previous findings as well as to facilitate the interpretation of these data by incorporating a wait-list control group. A limiting factor in the interpretation of our original study was the absence of a simultaneously studied control group. The inclusion of such a group is imperative to properly interpret the results of a study such as this to assess the effects of seasonal factors as well as interassay variability. The measures of immune system functioning chosen for this study were selected because previous studies suggested that they are responsive to certain types of stress and that they can be modulated by behavioural interventions similar to those employed in this study. The psychological parameters were chosen on the basis of their relationship to measures of health.

A secondary purpose of the study was to determine whether psychological changes might prove to be contingent on the behavioural interventions and correlated with immune changes. Additionally, the relationship between reductions in physiological arousal as measured by electromyography and immune changes was explored.

# 3 Methods

### 3.1 EXPERIMENTAL DESIGN

A fifteen-month study with two groups: (Group 1) immediate behavioural intervention, and (Group 2) a wait-list control was employed. Both groups underwent an initial three-week baseline period. During the six-month (24 weeks) period that followed, Group 1 was trained in the behavioural intervention methods, while Group 2 served as a control group for Group 1 — providing comparison data at equivalent points in time. At week 25 of the study Group 2, the wait-list control group, was crossed over to begin a sequence of behavioural training identical to that given to Group 1.

## 3.2 SUBJECTS

Thirteen breast cancer patients were recruited when they responded to newspaper advertisements announcing the study and from oncologists in the Washington, D.C. area. All patients had undergone a modified radical mastectomy and were lymph-node negative. No patients had undergone chemotherapy or radiation. (Prior to May 1988, patients with this diagnosis usually received a standardized treatment approach.) All of the patients had normal dietary habits. None had sleep disturbances or were psychotic. All patients were healthy with no evidence of organic conditions that might have altered endocrine or CNS functions. All patients were premenopausal (34–50 years old; $M = 44.6$ years). Pathology reports were obtained from their oncologists to confirm diagnoses, tissue type, and lymph node involvement.

## 3.3 PROCEDURE

Patients were initially screened by telephone for the study's criteria and randomly assigned to one of two experimental conditions: immediate treatment (Group 1, $n = 7$) or delayed treatment control (Group 2, $n = 6$). Patients in each group were brought to our Center on succeeding days for an explanation of the project and to complete informed consent procedures. All patients then provided three weekly baseline blood measures, and underwent psychological testing, and a computerized psychophysiological stress evaluation.

### 3.3.1 Blood samples

All blood samples were taken in the morning within two hours of the same time (10:00 a.m.) to control for diurnal variation. The blood samples consisted of 30 ml of blood drawn from the patient's arm (contralateral to the mastectomized side) into sterile sodium heparin tubes. Venepuncture was performed either by a registered nurse or a licensed phlebotomist. The schedule for collecting blood samples was as follows: fifteen blood samples were collected from patients in both groups during the first 24 weeks (six months) of the study. During the initial 12 weeks (months 1–3) patients in both groups provided 12 weekly blood samples. The first three blood samples comprised the baseline measure. During the subsequent nine weeks, Group 1 provided blood samples while undergoing behavioural training and Group 2 (the delayed treatment, 'control' group) provided weekly samples at corresponding points in time. In the 12 weeks that followed (months 4–6) patients in both groups provided three monthly blood samples. At month 6 of the study, Group 2 patients began training (identical to Group 1) and nine weekly samples were collected followed by three monthly follow-up samples post training. Group 1 patients continued to provide post-training monthly samples until the study's completion at month 15. This design allowed for both 'within-groups' and 'between-groups' comparisons.

### 3.3.2 Blood assays

All lymphocyte and NK-cell assays were carried out using fresh cells. Plasma was stored frozen for subsequent evaluation of antibody titres and protein bound cortisol levels (by radioimmunoassay) at the conclusion of the study. The immune assays performed included NK-cell cytotoxicity (that is 'NK-cell activity'), concanavalin A responsiveness (Con-A), mixed lymphocyte responsiveness (MLR), lymphocyte production of interleukin-2 (IL-2), titres of plasma IgG, IgA, and IgM, total white cell count as well as peripheral blood lymphocytes (PBL). Procedures used for these assays are described fully in our previous study (1b).

### 3.3.3 Psychological inventories

Several self-report, pencil-and-paper inventories were used to assess the patients' initial psychological status and emotional changes over time. These tests were administered at baseline and following training. Baseline psychological inventories were screened immediately after completion to eliminate those patients who might not reliably complete the study protocol. The criteria for exclusion included an invalid profile, or evidence of either psychotic patterns or extreme mood disorder. The inventories used included the Minnesota Multiphasic Personality Inventory (MMPI), the Millon Behavioural Health Inventory (MBHI), the Sarason Social Support Scale, the Rotter Locus of Control, and two quality of life instruments: the Affects Balance Scale (ABS) (14), and Greer's Mental Adjustment to Cancer (MAC) scale (15). These instruments were chosen because of their reliability and validity, relevance to cancer research, and sensitivity to therapeutic change.

### 3.3.4 Psychophysiological stress profile

Baseline measures of electromyographic activity, peripheral hand temperature, and skin conductance were made during a standard psychophysiological stress evaluation. These levels were used to evaluate biofeedback training effects.

### 3.3.5   Training

Following the initial three-week baseline period Group 1 was given a nine-week sequence of relaxation training, guided imagery, and EMG biofeedback training. All relaxation training was done in groups. The protocol was as follows. At training session one, patients were given a lecture on the immune system. They were then given group instruction in Jacobsonian relaxation. Following the session, patients were given an audio cassette tape and instructed to practise the relaxation exercise twice a day for the next week. At the second week, patients were introduced to a second relaxation exercise, 'Letting Go', developed by Lazarus (cited in Goldfried and Davison) (16) and were again instructed to practise twice daily using the audio tape. At the third week, guided imagery was introduced to the group using techniques developed at our Center and a second audio tape was given to the patients. Care was exercised to make the group meetings cordial but to minimize traditional group therapeutic effects. To do otherwise would unnecessarily complicate interpretation of the data.

The guided imagery tape used in the study began with a short segment on relaxation in which patients were asked to recall the feelings of relaxation experienced with their first tape. The imagery exercise then proceeded with a suggestion that they mentally place themselves in a relaxed setting where all things are possible. General guidelines were then given to patients regarding the immune system and the development of health promoting processes within their bodies. No specific imagery was suggested to the patients. We have found in our clinical experience that patients prefer the freedom to use their own imaginations to construct their imagery rather than having specific images suggested to them. We routinely use this procedure in all our studies.

At the fourth week, EMG biofeedback training began. Biofeedback sessions were held twice weekly. Each biofeedback session consisted of 500 seconds of stabilization and baseline, 1000 seconds of training and 100 seconds of rest. Biofeedback training continued until patients were able to achieve a frontal EMG level of $< 1.75$ microvolts/RMS for 200 seconds over two sessions. We have routinely used this criterion over the past five years at this Center. It is a relatively good index of a patient's ability to relax frontal muscle tension.

Throughout training and follow-up, patients were instructed to practice relaxation and guided imagery twice daily. Each Friday, patients sent in postcards documenting their frequency of practice and perceived quality of relaxation and imagery. Patients also used the postcards to document any acute illness, medication usage, medical treatment, and interpersonal or other changes in their lives. Because medication usage and other factors might affect immune measures, this information is critical. These data were used to facilitate training, for post hoc analyses, and to insure the quality of blood measures. Each month over the 15 months of the project, monthly brush-up sessions were held during which relaxation practice and help with imagery was provided. Patients made drawings of their imagery at these sessions which were scored according to the standardized Image-CA forms (17).

At week 25 (six months into the study), Group 2 patients began the nine-week behavioural intervention described above. As with Group 1, monthly post-training sessions were scheduled with patients in Group 2 to support continued practice of their new skills.

## 3.4 STATISTICAL ANALYSES

Due to the complexity and volume of the data, several levels and types of statistical procedures were used. A power analysis was carried out using variance estimates from our previous research with power set at 90 per cent for one-tailed tests at alpha equal to .05. Immune measures were initially subjected to a 2 × 2 analysis of variance (ANOVA) for repeated measures to test for training effects. T tests were used to assess biofeedback training effects with alpha rate adjusted to maintain the probability of type I error at .05. Bonferroni-adjusted probabilities (18) were also used to determine the use of the terms 'significant' and 'non-significant' in reporting results for individual immune assays. Separate analyses were carried out between immune measures and postcard data to determine whether any relation between frequency or perceived quality of relaxation existed. These data were also evaluated to determine whether immune changes were associated with acute illness or medication usage.

For the purpose of clarity the data are presented in two phases. Phase I covers the first six months of the study with between-groups comparisons for the experimental group (1) and the control group (2). In Phase II, baseline and post-treatment data for both groups 1 and 2 were pooled ($N = 13$) to assess the overall effects of training on the two groups combined. Phase II also presents 'within groups' comparisons for both groups.

# 4 Results

## 4.1 BETWEEN-GROUPS COMPARISON DURING FIRST SIX MONTHS

### 4.1.1 *Immune measures*

The between-groups effect for PBL comparing the Group 1 training period with the equivalent baseline period for Group 2 (delayed treatment control) was significant, $F(1, 37) = 23.356$, $p < .001$.

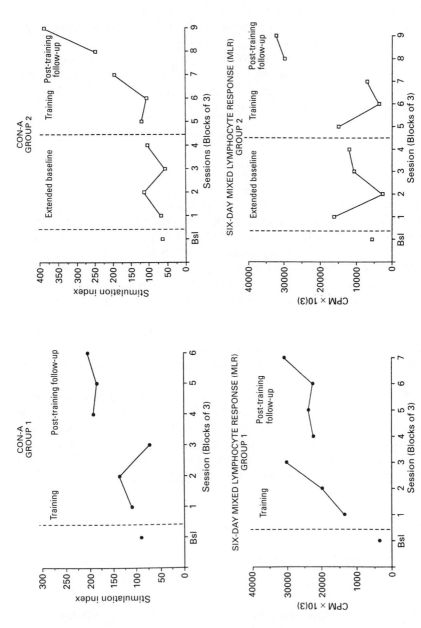

**Figure 1** Comparison of the course of weekly changes in Con-A (top), MLR (middle), and NK (bottom) for Group 1 and 2 during training of Group 1. The baseline data points represent the mean of three weekly samples for each group.

A significant 'between-groups' effect was found for the whole blood cell count (WBC) between the Group 1 training period and the equivalent baseline period for Group 2 ($F(1, 37) = 6.093, p < .02$). This effect was produced by a reduction in WBC for Group 2 while Group 1 remained unchanged. No significant correlation was found between WBC and cortisol values.

Figure 1, A–C, shows the course of 'between-groups' effects for T-cell and NK-cell measures. The between-groups effect was significant for Con-A, $F(1, 37) = 7.90, p < .008$. MLR 'between-groups' effects comparing Group 1 (experimental) with Group 2 (delayed treatment control) were also significant, $F(1, 37) = 9.43, p < .004$ (Figure 1, B). The 'between-groups' effect for NK-cell measures was not significant. A significant between-groups effect was found for IgG($F(1, 37) = 7.89, p < .008$). 'Between-groups' effects for antibody measures IgA and IgM were not significant.

A significant 'between-groups' effect ($F(1, 37) = 4.51, p < .04$) was found for cortisol. This effect was due to a downward trend in Group 1 values during training while Group 2 cortisol values rose slightly during the extended baseline.

## 4.2 OVERALL TRAINING EFFECTS AND WITHIN-GROUPS COMPARISON

### 4.2.1 *Immune measures*

The overall effect of treatment on PBL was significant, $F(1, 74) = 7.186$, $p < .009$. The main effects for WBC counts were not significantly different from baseline compared with training.

Con-A showed a significant overall treatment effect for Groups 1 and 2 combined ($F(1, 74) = 21.44, p < .001$). MLR main effects were also significant as a result of treatment, $F(1, 74) = 46.41, p < .001$, and the overall treatment effect on NK-cell activity[1] was significant, $F(1, 45) = 6.17$, $p < .017$.

The course of T-cell changes for each group (within-groups) is depicted in Figure 2, A–D. All T-cell measures changed significantly following training. Con-A data are presented as a stimulation index which reflect changes in Con-A responsiveness and not media values. These changes represent increases in the proliferative response, not reductions in background activity. A within-groups effect was significant for Group 1, $F(1, 40) = 4.33, p < .04$ and for Group 2, $F(1, 34) = 38.36, p < .001$. MLR within-groups comparisons were significant for both Group 1, $F(1, 40) = 20.99, p < .001$ and for Group 2, $F(1, 34) = 35.84, p < .001$ (Figure 2, C–D).

---

[1] NK results should be interpreted with caution as they are based on 70 per cent of the data. Thirty per cent of the NK values were lost due to a laboratory error. Losses were random, introducing no systematic bias by group or individual. The results are included here because they are consistent with our other measures and with other studies.

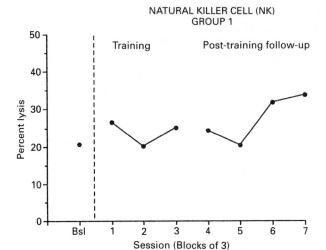

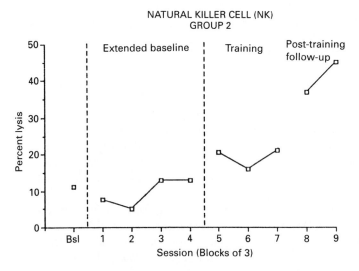

**Figure 2** The course of Con-A (top) and MLR (bottom) responsiveness for Group 1, experimental, and Group 2, delayed treatment, to behaviour intervention. For Group 1, data points 1, 2, and 3 represent blocks of three weekly blood samples during training; data points 4, 5, and 6 are blocks of three monthly samples during nine months of follow-up. For Group 2, data points 5, 6, and 7 are blocks of three weekly samples during training and data points 8 and 9 are blocks of three monthly, post-treatment samples.

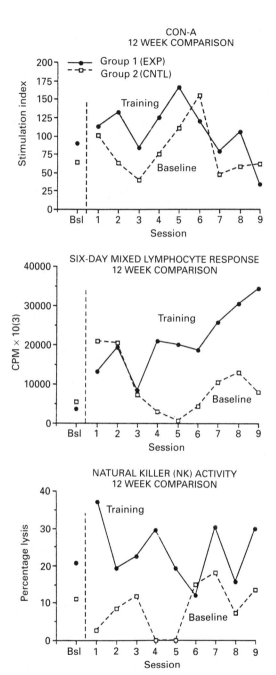

**Figure 3** The course of NK changes to behaviour intervention in Group 1, immediate treatment (left), and Group 2, delayed treatment control (right). For Group 1, data points 1, 2, 3, are blocks of three weekly samples during training and points 4, 5, 6, and 7 are blocks of three monthly, post-treatment, samples. For Group 2, data points 5, 6, and 7 are blocks of three weekly samples during training and data points 8 and 9 are blocks of three monthly, post-treatment samples.

The 'within-groups' effect on NK-cell activity is depicted in Figure 3. Group 1 baseline versus training effects were not significant $F(1, 26) = 3.83, p < .06$ nor were the 'within-groups' effects for Group 2, $F(1, 19) = 2.44, p < .134$ (Figure 3). Though these effects are non-significant within the criterion period, the data are presented because they do show long-term effects considered in the discussion section.

The only antibody measure to show a treatment effect that is ('within-groups') was that for IgM. A significant effect was found on this measure for Group 2, $F(1, 35) = 15.39, p < .001$. Other within-groups effects for IgM approached significance but fell short of the $p < .05$ level. IL-2 effects were significant for Group 2, $F(1, 34) = 9.90, p < .003$. Within-groups effects for all other measures were not significant.

An intercorrelation matrix constructed to assess interaction and biological consistency for the immune measures across all 13 subjects revealed considerable spread. MLR and Con-A values (Pearson's $r = .71$) demonstrated a strong relationship. The correlation between WBC and PBL was .64. Antibody measures showed several negative correlations with other assays: IgG and Con-A, $r = -.50$; IgA and IL-2, $r = -.48$; IgM and IL-2, $r = -.36$. The Pearson $r$ between antibody measures were as follows: IgA and IgG, $r = .03$; IgG and IgM = .35; and IgA and IgM = .41. Differences in half-lives of these immunoglobulins as well as specificity for antigens may have influenced these correlations.

### 4.3 BIOFEEDBACK TRAINING DATA

Biofeedback training effects were significant, $t(43) = 9.88, p < .003$ for both groups combined. Group 1 baseline-to-training effects were also significant, $t(27) = 6.96, p < .001$, as were Group 2 effects, $t(15) = 7.73, p < .001$. No significant between-groups effects were found with regard to training differences. Only one patient failed to reach the EMG biofeedback training criterion. This patient's reductions in EMG levels, however, were significant, $t(3) = 9.07, p < .003$.

### 4.4 POSTCARD DATA

Analysis of weekly postcard data showed that patients practiced relaxation eight to nine times per week immediately after the introduction of the first exercise. Weekly relaxation practice then increased to 11 times per week for four weeks. Practice frequency then returned to eight to nine times per week for the duration of the study. Patients consistently rated the quality of their relaxation higher than the quality of imagery. Quality of relaxation and imagery was rated on a scale of one to six representing a continuum of easy to difficult, respectively. Mean quality for relaxation was 2.5 while the mean quality for imagery was 3.8.

Incidences of colds and flu reported on the datacards showed a relationship with two immune measures, IL-2 and IgA. IL-2 values were found to be −.48 standard deviation units below the group mean, and IgA values were .47 standard deviations above the mean values at the time of reported illness.

## 4.5 PSYCHOLOGICAL DATA

None of the individual scales on any of the pencil-and-paper inventories showed statistically significant changes prior to or post training. These data are reported here because taken together they provide a global perspective on the effects of training. Post training MMPI scores showed decreases in Hypochondrias (Hs), Depression (D), and Hysteria (Hy) scales. These changes were 2.6, 3.8, and 2.5 t-score points, respectively. A two-point increase was also observed in the Ego Strength (ES) measure on the Wiggins Content scales.

The MBHI pre–post measures showed a decrease in 16 of the 20 scales.

The Affects Balance Scale (ABS) provides four measures of positive emotions (Joy, Contentment, Vigour, and Affection) and four measures of negative emotions (Anxiety, Depression, Guilt, and Hostility) and a composite score. Only Joy and Contentment values showed an increase among the positive scales in pre–post testing. Vigour and Affection showed slight decreases. Anxiety, Depression, Guilt, and Hostility values all showed slight decreases from pre-to-post testing. An improved composite score resulted from decreases in negative emotion scores rather than increases in positive emotions.

On the Mental Adjustment to Cancer (MAC) inventory, scores for the Fighting Spirit (FS) scale showed the largest increase (two t-score points). Scores for the other scales of the MAC, Helplessness–Hopefulness (HH), Anxious Preoccupation (AP), Fatalism (F), and Avoidance (A) were remarkably stable from pre-to-post-training. Of interest, however, were the strong correlations in the expected direction between HH and FS, Pearson's $r = -.78$, HH and F, $r = .75$, and F and AP, $r = .83$.

The Rotter Locus of Control measuring the internal and external locus of control showed almost no change (pretraining $M = 8.9$; post-training $M = 8.7$). From the beginning of the study the patients exhibited high internal control.

The Sarason Social Support Scale was modified to derive a measure of social support by collapsing several items into a single score with higher scores indicating greater support. The pretreatment mean was 51 while the post-treatment mean was 48.

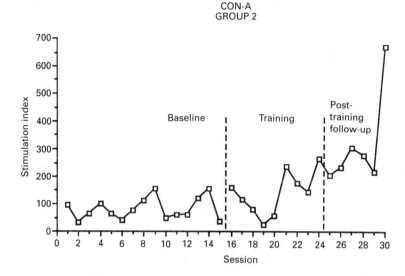

Figure 4   The course of Con-A changes for Group 2, delayed treatment control, during three phases of the study. All samples taken are depicted.


## 5  Discussion

Our results suggest that relaxation, imagery, and biofeedback training produce statistically significant effects primarily on T-cell populations and NK cells. Antibodies were minimally affected by the interventions programme. The findings of this study with breast cancer patients, who were 'healthy' at the time of training, replicate the findings of our earlier study with metastatic cancer patients (1). Our approach, therefore, appears to be applicable to patients at various stages of cancer.

The time course for immune changes in both studies was such that several weeks to months were required for changes to reach statistical significance. Figure 4 shows the course of Con-A changes for Group 2 for all blood samples collected over the 15 months of our present study. The shape of this curve is virtually isomorphic with the graph of Con-A changes in our first study. As noted for the present study, the increases in the stimulation index in the first study were also not artifacts produced by reductions in background cell proliferation. It is of interest to us that Spiegel and co-workers (19 and Chapter 4 of this volume) demonstrated increased mean survival time in advanced breast cancer patients following group therapy and that the group therapy effect required 20 months to develop. Therefore, it is possible that long-term-effects of behavioural interventions—whether relaxation, biofeedback, or group therapy — are cumulative. The immune system changes seen in our interventions and those observed by other researchers (3 and Chapter 11 of this volume) may be the basis for this increased survival time. Caution is warranted with respect to how much significance to give to NK measures as a recent study (20) found no relation between NK-cell activity and the stage of breast cancer. Furthermore, the manner in which a population of NK-cells behaves *in vitro* may not reflect their behaviour *In vivo*. Nonetheless, if our observations do reflect the enhanced ability of NK cells in our study population to lyse tumour cells *In vivo*, then incorporation of behavioural interventions into more traditional treatment protocols early in the process would be warranted.

One exception to the gradual changes seen in most of our immune measures was MLR. The MLR measures (important in tumour rejection) increased within the first two weeks of training. These changes were sustained for the remainder of the time during which measurements were taken; in this study it was 15 months. Other researchers have reported effects on T-cell and NK-cell populations (3, 7) that develop as rapidly as our MLR results. Since many of these studies were not conducted over the extended period of time (that is 15 months) of our study, it is not possible to ascertain whether the reported initial effects were maintained. It is not possible, therefore, to determine if the delayed time course for immune changes (for measures other than with MLR) is a phenomenon specific to our subject population and experimental conditions or to a more general aspect of immune system changes.

Our data also show that MLR is the most responsive index to behavioural interventions. Con A, a T-cell measure, was second. The reason for the differential responsiveness of these immune measures is not known at present.

From our biofeedback data it is evident that reduction in physiological arousal occurred contingent upon relaxation and biofeedback training. Both muscle tension and autonomic activity showed reductions. These changes began by the third week of training which in our protocol was the earliest point that psychophysiological measures were taken on patients following baseline. With the possible exception of MLR changes which began at week 2, it is clear that these psychophysiological reductions preceded the changes in immune parameters. Whether they were related causally to these changes has yet to be proven.

The relationship between reductions in arousal-related physiological activity and immune changes is apparently complex. Both our experimental and (delayed treatment) control group showed statistically significant decreases in physiological arousal as measured by EMG, skin temperature, and skin conductance. Group 1, the immediate treatment group, showed much larger immune responses than did Group 2, the delayed treatment control. If we interpret the physiological and the immune data together, it is clear that reductions in physiological arousal are not linearly related to changes in the immune system. Our speculation is that some psychological factor(s) may have influenced the performance of Group 2. Perhaps boredom or the psychological effect of providing blood samples over a six-month baseline period took its toll. Some Group 2 patients did express a growing impatience to begin the behavioural training sequence.

One potential mechanism whereby the relaxation training might have precipitated the immune system changes observed in this study would be via alterations in plasma levels of cortisol. Relaxation training has been shown to reduce cortisol output (21). Cortisol does have well-documented immunomodulatory effects with low doses stimulating and high doses inhibiting measures of immune system functioning (22). While a significant effect was seen between groups for cortisol during phase I of this study, Group 2 did not show a significant 'within-groups' effect after they underwent training. Since cortisol levels were not significantly reduced for both groups, possibly hormonal and/or autonomic, events were responsible for the observed changes. It is also possible that the amount of free cortisol, which was not measured in this study, that would have been available to act upon lymphocytes might have been elevated in proportion to total cortisol.

An analysis of the nature of the changes on the psychological inventories given pre- and post-treatment to our patients showed that the changes were primarily associated with anxiety reduction. To a lesser extent, scores on the scales measuring the positive emotions, Joy and Contentment, were increased. Levy and coworkers (23) have shown that the Joy scale of the ABS is an important prognostic indicator of survival time in breast cancer patients. Because significant immune effects on several measures were seen in our study with minimal increases in positive emotion scales, these effects may have derived from anxiety reduction rather than an increase in such positive emotions as joy. Our psychophysiological, psychological, and, possibly, cortisol measures suggest this may have been the case. It would be useful to know whether even larger changes could be produced if both significant anxiety reduction and positive emotional enhancement occurred simultaneously.

We have found both in clinical practice and over the course of several years of research in psychoneuroimmunology that patients find relaxation training easier than imagery training. Little change was seen in the patients' rating of relaxation and imagery quality over the course of treatment. Patients tended to persist with whatever quality rating they gave for the first week throughout the study. The frequency of practice and quality was highly correlated. It is clear from the data that patients were adhering to instructions to do daily practice. A post hoc analysis of the relationship between frequency and quality of relaxation and imagery and immune measures did not reveal any consistent relationship. This finding is probably due to the consistency of reported frequency and quality ratings producing a statistical artifact. Patients reported—and the data confirmed—that the effect of biofeedback training allowed them to practise imagery while maintaining a low level of physiological arousal.

A careful inspection of our social support data from the modified Sarason Scale indicated that the quality of support given to our patients improved over time even though the number of persons providing that support decreased. These changes led to lower support scores because number was weighted more heavily than quality. It is unclear whether this change in the quality of support was due to fewer persons actually being available to provide support or the result of our patients becoming more highly discriminating about those providing support. The improved quality of support would suggest that longer-term experience with the disease deepened interpersonal relationships. This change is of interest in view of the role that social interactions play in modulating the balance between health and disease. For example, a large epidemiological study has revealed that people who are married and/or have a large circle of friends have an increased life expectancy over people who are single (24).

We have noted with great interest the consistency of changes involving T-cell measures in response to behavioural interventions. T-cells are relatively more susceptible to subtle fluctuations in glucocorticoids and also bear receptors for catecholamines (25). Since most of the major immunological tissues are innervated by branches of the sympathetic nervous system and possibly the parasympathetic as well (26), this may be the mechanism whereby the behavioural interventions described in this study influenced the measures of the T-cell function. T-cells are capable of modulating other cell types within the immune compartments of the body (including B-cells) and so it is possible that all of the observed changes were a reflection of altered T-cell function. Given current knowledge, it would be presumptuous to formulate a precise mechanism whereby the relaxation and guided imagery protocol in the present study was found to influence measures of immune system functioning.

How can one conceptualize an interaction of emotions (origin, the CNS) and the immune system? (27). There is a growing body of literature suggesting that the immune system peptides are biologically active within the brain. Some of the biological effects include modulation of brain catecholamines which have been linked to a number of affective disorders, in addition to the control of immunomodulatory neuroendocrine circuits. Indeed, two recent studies have correlated circulating levels of thymosin alpha-1 with psychosocial constructs (28, 29). Thus, in addition to the behavioural interventions causing changes in the immune system there is the very real possibility that the immunological status of the individual might, in turn, influence cognitive functioning as well as the individual's behaviour. We infer that we are, at the very least, dealing with bidirectional cascading effects through which emotional and cognitive states influence all physiology, and physiological activities and states including those of the immune system. All these inter-actions subserve the interest of maintaining homeostasis for the organism.

As a cautionary note it is important to recognize that our study was designed not to demonstrate cause–effect relationships between the intervention and the specific immune parameters that were assessed, but rather to define cor-relations between certain indices of immune system functioning and this particular behavioural intervention. While it is difficult to interpret *in vitro* measures with respect to immunocompetence *in vivo*, the fact that there were significant correlations between these particular indices of the immune system and the behavioural intervention suggested that the intervention might be capable of either directly or indirectly modulating the immune system. Although causality is a possibility, further research would be required to firmly establish this relationship.

5.1 ACKNOWLEDGEMENTS

We wish to thank Douglas B. Coulson, Ph.D. for his expertise on the statistical analysis of the data. We would also like to thank Clay Steiner, M.D.; Janelle Oliver, M.S.; Maureen O'Grady, Ph.D.; and Rena Goetz, Ph.D., for their contribution to the performance of the assays. Finally, we thank both Sandy Bangham, R.N. and the medical laboratory staff at The Washington Clinic, Washington, D.C. for their services in performing phlebotomy.

# 6   References

1a.   Gruber, B. L., Hersh, S. P., Hall, N. R. S., Waletzky, L. R., Kunz, J. F., Carpenter, J. C. *et al.* (1993). Immunological responses of breast cancer patients to behavioural interventions. *Biofeedback Self Reg.*, **18**, 1–22.

1b.   Gruber, B. L., Hall, N. R., Hersh, S. P., and Dubois, P. (1988). Immune system and psychological changes in metastatic cancer patients using relaxation and guided imagery. *Scand. J. Behav. Ther.*, **17**, 25–46.

2.    Ader, R., Felten, D., and Cohn, N. (1991). *Psychoneuroimmunology.* Academic Press, New York.

3.    Kiecolt-Glaser, J. K., Glaser, R., Williger, D., Stout, J., Messick, G., Sheppard, S. *et al.* (1985). Psychosocial enhancement of immunocompetence in a geriatric population. *Health Psychols.*, **4**, 25–41.

4.    Friedmann, E., Ketcher, A. H., Thomas, S. A., Lynch, J.J., and Messent, P. R. (1983). Social interaction and blood pressure: Influence of animal companions. *J. Nerv. Ment. Dis.*, **171**, 461–465.

5.    Pennebaker, J. W., Kiecolt-Glaser, J. K., and Glaser, R. (1988). Disclosure of traumas and immune function: Health implications for psychotherapy. *J. Consult. Clin. Psychol.*, **56**, 239–245.

6.    Simon, H. B. (1991). Exercise and human immune function. In *Psychoneuro-immunology*, (ed. R. Ader, D. Felten, and N. Cohn), pp. 869–890. Academic Press, New York.

7.    Achterberg, J. and Lawlis, G. F. (1979). A canonical relationship between blood chemistries and psychological variables in cancer patients. *Multivar. Exp. Res.*, 41, 1–10.

8.    Basmajian, J. V. (1983). *Biofeedback: Principles and Practice for Clinicians*. Williams and Wilkens, Baltimore.

9.    Fotopoul, S. S. and Sunderland, W. P. (1978). Biofeedback in the treatment of psychophysiologic disorders. *Biofeedback Self Reg.*, 3 331–361.

10.   Schwartz, G. E. (1975). Biofeedback, self-regulation, and the patterning of physiological processes. *Am. Sci.*, 63, 314–324.

11.   Benson, H. (1983). The relaxation response and norepinephrine. *Integrat. Psychiat.*, 1, 15–18.

12.   Peavey, B. S., Lawlis, G. F., and Goven, A. (1985). Biofeedback-assisted relaxation: Effects on phagocytic capacity. *Biofeedback Self Reg.*, 10, 33–47.

13.   Jasnoski, M. L. and Kugler, J. (1987). Relaxation, imagery, and neuroimmuno-modulation. *Ann. N. Y. Acad. Sci.*, 496, 722–730.

14.   Derogatis, L. R., Abeloff, M. D., and Melisaratos, N. (1979). Psychological coping mechanisms and survival time in metastatic breast cancer. *JAMA*, 242, 1504–1508.

15.   Greer, S. (1983). Cancer and the mind. *Br. J. Psychiat.*, 143, 535–543.

16.   Goldfried, M. R. and Davison, G. C. (1976). *Clinical Behavior Therapy*, pp. 95–98. Holt, Rinehart and Winston, New York.

17.   Achterberg, J. and Lawlis, G. F. (1978). *Imagery of Cancer*. Institute for Personality and Ability Testing, Champaign, IL.

18.   Miller, R. (1981). *Simultaneous Statistical Inference*. Springer-Verlag, New York.

19.   Spiegel, D., Bloom, J. R., Kraemer, H. C., and Gottheil, E. (1989). Effect of psychosocial treatment on survival of patients with metastatic breast cancer. *Lancet*, 2, 888–891.

20.   Bonilla, F., Alvarez-Mon, M., Merino, F., and Espana, P. (1990). Natural killer activity in patients with breast cancer. *Eur. J. Gynaecol. Oncol.*, 11, 103–109.

21.   McGrady, A. V., Yonder, R., Tan, S. Y., Fine, T. H., and Woerner, M. (1981). The effect of biofeedback-assisted relaxation training on blood pressure and selected biochemical parameters in patients with essential hypertension. *Biofeedback Self Reg.*, 6, 343–353.

22.   Munck, A. and Guyre, P. M. (1991). Glucocorticoids and immune function. In *Psychoneuroimmunology*, (ed. R. Ader, D. Felten, and N. Cohn), pp. 447–486. Academic Press, New York.

23.   Levy, S. M., Herberman, R. B., Lippman M., and d'Angelo, T. (1987). Correlation of stress factors with sustained depression of natural killer cell activity and predicted prognosis in patients with breast cancer. *J. Clin. Oncol.*, 5, 348–353.

24.   Berkman, L. F. and Syme, S. L. (1979). Social networks, host resistance, and mortality: A nine year follow up study of Alameda County residents. *Am. J. Epidem.*, 109, 186–204.

25.   Hall, N. R. and Goldstein, A. L. (1983). Endocrine regulation of host immunity: The role of steroids and thymosins. In *Immune Modulation Agents and Their Mechanisms*, (ed. R. L. Fenichel and M. A. Chirigos), pp. 533–563. Marcel Dekker, New York.

26.   Felten, D. L., Felten, S. Y., Bellinger, D. L., Carlson, S. L., Ackerman, K. D., Madden, K. S. *et al.* (1987). Noradrenergic sympathetic neural interactions with the immune system: Structure and function. *Immunol. Rev.*, **100**, 225–260.

27.   Hall, N. R. and O'Grady, M. P. (1989). Regulation of pituitary peptides by the immune system: Historical and current perspectives. *Progr. Neuroendocrinimmun.*, **2**, 4–10.

28.   Hoon, E. F., Rand, K. H., Edwards, N. B., Hoon, P., Johnson, J., and Hall, N. R. (1991). A psychobehavioural model of genital herpes recurrence. *J. Psychosom. Res.*, **35**, 25–36.

29.   Aldwin, C. M., Spiro, A., Clark, G., and Hall, N. R. (1991). Thymic hormones, stress, and depressive symptoms in older men: A comparison of different statistical techniques for small samples. *Brain Behav. Immun.*, **5**, 206–218.

# 15

# Modulation of anti-tumour immunity by enkephalins

NICHOLAS P. PLOTNIKOFF AND ROBERT E. FAITH

## 1  Introduction

In recent years there has been increasing interest in the use of immunotherapy in the treatment of cancer. A large number of studies have shown that the immune system may play an important role in resistance to and/or recovery from neoplastic disease. It is hoped that anti-tumour immunity can be used to complement the effect of conventional treatments such as chemotherapy, radiotherapy, and/or surgery. Early studies in this area focused on a relatively small number of chemicals or treatment modalities that were known to influence immune function. More recently, a number of cytokines which modulate immune function have been identified and are being studied as adjuncts to cancer therapy. Methods are even being developed to introduce some of these agents into tumours by gene transfer.

The list of cytokines which modulate immune function is rapidly expanding. For the purposes of this discussion, the neuropeptides will be included as cytokines as many of them clearly modulate the function of immune cells. The list of cytokines known to modulate immune function includes the interleukins (IL-1 to IL-12), granulocyte-macrophage/colony-stimulating factor (GM-CSF), tumor necrosis factor-alpha (TNF alpha), transforming growth factor-beta (TGF beta), interferon-alpha (IFN alpha), interferon-gamma (IFN gamma), substance P, neurokinin A, neurotensin, bombesin, gastrin-releasing peptide, various opioids endorphins, enkephalins), somato-trophin, and somatostatin. The influence of a number of these compounds on tumour immunity has been investigated. Below, are a few examples of these studies.

The interleukins have been used extensively to boost anti-tumour immunity. In mice, systemic IL-1 in conjunction with local adjuvant therapy has been shown not only to produce primary tumour protection but also long lasting immunity to the tumour (1). Additionally, IL-1 has been shown to modify the ability of antigen-presenting cells to present tumour-associated antigens to lymphocytes (2). IL-2 is perhaps the most studied of the interleukins. IL-2 has been shown to augment tumour immunity, alone or in conjunction with other agents in both animal (3–8) and human (9–11) studies. IL-2 has just received FDA approval for the treatment of kidney cancer and is being studied for the treatment of melanoma and colon cancer (12). McBride *et al.* introduced the gene for murine IL-7 into a fibrosarcoma tumour by means of a retroviral-mediated gene transfer and showed this to result in a large increase in infiltra-tion of T-cells into the tumour, and later, the significant regression of the tumour (13).

IFN alpha has been shown to have clinical activity against hairy cell leukaemia as well as Kaposi's sarcoma (12, 14), whereas IFN gamma alters the presentation of tumour-associated antigens to lymphocytes by antigen-presenting cells (2). Watanabe used retrovirus-mediated gene transfer tech-niques to transfer the IFN gamma gene into murine tumour cells which then constitutively produced IFN gamma (15). When these cells were implanted into mice they usually lost their tumourigenicity due to specific and/or non-specific immune responses which were, most likely, augmented by the tumour-derived IFN gamma. GM-CSF, TNF alpha, and TGF beta have all been shown to modulate the presentation of tumour-associated antigens by antigen-presenting cells to lymphocytes (2, 16). A number of other cytokines and neuropeptides including substance P, neurokinin A, neurotensin, bombesin, gastrin-releasing peptide, endorphins, enkephalins, somatotrophin, and soma-tostatin have been shown to activate macrophages (17).

The enkephalins were originally described as the endogenous ligands for the morphine receptors in brain (18). We have recently shown that the enkephalins exhibit antidepressant, anti-anxiety, and anticonvulsant activities (19). In 1979, Wybran *et al.* (20) reported that normal human T-lymphocytes possess receptors for methionine-enkephalin (met-enkephalin), and subsequently the presence of opiate receptors on human phagocytic leukocytes was reported (21). Since the initial report of Wybran *et al.* a number of studies have shown that the enkephalins have an enhancing effect on various immune functions. The effects of enkephalins on host defence mechanisms which may play a role in resistance to, or recovery from, neoplastic disease are discussed below.

# 2  Animal studies

## 2.1  B16 MELANOMA

Murgo demonstrated an antitumour effect of met-enkephalin in 1985 (22). C57BL/6J mice were inoculated with B16-BL6 cells and then treated daily for 7 or 14 days with varying doses of met-enkephalin. Animals treated with a daily dose of 50 $\mu$g met-enkephalin showed significant inhibition of tumour growth. The antitumour effect of met-enkephalin was inhibited by naloxone, while naloxone alone had no significant effect on tumour growth. Our further studies confirmed these results and also demonstrated inhibition of metastasis of the B16-BL6 melanoma by met-enkephalin treatment in C57BL/6 mice (23, 24). These findings were independently confirmed by Scholar *et al.* (25).

## 2.2  L1210 LEUKAEMIA

$BDF_1$ mice were used to study the protective effects of met- and leucine-enkephalin (leu-enkephalin) against murine leukemia (26). Groups of mice were inoculated with either $1 \times 10^2$ or $1 \times 10^4$ L1210 tumour cells. Following the tumour inoculations, the low-tumour-dose animals were injected daily with 10 mg/kg body weight of either met- or leu-enkephalin, and the high-tumour-dose animals were injected daily with 30 mg/kg body weight of either met- or leu-enkephalin. Interestingly, the low-tumour-dose animals were significantly protected from tumour challenge by leu-enkephalin while the high-tumour-dose animals were significantly protected from tumour challenge by met-enkephalin.

2.3 NEUROBLASTOMA

Zagan and McLaughlin have performed a number of studies on the tumour growth inhibitory effects *in vitro* of several peptides. They have established that met-enkephalin is the most active tumour growth inhibitor *in vitro* of over twenty related peptides studied against the S20Y neuroblastoma cell line in culture (27). *In vivo*, met-enkephalin exhibited anti-tumour effects in mice at doses of 0.5 to 30 mg/kg body weight when given subcutaneously. In contrast, mice treated with leu-enkephalin or with [D-Ala$^2$, D-Leu$^5$]-enkephalin did not display any change in tumour growth when compared with untreated controls. A specific new receptor for met-enkephalin called the zeta receptor was proposed as a regulator of tumour growth (27).

2.4 FIBROSARCOMA

The murine fibrosarcoma cell line PYB6 was used by Srisuchart *et al.* to investigate the antitumour activities of enkephalins and enkephalin analogues (28). They transplanted PYB6 tumours into mice and treated them with either met-enkephalin, met-enkephalinamide, leu-enkephalin, or leu-enkephalin-amide. Surprisingly, met-enkephalin and met-enkephalinamide exhibited significant antitumour effects, while leu-enkephalin and leu-enkephalinamide had no antitumour activity against the PYB6 tumour line.

2.5 OVARIAN CANCER

*In vitro* studies were performed to explore the effects of opioid peptides on the immunocompetence of spleen cells from nude mice (29). Spleen cells were remixed and incubated with either alpha-endorphin, beta-endorphin, or met-enkephalin and then tested for their ability to lyse human ovarian cancer cells. Both beta-endorphin and met-enkephalin were shown to significantly increase the ability of spleen cells to lyse this form of tumour cell.

# 3   Human studies

3.1 LUNG CANCER

*In vitro* studies by Maneckjee and Minna (30) demonstrated the presence of opioid receptors on various types of human lung cancer cell lines using DAGO (a mu receptor agonist), DPDPE (a delta receptor agonist), and U-50,488H (a kappa receptor agonist). They found that these opioid agonists caused a concentration-dependent inhibition of tumour growth *in vitro*. The authors postulate that the endogenous opioids (enkephalins, endorphins, and dynorphins) represent another system of tumour suppression which may inactivate cancer cells. Wybran and Schandene (31) administered met-enkephalin intravenously to seven, newly diagnosed patients with lung cancer who had had no other therapy. They found an increase in the percentage of active T rosettes, OKT10+ cells, Leu11+ cells, and natural killer (NK) cell cytotoxicity. The effects on NK-cell activity were seen 24 hours following met-enkephalin infusion and declined by day six.

### 3.2 MELANOMA

Patients with advanced melanoma were treated with met-enkephalin over a period of several months at i.v. doses of 10 to 60 micrograms/kg body weight three times per week (32). These treatments resulted in significant increases in OKT8 cytotoxic/suppressor T-cells, and active T-cells positive for the OKT3, OKT11, and OKT4 cell markers.

### 3.3 KAPOSI'S SARCOMA (AIDS)

Plotnikoff *et al.* (32, 34) and Wybran *et al.* (33) have reported that treatment with met-enkephalin reduced the size and colouration of Kaposi's nodules in AIDS patients. In addition, met-enkephalin increased the number of cytotoxic T-cells (those carrying the CD3, CD4, and/or CD8 markers) and NK cells (those carrying the Leu 11 and Leu 19 markers); all of which are thought to be involved in tumour surveillance. Zunich and Kirkpatrick (35) studied the effects of met-enkephalin on immune functions in patients infected with the human immunodeficiency virus (HIV). They infused seven patients with 10 micrograms/kg body weight of met-enkephalin three times per week for up to three weeks. Changes in immune status of these patients were not consistent. The authors concluded 'that met-enkephalin appears to enhance temporarily selected immune responses in patients with HIV infection, however, in the schedule used in this study it was not clinically efficacious'.

## 4 Anti-tumor mechanisms–enhancement of natural killer cells, killer cells, cytotoxic T-cells, and macrophages

A large number of studies have shown that enkephalins have immunomodulatory properties. Wybran *et al.* (20) found significant increases in active T-cell rosettes following incubation with met-enkephalin. Plotnifoff, Miller, and Murgo (36); Miller, Murgo, and Plotnikoff (37–39); and Gilman *et al.* (40) found that the enkephalins and endorphins stimulate lymphocyte blastogenesis in rats and mice, and active T-cell rosettes in both normal volunteers and cancer patients. Hucklebridge *et al.* also reported that met-enkephalin enhanced the blastogenic response of human peripheral blood lymphocytes (41).

The function of phagocytic cells has been shown to be enhanced by the enkephalins. Both met- and leu-enkephalin were shown to modulate the release of superoxide anion release from unstimulated human polymorphonuclear cells and from polymorphonuclear cells stimulated with phorbol myristate acetate (42). Met-enkephalin has been reported to increase antibody-dependent cytotoxicity of rat peritoneal macrophages (43).

The enkephalins have been shown to have potent *in vitro* activity in elevating NK-cell numbers as well as functional activity against the target cells K562 and Molt4 cells. *In vitro* studies by Wybran and Schandene (31), Mathews *et al.* (44), Oleson and Johnson (45), and Faith *et al.* (46) have shown significant increases in human NK-cell activity following incubation with enkephalins in the range of $10^{-5}$ to $10^{-12}$ M. Gabrilovac *et al.* (47) have shown an interaction between alpha interferon and leu-enkephalin in the modulation of NK-cell activity of human peripheral blood lymphocytes. Recently Puente *et al.* (48) reported that only approximately half of the normal donors had significant increases in NK-cell activity following enkephalin treatment. This is similar to the findings of Faith *et al.* (46). Apparently, baseline NK values influence the results of enkephalin treatment. Thus, individuals with low NK baseline show an increase in activity following treatment with enkephalins or endorphins, while those with high NK baseline activity may show no effect or an actual decrease in activity following treatment.

Perhaps the most relevant *in vitro* study of the influence of enkephalins on NK-cell function was one conducted with peripheral blood lymphocytes from cancer patients. Both met- and leu-enkephalin were reported to increase NK-cell activity of cells from patients with a variety of cancers (49). The range of cancers in these patients included thyroid carcinoma, acute myelocytic leukaemia, small cell carcinoma of the lung, Hodgkins disease, chronic myelogenous leukaemia, breast cancer, ovarian cancer, gastric carcinoma, and lymphoma. The phenotypic NK-cell markers, Leu7, Leu11, and Leu19, were also reported to be increased by met-enkephalin treatment in normal volunteers and AIDS patients (34, 50). Finally, Wybran and Plotnikoff (51) found that met-enkephalin increased lymphokine-activated killer (LAK) cell activity with Daudi cells as the targets. Furthermore, IL-2 was synergistic with met-enkephalin in this system.

Other reported immunological effects of the enkephalins and endorphins include increase of cytotoxic T-lymphocytes in murine spleen cells following treatment (52). In lymphoma patients methionine- and leucine-enkephalin have been shown to increase the numbers of active T-cell rosettes (39). Dynorphin and leu-enkephalin were found to enhance tumouricidal activity against P815 murine mastocytoma cells by murine peritoneal macrophages (53).

## 5  Summary and conclusions

We believe that the enkephalins play a role in a central nervous system–endocrine–immune interrelationship in which dysfunctions in the immune system may be chronic, stress-related, and accompanied by perturbations in enkephalin levels in the adrenal glands, the primary source of enkephalins in the peripheral circulation (54). Large amounts of enkephalins, catecholamines, and steroids are secreted simultaneously from the adrenal glands during stress (55). It is well known that the central nervous system and behaviour can influence immune functions (56, 57). Behavioural states have been shown to influence the cerebrospinal fluid levels of endorphins (58). Recently, it has been shown that T-helper cells produce met-enkephalin (59), which completes the circuit between the central nervous system and the immune system where enkephalins are concerned. In view of these facts and the effects of the enkephalins reported herein, we believe that the enkephalins, together with a number of other factors, may play a central role in natural immunomodulation. Supplemental or replacement opioid therapy of patients with various diseases, such as cancer or viral infections may prove to be a new and extremely useful form of immunotherapy.

Since the enkephalins have been shown to have anti-tumour activities against B16 melanoma, neuroblastoma, fibrosarcoma, and L1210 leukaemia in rodents, it is highly probable that this cytokine will have clinical activity in cancer patients. The clinical studies reported to date were conducted in patients with advanced disease (melanoma, hypernephroma, and lung cancer). The clinical end-points used in these evaluations were solely immunological, that is, increases in cytotoxic T-cells and NK cells alone were measured. The large body of literature an NK- and killer cell activities has established the importance of these cell types in tumour surveillance and inhibition of metastasis. Two of the more interesting studies outlined earlier, were those showing that enkephaline increased NK-cell activity in peripheral blood lymphocytes from a variety of cancer patients (49), and inhibited metastasis of melanomas in mice (23). The study of NK-cell activity in the cancer patients was particularly interesting due to the fact that the patients were receiving heavy chemotherapy which is known to cause immunosuppression. The fact that met-enkephalin was active in these circumstances suggests that met-enkephalin could be clinically effective in combination with chemotherapeutic agents. One mechanism of this action may reside in the fact that the enkephalins have bone marrow stimulant activities similar to GM-CSF (60). We believe the future of cancer immunotherapy is bright and that the enkephalins will have a place in the developing therapeutic armamentarium.

# 6 References

1. Hornung, R. L., Kiertscher, S. H., and Mathews, H. L. (1992). Systemic IL-1 and adjuvant treatment of an experimental tumor. I. Immune status following tumor rechallenge. *Biotherapy*, **5**, 227–237.

2. Grabbe, S., Bruvers, S., and Granstein, R. D. (1992). Effects of immunomodulatory cytokines on the presentation of tumor associated antigen by epidermal Langerhans calls. *J. Invest. Dermatol.*, **99**, 66S–68S.

3. Akporiaye, E. T., Barbier, C. A., Stewart, C. C., and Bender, J. G. (1991). Gelatin sponge model of effector recruitment: tumoricidal activity of adherent and non-adherent lymphokine-activated killer cells after culture in interleukin-2. *J. Leukoc. Biol.*, **49**, 189–196.

4. Fearon, E. R., Pardoll, D. M., Itaya, T., Golumbek, P., Levitsky, H. I., Simons, J. W. *et al.* (1990). Interleukin-2 production by tumor cells bypasses T helper function in the generation of an antitumor response. *Cell*, **60**, 397–403.

5. Hornung, R. L., Back, T. C., Zaharko, D. S., Urba, W. J., Longo, D. L., and Wiltrout, R. H. (1988). Augmentation of natural killer activity, induction of IFN and development of tumor immunity during the successful treatment of established murine renal cancer using flavone acetic acid and IL-2. *J. Immunol.*, **141**, 3671–3679.

6. Steerenberg, P. A., DeJong, W. H., Geerse, E., Beuvink, A., Scheper, R. J., Denotter, W. *et al.* (1990). Major-histocompatibility-complex-class-II-positive cells and interleukin-2-dependent proliferation of immune T-cells are required to reject carcinoma cells in the guinea pig. *Canc. Immunol. Immunother.*, **31**, 297–304.

7. Stephenson, K. R., Perry-Lalley, D., Griffith, K. D., Shu, S., and Chang, A. E. (1989). Development of antitumor reactivity in regional draining lymph nodes from tumor-immunized and tumor-bearing murine hosts. *Surgery*, **105**, 523–528.

8. Woods, G., Kitagami, K., and Ochi, A. (1989). Evidence for an involvement of T4+ cytotoxic T-cells in tumor immunity. *Cell. Immunol.*, **118**, 126–135.

9. Zocchi, M.R., Ferrarini, M., and Rugarli, C. (1990). Selective lysis of the autologous tumor by delta TCS1+ gamma/delta+ tumor-infiltrating lymphocytes from human lung carcinomas. *Eur. J. Immunol.*, **20**, 2685–2689.

10. Okaneya, T. and Ogawa, A. (1990). Killer activities of peripheral blood mononuclear cells in patients with bladder cancer. *Jap. J. Urol.*, **81**, 532–537.

11. Bach, J. F. (1992). Cancer immunotherapy: from fundamental concepts to clinical applications. *Bull. Acad. Natl. Med.*, **176**, 867–871.

12. Klegerman, M. E. and Plotnikoff, N. P. (1993). Lymphokines and monokines. In *Biotechnology and Pharmacy*, (eds J. M. Pezzuto, M. E. Johnson, and H. R. Manasse, Jr.). Chapman and Hall, Now York.

13. McBride, W. H., Thacker, J. D., Comora, S., Economou, J. S., Kelley, D., Hogge, D, *et al.* (1992). Genetic modification of a murine fibrosarcoma to produce interleukin 7 stimulates host cell infiltration and tumor immunity. *Cancer Res.*, **S2**, 3931–3937.

14. Klegerman, M. E. and Plotnikoff, N. P. (1992). Proteins as biological response modifiers. In *Pharmaceutical Biotechnology*, (eds M. E. Klegerman and M. J. Groves). Interpharm Press, Buffalo Grove, Illinois.

15. Watanabe, Y. (1992). Transfection of interferon-gamma gene in animal tumors: a model for local cytokine production and tumor immunity. *Sem. Cancer Biol.*, **3**, 43–46.

16. Grabbe, S., Bruvers, S., Lindgren, A. M., Hosoi, J., Tan, K. C., and Granstein, R. D. (1992). Tumor antigen presentation by epidermal antigen-presenting cells in the mouse: modulation by granulocyte-macrophage colony-stimulating factor, tumor necrosis factor alpha, and ultraviolet radiation. *J. Leu. Biol.*, **52**, 209–217.

17. Hartung, H. P. (1988). Activation of macrophages by neuropeptides. *Brain Behav. Immun.*, **2**, 275–281.

18. Hughes, I., Smith, T. W., Kosterlitz, H. W., Fothergill, I. A., Morgan, B. A., and Morriss, H. T. (1975). Identification of two related pentapeptides from the brain with potent opiate agonist activity. *Nature*, **258**, 577–579.

19. Plotnikoff, N. P., Kastin, A. J., Coy, D. H., Christensen, C. W., Schally, A. V., and Sprites, M. A. (1976). Neuropharmacollogical actions of enkephalin after systemic administration. *Life Sci.*, **19**, 1283–1288.

20. Wybran, J., Appleboom, T., Famaly, J. P., and Govaerts, A. (1979). Suggestive evidence for receptors for morphine and methionine-enkephalin on normal human blood T-lymphocytes. *J. Immunol.*, **123**, 1068–1070.

21. Lopker, A., Abood, L. G., Hoss,, W., and Lionetti, F. J. (1980). Steroselective muscarinic acetylcholine and opiate receptors in human phagocytic leukocytes. *Biochem. Pharmacol.*, **29**, 1361–1365.

22. Murgo, A. J. (1985). Inhibition of B16-BL6 melanoma growth in mice by methionine-enkephalin. *J. Natl. Canc. Inst.*, **75**, 341–344.

23. Faith, R. E. and Murgo, A. J. (1988). Inhibition of pulmonary metastases and enhancement of natural killer cell activity by methionine-enkephalin. *Brain Behav. Immun.*, **2**, 114–122.

24. Murgo, A. J., Faith, R. E., and Plotnikoff, N. P. (1991). Enhancement of tumor resistance in mice by enkephalins. In *Stress and Immunity*, (eds N. P. Plotnikoff, A. J. Murgo, R. E. Faith, and J. Wybran), pp. 357–372. CRC Press, Boca Raton.

25. Scholar, E. M., Violi, L., and Hexum, T. D. (1987). The antimetastatic activity of enkephalin-like peptides. *Cancer Lett.*, **35**, 133–138.

26. Plotnikoff, N. P. and Miller, G. C. (1983). Enkephalins as immunomodulators. *Int. J. Immunopharmac.*, **5**, 437–441.

27. Zagon, I. S. and McLaughlin, P. J. (1991). The role of endogenous opioids and opioid receptors in human and animal cancer. In *Stress and Immunity*, (eds N. P. Plotnikoff, A. J. Murgo, R. E. Faith, and J. Wybran), pp. 43–355. CRC Press, Boca Raton.

28. Srisuchart, B., Fuchs, B. A., Sikorski, E. E., Munson, A. E., and Loveless, S. E. (1989). Antitumor activity of enkephalin analogues in inhibiting PYB6 tumor

growth in mice and immunological effects of methionine enkephalinamide. *Int. J. Immunopharmac.*, **11**, 487–500.

29. Kita, T., Kikuchi, Y., Oomori, K., and Nagata, I. (1992). Effects of opioid peptides on the tumoricidal activity of spleen cells from nude mice with or without tumors. *Cancer Detect. Prev.*, **16**, 211–214.

30. Maneckjee, R. and Minna, J. D. (1990). Opioid and nicotine receptors affect growth regulation of human lung cancer cell lines. *Proc. Natl. Acad. Sci.*, **87**, 3294–3298.

31. Wybran, J. and Schandene, L. (1986). Some immunological effects of methionine-enkephalin in man: potential therapeutic use. In *Leukocytes and Host Defense*, (eds J. J. Oppenheim and D. M. Jacobs), pp. 205–212. Alan R. Liss, Inc., New York.

32. Plotnikoff, N. P., Miller, G. C., Nimeh, N., Faith, R. E., Murgo, A. J., and Wybran, J. (1987). Enkephalins and T-cell enhancement in normal volunteers and cancer patients. *Ann. N. Y. Acad. Sci.*, **496**, 608–619.

33. Wybran, J., Schandene, L., Van Vooren, J. P., Vandermoten, G., Latinne, D., Sonnet, J. *et al.* (1987). Immunologic properties of methionine-enkephalin and therapeutic implications in AIDS, ARC, and cancer. *Ann. N. Y. Acad. Sci.*, **496**, 108–114.

34. Plotnikoff, N. P., Wybran, J., Nimeh, N. F., and Miller, G. C. (1986). Methionine enkephalin: enhancement of T-cells in patients with Kaposi's sarcoma, AIDS, and lung cancer. In *Enkephalis and Endorphins: Stress and the Immune System*, (eds N. P. Plotnikoff, R. E. Faith, A. J. Murgo, and R. A. Good), pp. 425–429. Plenum Press, New York.

35. Zunich, K. M. and Kirkpatrick, C. H. (1988). Methionine-enkephalin as immunomodulator therapy in human immunodeficiancy virus infections: clinical and immunological effects. *J. Clin. Immunol.*, **8**, 95–102.

36. Plotnikoff, N. P., Miller, G. C., and Murgo, A. J. (1982). Enkephalins-endorphins: immunomodulators in mice. *Int. J. Immunopharmac.*, **4**, 336–341.

37. Miller, G. C., Murgo, A. J., and Plotnikoff, N. P. (1982). The influence of leucine and methionine enkephalin on immune mechanisms in humans. *Int. J. Immunopharmac.*, **4**, 367–375.

38. Miller, G. C., Murgo, A. J., and Plotnikoff, N. P. (1984). Enkephalins—enhancement of active T-cell rosettes from normal volunteers. *Clin. Immunol. Immunopathol.*, **31**, 132–137.

39. Miller, G. C., Murgo, A. J. and Plotnikoff, N. P. (1983). Enkephalins—enhancement of active T-cell rosettes from lymphoma patients. *Clin. Immunol. Immunopathol.*, **26**, 446–451.

40. Gilman, S. C., Schwartz, J. M., Milner, R. J., Bloom, F. E., and Feldman, J. D. (1982). B-endorphin enhances lymphocyte proliferative responses. *Proc. Natl. Acad. Sci.*, **79**, 4226–4230.

41. Hucklebridge, F. H., Hudspith, B. N., Muhamed, J., Lydyard, P. M., and Brostoff, J. (1989). Methionine-enkephalin stimulates in vitro proliferation of human peripheral lymphocytes via delta-opioid receptors. *Brain Behav. Immun.*, **3**, 183–189.

42. Marotti, T., Sverko, V., and Hrsak, I. (1990). Modulation of superoxide anion

release from human polymorphonuclear cells by met- and leu-enkephalin. *Brain Behav. Immun.*, **4**, 13–22.

43. Foris, G., Medgyesis, A., Gyimesi, E., and Hauck, M. (1984). Met-enkephalin induced alterations of macrophage function. *Mol. Immun.*, **21**, 747–750.
44. Mathews, P. M., Froelich, C. J., Sibbitt, W. L., Jr., and Bankhurst, A. D. (1983). Enhancement of natural cytotoxicity by B-endorphin. *J. Immunol.*, **130**, 1658–1662.
45. Oleson, D. R. and Johnson, D. R. (1989). Regulation of human natural cytotoxicity by enkephaline and selective opiate agonists. *Brain Behav. Immun.*, **2**, 171–186.
46. Faith, R. E., Liang, H. J., Murgo, A. J., and Flotnikoff, N. P. (1984). Neuroimmunomodulation with enkephalins: enhancement of human natural killer (NK) cell activity in vitro. *Clin. Immunol. Immunopathol.*, **31**, 412–418.
47. Gabrilovac, J., Martin-Kleiner, I., Ikic-Sutlic, M., and Osmak, M. (1992). Interaction of Leu-enkephalin and alpha-interferon in modulation of NK-activity of human peripheral blood lymphocytes. *Ann. N.Y. Acad. Sci.*, **650**, 140–145.
48. Puente, J., Maturana, P., Miranda, D., Navarro, C., Wolf, M. E., and Mosnaim, A. D. (1992). Enhancement of human natural killer cell activity by opioid peptides: similar response to methionine-enkephalin and beta-endorphin. *Brain Behav. Immun.*, **6**, 32–39.
49. Faith, R. E., Liang, H. J., Plotnikoff, N. P., Murgo, A. J., and Nimeh, N. F. (1987). Neuroimmunomodulation with enkephalins: in vitro enhancement of natural killer cell activity in peripheral blood lymphocytes from cancer patients. *Nat. Immun. Cell Growth Regul.*, **6**, 88–98.
50. Plotnikoff, N. P., Miller, G. C., Solomon, S., Faith, R. E., Edwards, L., and Murgo, A. J. (1986). Methionine enkephalin: immunomodulator in normal volunteers (in vivo). In *Enkephalins and Endorphins: Stress and the Immune System*, (eds N. P. Plotnikoff, R. E. Faith, A. J. Murgo, and R. A. Good), pp. 399–405. Plenum Press, New York.
51. Wybran, J. and Plotnikoff, N. P. (1989). Enhancement of immunological mechanisms, inuluding LAK induction, by methionine enkephalin. *Proceedings of the 7th Int. Cong. Immunol.* Berlin.
52. Carr, D. J. J. and Klimpel, G. R. (1986). Enhancement of the generation of cytotoxic T-cells by endogenous opiates. *J. Neuroimmun.*, **12**, 75–87.
53. Foster, J. S. and Moore, R. N. (1987). Dynorphin and related opioid peptides enhance tumoricidal activity mediated by murine peritoneal macrophages. *J. Leuk. Biol.*, **42**, 171–174.
54. Hanbauer, I., Kelly, G.D., Saiani, L., and Yang, H. Y. T. (1982). Met[1]-enkephalin-like peptides of the adrenal medulla: release by nerve stimulation and functional implications. *Peptides*, **3**, 469–473.
55. Amir, S., Brown, Z. W., and Amit, Z. (1980). The role of endorphins in stress: evidence and speculation. *Neurosci. Biobehav. Res.*, **4**, 77–86.
56. Stein, M., Schiavi, R.C., and Comerino, M. (1976). Influence of brain and behavior on the immune system. *Science*, **191**, 435–439.
57. Ader, R. (1981). *Psychoneuroimmunology.* Academic Press, New York.
58. Pickar, D., Naber, D., Post, R. M., Van Kammon, D. P., Bellenger, J., Kalin,

N. *et al.* (1981). Measurement of endorphins in CFS. Relationship to psychiatric diagnosis. *Mod. Probl. Pharmacopsychiatry*, **17**, 246–262.

59. Zurawski, G., Benedik, M., Kamb, B. J., Abrams, J. S., Zurawski, S. M., and Lee, T. D. (1986). Activation of mouse T-helper cells induces abundant prepro-enkephalin in RNA synthesis. *Science*, **232**, 772–775.
60. Petrov, R. V. and Zakharova, L. A. (1991). Physiological stress and immune response: myelo-peptides. In *Stress and Immunity*, (eds N. P. Plotnikoff, A. J. Murgo, R. E. Faith, J. Wybran), pp. 399–408. CRC Press, Boca Raton.

# 16

# Tumour cell strategies for escaping immune control: implications for psychoimmunotherapy

## S. SOMERS AND P. J. GUILLOU

## 1   Introduction

Immunological mechanisms for the control of neoplastic cells have assumed considerable significance with the development of immuno-therapeutic strategies for the treatment of certain malignant diseases. The impetus for this advance was brought about by the exponential increase in knowledge of the cellular and molecular mechanisms of immune activation in the early 1980s. A better understanding of the effects which follow the action of specific cytokines on immune cells has shed light upon the interactions between the immune system and the tumour cell population. The experimental demonstration of immune responses, in a variety of animal tumour models and some human tumours, raises a number of significant questions. If an immune response to autologous tumour exists, why do the available effector mechanisms for tumour destruction fail in most patients? Furthermore, if immunological means of eliminating circulating tumour cells exist, why do metastases occur? Whilst the diversity of anti-tumour immune responses appears to present a formidable array of potential mechanisms for tumour destruction, more recent evidence suggests that tumour cells may evade and subvert these responses in order to survive.

## 2  Immune suppression in cancer patients

The influence of tumour burden upon the generation of an effective immune response had received little experimental attention until 1942 when Blumenthal (1) showed that mice bearing mammary tumours accepted transplants more readily than did healthy animals. Similarly, Browning (2) and Gorer (3) demonstrated that tumour-bearing animals were more susceptible to bacterial infections than healthy animals. In addition, a number of workers showed that animals subjected to procedures which reduced their immunological responses to antigenic stimuli exhibited enhanced tumour gowth and an increased incidence of metastases (4, 5, 6). Moore (7) extended these observations to tumour-bearing patients receiving cytotoxic therapy. Using delayed hypersensitivity responses as an alternative *in vivo* measurement of immune competence, it has been demonstrated that the presence of a tumour and even the extent of the tumour burden could influence the response to tuberculin (8) or to 2–4 dinitrochlorobenzene (9).

Whilst generalized immune suppression has been found in patients with advanced tumours, the identification of specific immunological defects in tumour-bearing patients has yielded more useful information. Monson *et al.* (10) showed that peripheral blood lymphocytes from patients with gastrointestinal cancer exhibited decreased IL-2 production on mitogenic stimulation and that this effect was not the result of a change in circulating T-lymphocyte subsets. This study was followed by the description of impaired IL-2-induced LAK effector generation in patients with advanced but not localized cancer, indicating a tumour bulk-related effect on host immune responses (11). Hakim (12) demonstrated that in patients with a variety of tumours, peripheral blood lymphocytes failed to express both mRNA and peptides for functional IL-2 receptors.

Many studies over the past 20 years have demonstrated the inhibitory effects of serum from cancer patients on the stimulation of lymphocytes by non-specific mitogens (13–16). These findings are supported by the concomitant description of impaired lymphocyte responsiveness in tumour-bearing humans (17–19), indicating an immunosuppressive environment in these patients.

With the advent of clinical immunotherapy, investigators have looked specifically at the function of IL-2-dependent immune responses in cancer patients. A thorough study by Shiiba *et al.* (20) described the suppression of *in vitro* LAK activation by autologous serum in patients with gastric cancer. Patients with suppressive serum also possessed peripheral blood mononuclear cells (PBMC) with impaired responses to IL-2. The suppressive effect could be partially reversed *in vitro* by the addition of interferon-gamma (IFN-γ) to the LAK culture, but was not characterized further. Subsequent description of suppressive serum factors from patients with melanoma (21) and squamous carcinoma of the head and neck (22) have provided further evidence for the existence of humoral immunosuppressive factor(s) associated with the presence of malignant disease.

# 3   Mechanisms for the failure of anti-tumour immune responses

## 3.1   TUMOUR HETEROGENEITY

The development of a tumour involves the progressive phenotypic diversification of constituent tumour cells in order to conform to selection pressures operative in a particular host environment. An established tumour deposit may, therefore, evolve in an environment where immunological responses exert a selection pressure which eliminate those tumour cells that elicit an immune response. Tumour cells that acquire the capacity to evade immune recognition or inactivate immune responses will, therefore, succeed in the establishment of clinical tumour deposits (for review, see ref. 23).

## 3.2   TOLERANCE OF SELF ANTIGENS

Tolerance, the process whereby self antigens are recognized, and not subjected to reaction by immune effector mechanisms, occurs physiologically in the neonatal period. This process, though intended to limit immune auto-reactivity, may explain why embryonic or fetal antigens that are expressed on adult malignant cells (for example CEA, alpha-fetoprotein) may be weak inducers of immune responses *in vivo*. The work of Morton (24, 25) demonstrated the acquisition of immunological tolerance to mammary tumour viral antigens by mice neonatally infected through nursing with infected mothers. Significantly, these studies also described the decreased resistance of neonatally tolerized mice to the gowth of mammary carcinoma in adult life. The involvement of immunological tolerance in human malignant disease remains uncertain.

### 3.3 ROLE OF MHC CLASS I EXPRESSION

Alteration of MHC class I antigen expression, usually a reduction or loss of these molecules, provides a mechanism whereby some tumour cells may escape recognition by the host MHC-dependent lymphocyte anti-tumour responses. These mechanisms could account for the loss of reactivity against those tumours that require obligatory antigen expression for maintenance of the malignant phenotype, such as those virally induced tumours which escape killing by MHC class I restricted cytotoxic T-lymphocytes (26). Murine cells transformed with SV40 and adapted for growth *in vivo*, exhibited a loss of H-2K (murine MHC class I equivalent), became resistant to SV40 specific cytotoxic T-lymphocytes and failed to induce a specific T-lymphocyte response *in vivo* (27).

Certain human tumours show a consistent reduction in MHC class I antigen expression. Choriocarcinoma cells lack MHC class I expression, though this may be unrelated to immune escape and simply relate to retention of the class I-negative phenotype of the trophoblast cells (28). Human small cell lung carcioma (29) and neuroblastoma (30) also show consistent loss of MHC class I expression.

Studies on the more common human tumours of breast (31, 32), colon (33) and melanoma (34) have failed to demonstrate a consistent and generalized loss of MHC class I antigen expression, although a relative reduction in the expression of these antigens may provide a protective element for certain subpopulations of cells. Heterogeneity of MHC antigen expression within individual human tumour deposits may account for the lack of convincing data.

### 3.4 BLOCKING FACTORS

Existence of tumour-derived blocking factors has been inferred from the observation that the effective *in vitro* cytolytic action of lymphocytes from tumour-bearing individuals can be blocked by the addition of allogeneic sera (35–36). Though the specificity of the lymphocytes and sera tested remained unknown, antibody-tumour antigen complexes and shed antigen (37) have been implicated in this blocking phenomenon. Furthermore, experimentally constructed complexes of tumour antigen and antibody can induce T-lymphocytes *in vitro* with suppressor activity (38), indicating another possible blocking mechanism.

These effects are difficult to investigate *in vivo*. It is not known whether blocking factors act primarily in the tumour locality or systemically. Local blocking of immune responses may play a role in the phenomenon of 'concomitant immunity' (39) where local factors appear to protect the primary tumour from immune attack even though the host may reject tumour inocula at distant sites. Conversely, some investigators have postulated direct stimulation of tumours by immune responses against tumour antigens (40).

Endogenous blocking factors may be diverse in their origin. Studies have demonstrated elevated levels of soluble $\beta$2-microglobulin in patients with carcinoma of the breast (41), lung, and prostate (42). Soluble molecules capable of interacting with MHC receptors on lymphocytes may impair specific anti-tumour responses. Similarly monomeric IgG has been shown to influence NK-cell cytotoxicity (43). Thus, a humoral anti-tumour immune response involving the production of IgG may block innate anti-tumour immune responses.

### 3.5 SUPPRESSOR T-LYMPHOCYTE GENERATION

The existence of suppressor T-lymphocyte networks in experimental tumour models has been described by a number of workers (44–47). These studies identify both specific and non-specific suppressor T-lymphocytes that are induced in tumour-bearing hosts and act to inhibit *in vitro* assays of immune response. Early human work identified a 'tumour promoting' suppressor cell population in melanoma (48) and osteosarcoma (49). Re-activation of suppressor T-lymphocytes isolated from human tumours by co-culture with autologous tumour cells has been suggested in bladder, lung, and renal carcinoma (50). In a human malignant paraganglioma, Mukherji *et al.* (51) accomplished the isolation of a T-helper lymphocyte clone from the primary tumour and a T-suppressor lymphocyte clone from a tumour-invaded lymph node. Cozzolino *et al.* (52) showed that lymphocytes derived from tumour-draining lymph nodes could be induced to proliferate in response to autologous tumour cells only when cells bearing the OKM-1 (monocyte/macrophage) and Leu-7 (CD57/HNK1) antigens were removed and the culture supplemented with exogenous interleukin-2 (IL-2). A study in melanoma patients showed that lymphocytes from lymph nodes close to tumour deposits responded poorly to Con-A *in vitro* when compared to lymph node lymphocytes from more distant nodes (53). This effect was partly due to the presence of suppressor T-lymphocyte activity.

Evidence from experimental tumours has shown that suppressor cells, when present in tumours can be eliminated by treatment with cytotoxic agents such as cyclophosphamide (54). This effect has been utilized in the design of some immunotherapeutic protocols. The existence of T-lymphocyte regulatory networks in tumour-immune interactions would seem probable, however, their functional role as *in vivo* modulators of anti-tumour immune responses remains to be determined.

## 3.6 PROSTAGLANDINS

The role of prostaglandins, particularly prostaglandin $E_2$, in the suppression of a wide variety of immune responses has been extensively documented (55; for review see ref. 56) and has been linked with tumour-mediated immunosuppression (57, 58, 59). In an attempt to reverse these immunosuppressive effects, Tilden and Balch (60) described the enhancement of immunocompetence in melanoma patients by treatment with the cyclooxygenase inhibitor, indomethacin. The use of indomethacin treatment *in vitro* and *in vivo* has been shown to increase LAK-effector activity generated from spleen cells of tumour-bearing mice (56). The *in vitro* augmentation of IL-2 induced LAK activity derived from PBMC can be achieved by depleting PBMCs of their adherent cell population prior to IL-2 stimulation (61). This effect was attributed to the removal of prostaglandin-secreting monocytes.

Maxwell *et al.* (62) showed that macrophages infiltrating colonic tumours exihibited enhanced prostaglandin $E_2$ production. This mechanism may be more appropriate than direct tumour cell secretion of prostaglandins since this study would suggest that tumour resident macrophages may interact with, and become stimulated by, the disordered tumour microenvironment. The relative suppression of immune responsiveness has been postulated to derive from excess prostaglandin secretion by monocytes (63). In this study the addition of indomethacin to phytohaemagglutinin or IL-2 stimulation assays of cancer patients' peripheral blood lymphocytes caused an increase in lymphocyte response. This result has been further refined by Itoh *et al.* (64) who demonstrated that a serum-borne and monocyte-dependent suppressor of LAK-effector induction in melanoma patients was not reversible by indomethacin.

## 3.7 TUMOUR-MEDIATED IMMUNOSUPPRESSION

The relationship between immunosuppression and tumour bulk lends itself to the hypothesis that the tumour may be the source of immunosuppressive factors (for review see ref. 65).

In an attempt to define further the effect of tumour burden on IL-2 responsiveness, Ting *et al.* (66) attempted to generate activated killer cells from spleen cells of tumour-bearing mice. These studies showed that the presence of tumour cells could trigger the activation of LAK precursors, but the same tumour cells could also prevent the full differentiation of these lymphocytes into anti-tumour effectors. Small amounts of irradiated tumour cells were also found to suppress IL-2-induced activation of lymphocytes *in vitro*.

The attempted generation of sensitized lymphocytes from mice bearing a weakly immunogenic tumour was not possible, indicating a suppressive effect of the tumour bearing host (67). Following an *in vitro* sensitization regimen, however, these cells could be induced to develop cytolytic responses. These results were confirmed and expanded upon by the elegant murine studies of Gregorian and Battisto (68, 69) utilizing the Renca murine renal carcinoma system. In this work, the authors showed that the *in vitro* generation of LAK effectors from mice bearing 3 week-established Renca tumours was negligible compared to normal control mice. Similar findings for the generation of cytotoxic T-lymphocytes and delayed-type hypersensitivity responses were recorded. Multiple mechanisms for this suppressive effect were found to arise from suppressive splenic lymphocytes and prostaglandin-secreting splenic macrophages and of greater significance, the Renca tumour cells. The exact mechanism of suppression caused by the Renca cells was not investigated further. Recent work by Sondak *et al.* (70) has shown that the generation of anti-tumour T-lymphocytes is impaired from animals bearing visceral metastases, though the mechanisms for this effect also remain to be identified.

# 4 Tumour cell-derived immunosuppressive factors

The demonstration that host immunosuppression in patients with cancer is related to bulk of malignant disease lends considerable weight to the hypothesis that tumour cells may be directly responsible for this phenomenon. Determination of the mechanisms for this effect *in vivo* are technically difficult. However, a number of *in vitro* strategies have been used to investigate this phenomenon.

## 4.1 TUMOUR CELL-DERIVED MOLECULES KNOWN TO HAVE IMMUNO-SUPPRESSIVE ACTIONS

### 4.1.1 *Transforming growth factor-beta*

Tumour cells are known to secrete a variety of protein growth factors that may be necessary for continued proliferation and maintenance of the malignant phenotype (71, 72).

Transforming growth factor-$\beta$ (TGF-$\beta$) and related peptides may be found in tumours (72), serum (73), and platelets (74), and have multiple, diverse effects on both normal and malignant cells (75). Under certain conditions, tumour cells may secrete TGF-$\beta$ as an autocrine growth factor which may interact with other growth factors to maintain proliferation, differentiation, and the transformed phenotype (72). Knabbe *et al.* (76) showed that secretion of TGF-$\beta$ by the MCF-7 breast cancer cell line was increased by treatment with anti-oestrogens and that the secreted TGF-$\beta$ was responsible for the gowth inhibitory effects. Expression of TGF-$\beta$ mRNA has been found in a wide variety of human tumour specimens.

In addition to these tumour-directed effects, TGF-$\beta$ has been found to possess potent immunomodulatory properties. The *in vitro* generation of LAK cells can be inhibited by co-culture with TGF-$\beta$ (77, 78) as can the generation of mitogen-induced T-cell responses (77), interferon-activated NK-cell activity (79) and mitogen-induced B-cell immunoglobulin secretion (80). Activation of both T- and B-lymphocytes leads to the expression of TGF-$\beta$ by these cells and may represent a non-specific, autocrine, inhibitory cytokine system limiting immunological activation (81, 77). The nature and physiology of this peptide has been reviewed by Sporn *et al.* (75).

The demonstration that primary human glioblastoma cells secrete TGF-$\beta$ (82) has suggested one mechanism whereby tumour cell-derived growth factors could subvert the generation of an immunologically mediated therapeutic response *in vivo*. This mechanism is further supported by the finding that transfection of a highly immunogenic experimental tumour with cDNA for TGF-$\beta$ enables the tumour cells to escape immune surveillance when implanted into immunocompetent mice (83).

## 4.1.2   Retroviral proteins

The involvement of virus and viral products in the tumour–host interaction has been postulated by a number of workers. Retroviral envelope protein, p15E, has been found in murine and feline leukaemia viruses and appears to be one mediator of immune dysfunction associated with retroviral infection (84). The p15E protein has also been found in various non-infected tumour cell lines and its thought to derive from endogenous retroviral sequences present in mammalian DNA (85, 86). Inoculation of mice with retrovirus or the hydrophobic 19 kD molecule p15E, causes suppression of inflammatory immune responses (84). In addition, *in vitro* inhibition of lymphocyte, mono-cycte, and NK-cell responses was observed after treatment with the p15E analog CKS-17, including interferon-induced NK-cell activity. However, lymphocyte responses to IL-2 were unaffected (87). Cell surface binding of p15E has been confirmed on a number of lymphoid origin human cell lines (88), further supporting an immunomodulatory role in *in vivo*. P15E has not shown any tumour mitogenic or inhibitory effects and has not shown enhancement of tumourigenesis in infected cells (89). Molecular analysis has identified mRNA for p15E in primary human colorectal and gastric cancers, indicating the potential for this molecule to mediate immune suppression in such patients (90).

## 4.2 IMMUNOSUPPRESSIVE MOLECULES DERIVED FROM TUMOUR EXTRACTS

Primary tumour cell culture experiments, though technically demanding, have enabled the investigation of *in vitro* interactions between human tumour cells and lymphocytes. A number of workers have identified immunosuppressive moieties derived from cultures or extracts of fresh human tumours. A summary of these factors is shown in Table 1.

Extraction of soluble components from fresh human colonic tumour cells permitted Remacle-Bonnet *et al.* (91) to identify a soluble suppressor material of approximately 70 kD molecular weight, unrelated to CEA or alpha-fetoprotein. This material did not induce proliferation in normal resting lymphocytes, inhibited lectin-induced lymphocyte blastogenesis, and was not present in normal tissues. Similar experiments extracting factors from human lung (92) and oesophageal (93) tumours identified the presence of factors which suppressed lymphocyte activation. Using extracts from bovine ocular squamous carcinoma, Nelson *et al.* (94) demonstrated the non-specific suppressive nature of this factor in murine test models. The active component was estimated to be of 10–37 kD molecular weight. Roth and co-workers thoroughly investigated the immunosuppressive component of a soft tissue sarcoma extract that potently inhibited lectin induced lymphocyte proliferation (95, 96). The 70 kD factor with a pI of 7.6–7.8 could be inactivated by chemical reduction and treatment with extremes of pH. The factor was shown to have determinants which bound to both anti-MHC-DR framework and anti-IgM $\mu$ chain antibodies, although the study did not demonstrate the degree of MHC class 2 expression in the original tumour specimen from which the extract was derived. Roth's group also identified tumours which did not produce immunosuppressive factors and established that extracts from normal tissues were similarly non-suppressive in nature.

Isolation of an immunosuppressive factor from the malignant ascites of colorectal cancer patients was achieved by Medoff *et al.* (97). This factor suppressed stimulation by phytohaemagglutinin of peripheral blood lymphocytes and was found to be stable to both heat and extremes of pH. The factor had an apparent isoelectric point of 3.4 and a molecular weight of 50 kD.

Despite the above research, few of these molecules have been characterized and identified to the molecular level. This may in part be due to the technical difficulties involved in the purification of molecules from human tumour samples, which by their nature are composed of heterogeneous tissues. In order to overcome these problems, workers have attempted to isolate immuno-suppressive substances from human tumour cell lines maintained *in vitro*.

**Table 1** Immunosuppressive factors derived from tumour extracts

| Author | Year | Source | MW (kDa) | pI | DIG | °C | pH | RED | Suppressive effects |
|---|---|---|---|---|---|---|---|---|---|
| Remacle-Bonnet et al. (91) | 1978 | Human Ca colon | 70 | | | | | | PHA induced T-cell mitogenesis |
| Mohagheghpour et al. (93) | 1979 | Human Ca oesophagus | 75 | | U | | U | | PHA induced T-cell mitogenesis |
| Hess | 1979 | Ovarian ascites | 50–100 | | | U | S | | Lectin induced T and B-cell responses |
| Roth et al. (96) | 1983 | Human liposarcoma | 70 | 7.7 | U | U | S | U | PHA/PWM/ConA induced T-cell mitogenesis |
| Fontana | 1984 | Human glioblastoma | 97 | 4.6 | U | | | | IL-2 dependent T-cell proliferation |
| Medoff et al. (97) | 1986 | Colonic ascites | 50 | 3.4 | | S | S | S | PHA induced T-cell mitogenesis |
| Nelson et al. (94) | 1987 | Bovine sq. carcinoma | 10–37 | | U | S | S | S | In vivo murine tumour rejection inhibition assay |

MW = Molecular weight; pI = Isoelectric point; DIG = Proteolytic digestion; °C = Heat sensitivity; pH = pH sensitivity; S = Stable; U = Unstable.

4.3 IMMUNOSUPPRESSIVE MOLECULES DERIVED FROM HUMAN TUMOUR
CELL LINES

The establishment of continuous cultures of human tumour cells has facilitated the investigation of tumour cell products with immunosuppressive activity, since these cultures represent a pure tumour cell source for any derived molecules. Numerous workers have, over the past decade investigated these *in vitro* tumour-derived 'factors' with variable success. However, few have exploited the availability of purified or recombinant IL-2 as a means of accurately characterizing their suppressive effects. These results are discussed in more detail below and are summarized in Table 2.

In 1980, Werkmeister *et al.* (98) identified the presence of a factor in the supernatant of melanoma and bladder cell lines that inhibited normal lymphocyte stimulation with phytohaemagglutinin. Production of this factor was related to the number of tumour cells in culture and increased with the time allowed for generation. Blockade of protein synthesis by cycloheximide inhibited elaboration of the factor. DNA and RNA synthesis was not required for production. The factor appeared to be potently suppressive but was not further characterized.

Whitehead and Kim (99) characterized an inhibitor of mitogenic lymphocyte stimulation in the supernatant of the SKCO-1 colonic carcinoma cell line. This factor was heat and UV radiation stable and had a molecular weight greater than 100 kD.

Hersey *et al.* (100) isolated a factor which from the MM200 melanoma cell line suppressed IL-2 induced lymphocyte proliferation. The MM200 factor was found to have a molecular weight of approximately 44 kD and was not susceptible to digestion with trypsin or pronase. The MM200 melanoma product was also found to inhibit IL-1 secretion by macrophages in response to lipopolysaccharide, indicating a non-IL-2 specific effect (101).

Putnam and Roth (102) described a heat stable, acid-labile glycoprotein derived from murine melanoma which inhibited lymphocyte proliferative responses to both lectins and IL-2. However, the molecular weight of the murine melanoma factor was only in the order of 10–12 kD.

Using the HT-29 colonic carcinoma line, Ebert *et al.* (103) identified a soluble factor in the tumour cell conditioned medium of approximate molecular weight 56 kD and isoelectric point 7.9. The HT-29 factor could reversibly block *in vitro* mitogen-induced lymphocyte proliferation and production of IL-2, but did not regulate CD25 expression on T-lymphocytes. Physicochemical manipulation showed sensitivity to endopeptidases, extremes of pH, and temperature greater than 56 °C. These findings were reproduced by Pommier *et al.* (104) who studied the suppressive activity of HT-29 supernatants which mediated strong *in vitro* suppression of lectin-induced

Table 2 Immunosuppressive factors derived from tumour cell line-conditioned culture medium

| Author | Year | Source | MW (kDa) | pI | DIG | °C | pH | Suppressive effects |
|---|---|---|---|---|---|---|---|---|
| Whitehead and Kim (99) | 1980 | SKCO-1, colon | 45 100 | | S | S | | ConA/PHA T-cell mitogenesis |
| Werkmeister et al. (98) | 1980 | MM200, melanoma | 70 140 200 | 4.2 7.4 | S | U | | T-cell mitogenesis |
| Farram et al. (101) | 1982 | MM200, melanoma | 1–10 | | | | | Macrophage IL-1 production |
| Hersey et al. (100) | 1983 | MM200, melanoma | 7 44 | | S | S | | PHA T-cell mitogenesis and IL-2 production |
| Fujiwara et al. (107) | 1987 | U937, histiocyte | 85 | | | | | PHA T-cell mitogenesis, IL-2 production and CD25 expression |
| Ebert et al. (103) | 1987 | HT-29, colon | 56 | 7.9 | | U | U | PHA T-cell mitogenesis and IL-2 production |
| Romeo and Mizel | 1989 | A673, rhabdomyosarcoma | 25 | 9.5 | | | S | PHA T-cell mitogenesis |
| Muraki et al. (105) | 1989 | KU2, renal | | | | U | | PHA T-cell mitogenesis and IL-2 production |
| Sugimura et al. (108) | 1990 | U-937, histiocyte | 45 | 4.5 | | U | U | PHA T-cell mitogenesis and IL-2 production |
| Serrano et al. (110) | 1990 | CAP-2, lung | 8–12 | | | | | Increased target resistance to NK lysis, but not to LAK lysis |

MW = Molecular weight; pI = Isoelectric point; DIG = Proteolytic digestion; °C = Heat sensitivity; pH = pH sensitivity; S = Stable; U = Unstable lymphocyte proliferation. Rather than proceeding to physicochemical characterization of the HT-29 factor, this group convincingly demonstrated the *in vivo* suppressive effects of the HT-29 factor in murine models of delayed-type hypersensitivity responses and rejection of immunogenic fibrosarcoma.

Renal carcinoma supernatants from the cell line, KU-2 factor have also yielded suppressive activity in assays of lectin-induced lymphocyte proliferation (105). The KU-2 factor was heat sensitive to temperatures over 56 °C and was non-dialysable.

Fujiwara and colleagues have isolated and characterized a lymphocyte blastogenesis inhibitory factor from the U-937 human histiocytic lymphoma cell line (106, 107). These authors described a factor capable of blocking IL-1, IL-2, and phytohaemagglutinin-induced lymphocyte responses in addition to decreasing T-lymphocyte transferrin receptor expression. The factor was non-dialysable, inactivated by heating ( > 56 °C) and exposure to extremes of pH, with a molecular mass of approximately 85 kD. Further work on this factor has demonstrated that it has anti-mitogenic effects on a number of human tumour cell lines of both lymphoid and non-lymphoid origin, suggesting a range of potential target cells for this molecule (108, 109).

Induction of resistance to NK-mediated lysis has been shown by treatment of K562 target cells with CAP-2, a soluble factor derived from human lung tumours (110). Characterization of the CAP-2 factor identified a protein with a mass of 8 to 12 kD, which did not diminish the generation of LAK effectors or of activated macrophages *in vitro*.

Few of the suppressive moieties described by the above workers have been investigated using the inhibition of IL-2-activated non-NMC-restricted lymphocytotoxicity as an assay system. This cytokine is thought to be central to immunological activation of both innate and adaptive immune responses against tumour cells. These responses form the basis of therapeutic strategies incorporating interleukin-2-based immunotherapy.

A series of experiments in our laboratories have demonstrated the capacity of a number of *in vitro* maintained human tumour cell lines to actively secrete soluble factors which can potently suppress the activation of healthy-donor peripheral blood lymphocytes into lymphokine-activated killers (LAK) by IL-2 (Figure 1). In these experiments, peripheral blood mononuclear cells from healthy volunteers were isolated and cultured at a concentration of $1.5 \times 10^6$ lymphocytes/ml in RPMI 1640 medium with 10 per cent fetal calf serum. After 3 days incubation, the activated lymphocytes were harvested and assayed for anti-tumour cytotoxicity in a 4 hour $Cr^{51}$ release cytotoxicity assay against NK effector-resistant tumour cell targets. To this assay system were added the samples of serum-free tumour cell culture supernatants to test for suppressive activity. A detailed description of the methods can be found in the paper by Somers *et al.* (111).

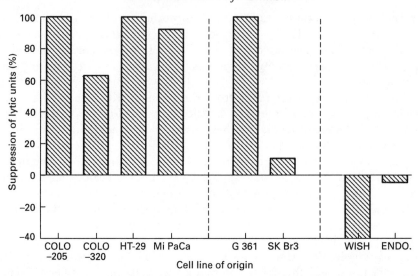

**Figure 1** Serum-free supernatants conditioned by a number of different cell lines and 'non-malignant' cells were used at a concentration of 20 per cent v/v in culture medium to treat cultures of healthy human peripheral blood lymphocytes and IL-2 for 3 days.

Tumour cell lines of gastrointestinal and melanoma cell origin were consistently suppressive. However, supernatants derived from breast carcinoma cells or non-malignant cell lines (WISH: human amnion cell line or primary cultures of primary cultures of normal human endothelial cells) did not suppress lymphocyte activation induced by IL-2. The results of dose–response experiments demonstrated the suppressive effects of serum-free human tumour cell supernatants when included in the assay culture system. Concentrations as low as 5 per cent (v/v) serum-free supernatant in culture medium inhibited IL-2-induced LAK effector generation and pronounced suppression of LAK generation was seen with concentrations of 10 per cent and 20 per cent (Figure 2). Serum-free supernatants from the previously determined non-suppressive cell lines failed, however, to suppress the generation of LAK cytotoxicity at concentrations as high as 50 per cent.

The inhibitory effects of supernatants from the cell lines, COLO 205 (colonic carcinoma), G-361 (malignant melanoma), and MiaPaCa (pancreatic carcinoma) on the proliferation of IL-2 activated lymphocytes was assessed by uptake of $^3$H-thymidine (Figure 3). Inhibition of lymphocyte proliferation in response to IL-2 was significantly diminished only at supernatant concentrations of 10 per cent and above. The MiaPaCa cell supernatant, only moderately suppressive of LAK effector generation, failed to show substantial suppression of PBMC proliferation in response to IL-2.

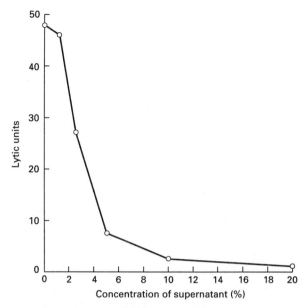

**Figure 2** Effects of increasing doses of serum-free supernatant of G-361 cells on the generation of the LAK-effector cytotoxicity in 3 day, IL-2-stimulated lymphocyte cultures. Lymphocytes were assayed using a 4-hour[51] chromium release assay.

Mature IL-2-induced LAK effector cytotoxic function was not affected by the presence, in the 4 hour $Cr^{51}$ release cytotoxicity assay, of up to 40 per cent serum-free tumour cell supernatant. Furthermore, suppression was not specific for the origin of the suppressive factor. Thus, G-361-derived supernatant suppressed the induction of LAK effector cytotoxicity against any other LAK effector target cell line when tested in a 4 hour [51]-chromium release cytotoxicity assay.

The successful generation of a lymphocyte proliferative response in a 6 day, two-way, allogeneic, mixed culture of lymphocytes from healthy donors is shown in the control cultures of Table 3. Addition of tumour cell supernatants from a number of different cell types resulted in profound suppression of lymphocyte blastogenesis as reflected by decreased $^{3}$H-thymidine incorporation. A distinct, dose-dependent suppressive effect was observed for each of the tumour cell line-derived supernatants, supporting the existence of a soluble tumour-derived suppressive moiety. This indicates that the tumour-derived suppressive moiety can inhibit lymphocyte proliferation triggered by non-self MHC interactions, in addition to MHC-independent responses triggered by

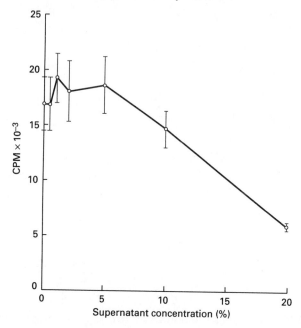

**Figure 3** Effects of increasing doses of serum-free supernatant of COLO 320 cells on the induction of lymphocyte proliferation by IL-2 in 3-day cultures was investigated using a $^3$H-thymidine incorporation assay.

**Table 3** Effects of various supernatants on $^3$H-thymidine incorporation in a two way mixed lymphocyte reaction

| Supernatant origin | Control no. supernatant | 10% supernatant | 20% supernatant | 40% supernatant | Suppression (%) |
|---|---|---|---|---|---|
| | Results in CPM $\times$ 10$^{-3}$ (mean of 4 wells) | | | | |
| G-361 | 47049 | 11678 | 5133 | 935 | 89.1 |
| COLO 205 | 49602 | 2904 | 1008 | 366 | 97.9 |
| COLO 320 | 43651 | 15888 | 7196 | 2404 | 83.5 |

exogenous IL-2. Failure of healthy lymphocytes to respond when challenged with non-self MHC antigens would indicate a mechanism of lymphocyte suppression which influences a fundamental common point in lymphocyte activation.

Figure 4 shows data indicating that the inhibitory effects of the tumour cell line supernatants are temporally related to the time of addition in culture. Significant inhibition of LAK effector generation occurred only when the

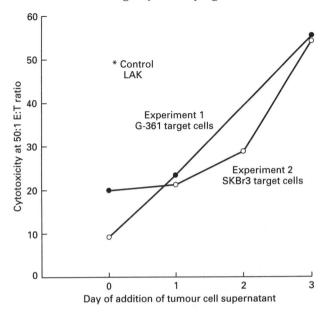

**Figure 4** This figure shows the effects of delayed addition of tumour cell (G-361 cells) supernatant to the IL-2-stimulated lymphocyte cultures. Cultures to which supernatant had been added within 48 hours of initiation showed marked suppression of IL-2-induced LAK-effector cytotoxicity. Delayed addition of supernatant beyond 48 hours resulted in little or no suppression. All assays were performed simultaneously on day 3.

supernatant was present within the first 48 hours of culture, there being no suppression when the addition of supernatant was delayed until the third day of culture.

Interferon-gamma (IFN-$\gamma$) is a fundamental regulatory cytokine in immune activation pathways (112). The autocrine secretion of IFN-$\gamma$ is an obligatory step in the differentiation of lymphocytes into LAK effectors (113). Activation of peripheral blood lymphocytes with either phytohaemagglutinin or IL-2 leads to proliferation and secretion of IFN-$\gamma$. In a series of experiments designed to investigate the effects of the serum-free tumour cell supernatants on lymphocyte activation, we determined that addition of tumour cell supernatants to IL-2 or phytohaemagglutinin-activated PBMC caused a dose-dependent reduction in proliferation (as measured by $^3$H-thymidine uptake) and IFN-$\gamma$ secretion (as measured by immunoradiometric assay of culture supernatants). A representative of three experiments with identical results is shown in Table 4. Secretion of IFN-$\gamma$ is a relatively early event in the activation of lymphocytes, mRNA transcripts being present after only 4 hours

**Table 4** Effects of tumour cell supernatants on IL-2 or mitogen-induced proliferation and interferon-$\gamma$ production

| Culture | Interferon-$\gamma$ (Units ml$^{-1}$) | Proliferation (CPM $\times$ 10$^{-3}$ $\pm$ SEM) |
|---|---|---|
| Control—No Supernatant | <1 | 423 ± 161 |
| Control—50% MiaPaCa Sup | <1 | 432 ± 116 |
| Control—25% MiaPaCa Sup | <1 | 443 ± 111 |
| Control—12.5% MiaPaCa Sup | <1 | 285 ± 185 |
| Control—6.25% MiaPaCa Sup | <1 | 329 ± 89 |
| IL-2 (1000 U ml$^{-1}$) control | 110 | 19724 ± 789 |
| IL-2 + 50% MiaPaCa Sup | 51 | 12808 ± 912 |
| IL-2 + 25% MiaPaCa Sup | 62 | 16408 ± 267 |
| IL-2 + 12.5% MiaPaCa Sup | 78 | 17929 ± 2522 |
| IL-2 + 6.25% MiaPaCa Sup | 67 | 17467 ± 2285 |
| PHA (5 $\mu$g ml$^{-1}$) control | 520 | 64671 ± 5895 |
| PHA + 50% MiaPaCa Sup | 195 | 37957 ± 2096 |
| PHA + 25% MiaPaCa Sup | 230 | 67054 ± 4676 |
| PHA + 12.5% MiaPaCa Sup | 402 | 66465 ± 3053 |
| PHA + 6.25% MiaPaCa Sup | 360 | 60930 ± 3522 |
| Control—No Supernatant | <1 | 375 ± 30 |

stimulation with IL-2 (114). From the information gained in the above experiments we would consider that the supernatant suppressive factor must act at a critical point in a common lymphocyte activation pathway, and may reflect an 'activation paralysis' of healthy peripheral blood lymphocytes treated with supernatant.

In order to determine whether tumour cells constitutively secrete the active moiety present within the supernatant, experiments were undertaken to block cellular metabolic activity. In addition, treatment of tumour cells with interferons may enhance antigen expression and may influence secretion of certain factors leading to alteration of suppressive factor production.

Inhibition of tumour cell protein synthesis bv incubation of suppressive tumour cells with 10 $\mu$g ml$^{-1}$ cycloheximide markedly inhibited the production of a suppressive supernant as shown in Figure 5. In addition, inhibition of RNA and DNA synthesis by actinomycin and mitomycin-C respectively (as confirmed by the reduced uptake of radio-labelled uridine and thymidine respectively by the tumour cells) was also effective in impairing the production of the LAK-effector suppressive factors present in the tumour cell supernatant.

Treatment of a suppressive tumour cell line with either IFN-$\alpha$ or IFN-$\gamma$ for 48 hours was carried out prior to inclusion into IL-2-stimulated lymphocyte cultures as described above. The results shown in Table 5 indicate that pretreatment with IFN-$\gamma$ but not IFN-$\alpha$ enhances the capacity of G-361 melanoma cells to secrete the soluble suppressive factor(s).

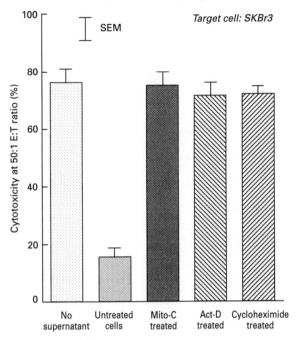

**Figure 5** Treatment of tumour cells with Mitomycin-C, Actinomycin-D, and Cyclo-heximide inhibited DNA, RNA, and protein synthesis respectively (data not shown). When tumour cells were so treated for 12 hours prior to the harvest of a serum-free supernatant, it resulted in the abrogation of suppressive factor production as determined by assay of LAK-effector generation in the presence of treated tumour cell supernatant.

A series of further experiments were undertaken to determine some of the physicochemical characteristics of the tumour-derived suppressive factor (TDSF) obtained from the G-361 human malignant melanoma cell line. In order to confirm the validity of our methodology, we conducted parallel experiments on samples of TDSF and TGF-$\beta$. In this way, dissimilarity between the active component of TDSF and the known tumour-derived immunosuppressive cytokine TGF-$\beta$ could be demonstrated.

When TDSF samples were treated with 2 mM 2-mercapto-ethanol and then re-equilibrated with serum-free medium, the capacity of treated TDSF to suppress the generation of IL-2-induced LAK-effector cytotoxicity was unaffected. In contrast, treatment of TGF-$\beta$ under identical conditions led to complete loss of suppressive activity, confirming the published susceptibility of TGF-$\beta$ to reduction. The data from three identical experiments is shown in Figure 6.

*S. Somers and P. J. Guillou*

**Table 5** Effects of pretreatment of tumour cell lines with recombinant human interferons on tumour cell-mediated suppression of LAK-effector induction

| Effector cells | Cytotoxicity (%) at Effector: Target ratio | | | |
|---|---|---|---|---|
| | 50:1 | 12:1 | Lytic units | Suppression (%) |
| **Experiment 1** | | | | |
| LAK control | 76.8 | 57.3 | 146.5 | – |
| LAK:G361 | 55.8 | 18.9 | 51.3 | 65.0 |
| LAK:G361 + IFN$\alpha$ ($10^2$ U/ml) | 48.8 | 20.0 | 44.8 | 69.4 |
| LAK:G361 + IFN$\alpha$ ($10^3$ U/ml) | 52.0 | 20.7 | 47.5 | 67.6 |
| LAK:G361 + IFN$\gamma$ ($10^2$ U/ml) | 50.7 | 21.4 | 49.7 | 66.1 |
| LAK:G361 + IFN$\gamma$ ($10^3$ U/ml) | 31.6 | 10.6 | 16.8 | 88.5 |
| **Experiment 2** | | | | |
| LAK control | 29.8 | 13.5 | 14.3 | – |
| LAK:G361 | 19.7 | 6.2 | 3.4 | 76.2 |
| LAK:G361 + IFN$\alpha$ ($10^2$ U/ml) | 20.1 | 6.8 | 3.6 | 74.8 |
| LAK:G361 + IFN$\alpha$ ($10^3$ U/ml) | 17.9 | 5.7 | 2.8 | 80.4 |
| LAK:G361 + IFN$\gamma$ ($10^2$ U/ml) | 12.1 | 4.9 | 0.3 | 98.1 |
| LAK:G361 + IFN$\gamma$ ($10^3$ U/ml) | 12.0 | 4.6 | 0.3 | 98.1 |

NB G361 tumour cells used as LAK-effector targets throughout.

The stability of TGF-$\beta$ following denaturation with 8M urea has been described by Assoian *et al.* (74). Treatment of TDSF by denaturation using 6M urea under the same conditions resulted in loss of the suppressive effects of this molecule as shown by the data in Figure 7. Identical treatment of TGF-$\beta$ did not affect the immunosuppressive capacity of this molecule in simultaneous experiments.

Treatment of TDSF with a range of pH environments demonstrated that the suppressive activity was lost following exposure to conditions below pH 4 and above pH 11.5 (Figure 8). In contrast, when TGF-$\beta$ was subjected to the same experimental conditions, slight enhancement of its suppressive activity was observed at a pH of less than 3.

Molecular weight estimation of the TDSF active component was performed by gel exclusion chromatography. Bioassay of sequential fractions from the gel exclusion column revealed that the suppressive activity was eluted in the fraction collected between 10–10.5 minutes from the initiation of the run (Figure 9). A molecular weight standards curve for the same column indicates that the TDSF suppressive activity corresponds to a relative molecular weight of between 69–87 kD.

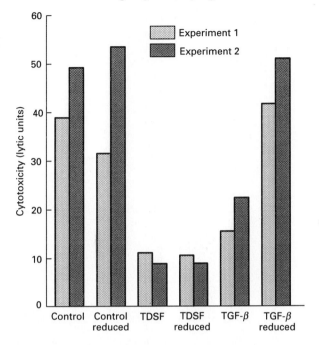

**Figure 6** Effect of reduction by 2-mercaptoethanol on the suppressive effects of TDSF and TGF-$\beta$. Sample of the TDSF and TGF-$\beta$ were placed in sections of dialysis tubing and subjected to reduction by immersing overnight in excess 2 mM 2-mercaptoethanol. Dialysis in serum-free medium for a further 24 hours allowed excess 2-mercaptocathanol to diffuse from the samples and allowed their inclusion in the LAK-effector generation assay. Control samples using serum-free medium were included with each experiment.

# 5  Conclusions: implications for psychoimmunotherapy

Over the past twenty years, *in vitro* and some *in vivo* experiments have shown a role for immune cells in the mediation of tumour cell destruction. More recently, attention has been focused on the IL-2-mediated enhancement of both innate (LAK) and adaptive (T-lymphocyte) anti-tumour responses as a possible therapeutic means. However, despite these host defence mechanisms, it would appear that tumour cells may adapt in such a way as to evade or subvert immunological responses directed against them. The secretion of factors by tumour cells may be one possible mechanism by which tumour cells gain advantage over anti-tumour immune responses present within the host. It must be admitted that the generalized immunosuppression seen in patients with advanced cancer may not be solely due to tumour-derived factors. The

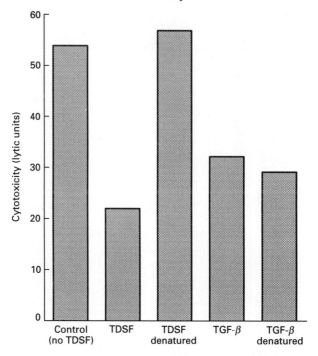

**Figure 7** Effects of denaturation with 6 M urea on the suppressive effects of TDSF and TGF-β. Samples of the TDSF and TGF-β were placed in sections of dialysis tubing and subjected to denaturation by immersing overnight in excess 6 M urea solution. Dialysis in serum-free medium for a further 24 hours allowed excess urea to diffuse from the samples and allowed their inclusion in the LAK-effector generation assay. Control samples using serum-free medium were included with each experiment.

possibility, therefore, exist that in those patients with immune defects, enhancement of immune defences may improve the capacity to neutralize susceptible tumour cells. In this hypothesis, consideration must be given to the possible capacity of tumour cells to undergo progression and to evolve further evasion mechanisms including immunoresistance and loss of antigenicity.

There is, as yet no information on the influence which psycho-neurological and neuro-endocrinology parameters have on these important interactions. If we are to maximally capitalize on these delicate balances which exist *in vivo*, more information is urgently needed on the interrelationships between the psycho-neurological aspects of tumour immunity and tumour progression. Further work to determine the *in vivo* tumour–host immune system relationship, in particular the role of tumour-derived suppressive factors, is necessary for the logical design of immunologically based cancer treatments.

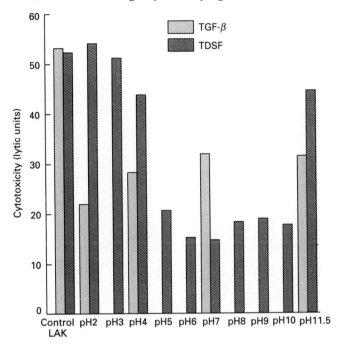

**Figure 8** Effect of pH treatment on the suppressive effect of TDSF and TGF-$\beta$. Samples of the TDSF and TGF-$\beta$ were placed in sections of dialysis tubing and subjected to conditions of varying pH by immersing overnight in excess phosphate buffered saline at a specific pH. Dialysis in serum-free medium for a further 24 hours allowed equilibration to neutral pH and allowed the inclusion of samples in the LAK-effector generation assay. Control samples using serum-free medium were included with each experiment.

# 6 References

1. Blumenthal, H. T. (1942). Homotransplantation of spontaneous tumours into mice bearing spontaneous tumours. *Cancer Res.*, **2**, 56–58.
2. Browing, P. M. H. (1947). Report of the British Empire Cancer Campaign. 1947, **24**, 177–193.
3. Gorer, P. A. (1948). The significance of studies with transplanted tumours. *Br. J. Cancer*, **2**, 103–107.
4. Pomeroy, T. C. (1952). Studies of mechanisms of cortisone-induced metastasis of transplantable mouse tumours. *Cancer Res.*, **14**, 201–214.
5. Zeidman, I. (1957). Metastasis: A review of recent advances. *Cancer Res.*, **17**, 157–166.
6. Moore, G. E. and Kondo, T. (1958). Study of adjuvant cancer chemotherapy by model experiments. *Surgery*, **44**, 199–225.

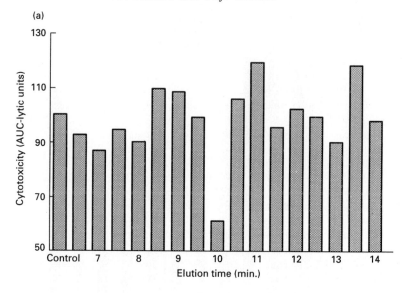

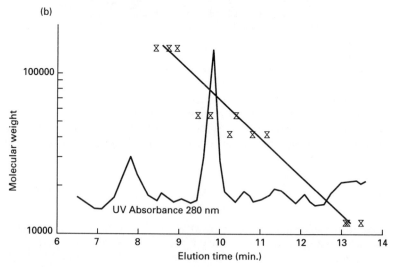

**Figure 9** Molecular weight estimation of TDSF. (a) A concentrated sample of G-361 derived suppressor factor was loaded on to a gel exclusion column which had been pre-run with molecular weight standards. Aliquots of eluate were then collected at 30 second intervals, dialysed in excess serum-free medium for 6 hours, then included in LAK-effector generation assays to determine which of them contained the suppressive moiety. (b) A molecular weight standard curve was constructed and correlated with the data in part (a). From this it can be seen that the suppressive fraction eluted after 10 minutes, which corresponds to a molecular weight band of approximately 69–87 kDa and is associated with a peak of protein on the UV absorbance chromatogram.

7. Moore, G. E. (1958). Personal communication quoted by Grace, J. T. and Kondo, T. Investigations of host resistance in cancer patients. *Ann. Surg.*, **148**, 633–641.

8. Hughes, L. E. and MacKay, W. D. (1965). Suppression of the tuberculin response in malignant disease. *Br. Med. J.*, **ii**, 1346–1348.

9. Kelly, W. D., Good, R. A., and Varco, R. L. (1958). Anergy and skin homograft survival in Hodgkins disease. *Surg. Gynaecol. Obstet.*, **107**, 565–570.

10. Monson, J. R. T., Ramsden, C. W., and Guillow, P. J. (1986). Decreased interleukin-2 production in patients with gastrointestinal cancer. *Br. J. Surg.*, **73**, 483.

11. Monson, J. R. T., Ramsden, C. W., Giles, G. R., Brennan, T. G., and Guillou, P. J. (1987). Lymphokine activated killer (LAK) cells in patients with gastrointestinal cancer. *Gut*, **28**, 1420–1425.

12. Hakim, A. A. (1988). Peripheral blood lymphocytes from patients with cancer lack interleukin-2 receptors. *Cancer*, **61**, 689–701.

13. Silk, M. R. (1967). Effect of plasma from patients with carcinoma on *in vitro* lymphocyte transformation. *Cancer*, **20**, 2088–2093.

14. Sample, W. F., Gertner, H. R., and Cheretien, P. B. (1971). Inhibition of phytohaemagglutinin induced *in vitro* lymphocyte transformation by serum from patients with carcinoma. *J. Natl. Cancer Inst.*, **46**, 1291–1297.

15. Brooks, W. H., Netsky, M. G., Normansell, D. E., and Horwitz, D. V. (1972). Depressed cell mediated immunity in patients with primary intracranial tumours. *J. Exp. Med.*, **136**, 1631–1633.

16. Glasgow, A. H., Menzoian, J. O., Nimber, R. B., Cooperband, S. R., Schmid, K., and Mannick, J. A. (1974). Immunosuppressive peptide fraction in the serum of cancer patients. *Surgery*, **76**, 35–39.

17. Whittaker, M. G., Rees, K., and Clark, C. C. G. (1971). Reduced lymphocyte transformation in breast cancer. *Lancet*, **i**, 892–893.

18. Sucie-Foca, N., Buda, J., and McManus, J. (1973). Impaired responsiveness of lymphocytes and serum inhibitors factors in patients with cancer. *Cancer Res.*, **33**, 2373–2377.

19. Golub, S. H., O'Connell, T. X., and Morton, D. L. (1974). Correlation of *in vitro* and *in vivo* assays of immunocompetence in cancer patients. *Cancer Res.*, **34**, 1834–1837.

20. Shiiba, K., Suzuki, R., Kawakami, K., Ohuchi, A., and Kumagai, K. (1986). Interleukin 2-activated killer cells: generation in collaboration with interferon-γ and its suppression in cancer patients. *Cancer Immunol. Immunother.*, **21**, 119–128.

21. Itoh., K., Tilden, A. B., and Balch, C. M. (1985). Role of interleukin 2 and a serum suppressor factor on the induction of activated killer cells for autologous human melanoma cells. *Cancer Res.*, **45**, 3173–3178.

22. Bugis, S. P., Lotzova, E., Savage, H. E., Hester, J. P., Racz, T., Sacks, P. G. (1990). Inhibition of lymphokine-activated killer cell generation by blocking factors in sera of patients with head and neck cancer. *Cancer Immunol. Immunother.*, **31**, 176–181.

23. Fidler, I. J. and Hart, I. R. (1982). Biological diversity in metastatic neoplasms: Origins and implications. *Science*, **217**, 998–1003.

24. Morton, D. L. (1968). Acquired immunological tolerance and carcinogenesis by the mammary tumour virus. I. Influence of neonatal infection with the mammary tumour virus on the growth of spontaneous mammary adenocarcinomas. *J. Natl. Cancer Inst.*, **42**, 311–320.

25. Morton, D. L., Goldman, L., and Wood, D. A. (1968). Acquired immunological tolerance and carcinogenesis by the mammary tumour virus. II. Influence of neonatal infection with the mammary tumour virus on the growth of spontaneous mammary adenocarcinomas. *J. Natl. Cancer Inst.*, **42**, 321–329.

26. Doherty, P. C., Knowles, B. B., and Wettstein, P. J. (1984). Immunological surveillance of tumours in the context of major histocompatability complex restriction of T-cell function. *Adv. Cancer Res.*, **42**, 1–65.

27. Gooding, L. R. (1982). Characterisation of a progressive tumour from CH3 fibroblasts transformed *in vitro* with SV40 virus. Immunoresistance *in vivo* correlates with phenotypic loss of $H2K^k$. *J. Immunol.*, **129**, 1306–1311.

28. Trowsdale, J., Travers, P., Bodmer, W. F., and Patillo, R. A. (1980). Expression of HLA-A,-B and -C and $\beta_2$-microglobulin antigens in human choriocarcinoma cell lines. *J. Exp. Med.*, **152**, 11s–17s.

29. Doyle, A., Martin, W. J., Funa, K., Gadzar, A., Carney, D., Martin, S. E. *et al.* (1985). Markedly decreased expression of class 1 histocompapability antienens, protein, and mRNA in human small-cell lung cancer. *J. Exp. Med.*, **161**, 1135–1151.

30. Lampson, L. A., Fisher, C. A., and Whelan, J. P. (1983). Striking paucity of HLA-A, B, C and $\beta_2$-microglobulin on human neuroblastoma cell lines. *J. Immunol.*, **130**, 2471–2478.

31. Travers, P. J., Arklie, J. L., Trowsdale, J., Patillo, R. A., and Bodmer, W. F. (1982). Lack of expression of HLA-ABC antigent in choriocarcinoma and other human tumour cell lines. *Natl. Cancer Inst. Monogr.*, **60**, 175–180.

32. Natali, P. J., Giacomini, P., Bigotti, A., Imai, K., Nicotra, M. R., Ng, A. K. *et al.* (1983). Heterogeneity in the expression of HLA and tumour associated antigens by surgically removed and cultured breast carcinoma cells. *Cancer Res.*, **43**, 660–668.

33. Stein, B., Momberg, F., Schwarz, V., Schlag, P., Moldenhauer, G., and Moller, P. (1988). Reduction or loss of HLA-A,B,C antigens in colorectal carcinoma appears not to influence survival. *Brit. J. Cancer*, **57**, 364–368.

34. Ruiter, D. J., Bergman, W., Welvaart, K., Scheffer, E., van Volten, W. A., Russo, C. *et al.* (1984). Immunohistochemical analysis of malignant melanomas ani nevocellular nevi with monoclonal antibodies to distinct monomorphic determinants of HLA antigens. *Cancer Res.*, **44**, 3930–3935.

35. Hellstrom, K. E. and Hellstrom, I. (1974). Lymphocyte-mediated cytotoxicity and blocking serum activity to tumour antigens. *Adv. Immunol.*, **18**, 209–277.

36. Hellstrom, K. E., Hellstrom, I., and Nepom, J. T. (1977). Specific blocking factors—are they important? *Biochim. Biophys. Acta*, **473**, 121–148.

37. Baldwin, R. W., Embleton, M. J., and Price, M. R. (1973). Inhibition of lymphocyte cytotoxicity for human colon carcinoma by treatment with solubilised tumour membrane fractions. *Int. J. Cancer*, **12**, 84–92.

38. Rao, V. S., Bennett, J. A., Shen, F. W., Gershon, R. K., and Mitchell, M. S.

(1980). Antigen-antibody complexes generate Lyt-1 inducers of suppressor cells. *J. Immunol.*, **125**, 63–67.

39. Gorelik, E. (1983). Concomitant tumour immunity and the resistance to a second tumour challenge. *Adv. Cancer Res.*, **39**, 71–120.

40. Lamon, E. W. (1977). Stimulation of tumour cell growth *in vitro*: A critical evaluation of immunologic specificity. *J. Natl. Cancer Ins.*, **59**, 769–774.

41. Klein, B., Klein, T., Figer, A., Bleiberg, M., Shapira, J., Loven, D. *et al.* (1991). Soluble histocompatability antigen class I in breast cancer patients in relation to tumour burden. *Cancer*, **67**, 2295–2299.

42. Forbes, M. A., Cox, A. M., and Cooper, E. H. (1988). A method to detect the *in vitro* modification of serum beta-2 microglobulin in health and disease. *Clin. Chim. Acta*, **177**, 88–99.

43. Sulica, A., Gherman, M., Manciulea, M., Galatiuc, C., and Herberman, R. B. (1989). Regulation of human natural cytotoxicity by IgG. III. Interaction between negative regulation by monomeric IgG and positive regulation by interferons of different types. *Nat. Immun. Cell Growth Regul.*, **8**, 266–278.

44. Fujimoto, S., Greene, M. I., and Semon, A. H. (1976). Regulation of the immune response to tumour antigen. I. Immunosuppressor cells in tumour bearing hosts. *J. Immunol.*, **116**, 791–799.

45. Fujimoto, S., Greene, M. I., and Semon, A. H. (1976). Regulation of the immune response to tumour antigen. II. The nature of immunosuppressor cells in tumour-bearing hosts. *J. Immunol.*, **116**, 800–806.

46. Treves, A. I., Cohen, L. R., and Feldman, M. (1976). Suppressor factor secreted by T-lymphocytes from tumour-bearing mice. *J. Natl. Cancer Inst.*, **57**, 709–713.

47. Elgert, K. D. and Farrar, W. L. (1978). Suppressor cell activity in tumour-bearing mice. I. Dualistic inhibition by suppressor T-lymphocytes and macrophages. *J. lmmunol.*, **120**, 1345–1441.

48. Werkmeister, J., Phillips, G., McCarthy, W., and Hersey, P. (1981). Suppressor cell activity in melanoma patients-II, concanavalin A-induced suppressor cells in relation to tumour gowth and suppressor T-cell subsets. *Int. J. Cancer*, **28**, 1–9.

49. Yu, A., Watts, H., Jaffe, N., and Parkman, R. (1977). Concomitant presence of tumour-specific cytotoxic and inhibitor lymphocytes in patients with osteogenic sarcoma. *N. Engl. J. Med.*, **297**, 121–127.

50. Akiyama, M., Bean, W., Sadamoto, K., Takahashi, Y., and Brankovan, V. (1983). Suppression of the responsiveness of lymphocytes from cancer patients triggered by co-culture with autologous tumor-derived cells. *J. Immunol.*, **131**, 3805–3090.

51. Mukherji, B., Guha, A., Loomis, R., and Ergin, M. T. (1987). Cell-mediated amplification and down regulation of cytotoxic immune response against autologous human cancer. *J. Immunol.*, **138**, 1987–1991.

52. Cozzolino, F., Torcia, M., Carossino, A. M., Giordani, R., Selli, C., Talini, G. *et al.* (1987). Characterization of cells from invaded lymph nodes in patients with solid tumors. Lymphokine requirement for tumor specific lymphoproliferative response. *J. Exp Med.*, **166**, 303–318.

53. Hoon, S. B., Bowker, R. J., and Cochran, A. J. (1987). Suppressor cell activity in melanoma-draining lymph nodes. *Cancer Research*, **47**, 1529–1533.

54. Scott, M. T. (1982). Tumour-induced specific suppression; a limitation to immunotherapy. *Immunol. Today*, **3**, 8–9.

55. Rappaport, R. S. and Dodge, G. R. (1982). Prostaglandin E inhibits the production of human interleukin 2. *J. Exp. Med.*, **155**, 943–948.

56. Eisenthal, A. (1990). Indomethacin up-regulates the generation of lymphokine-activated killer-cell activity and antibody-dependent cellular cytotoxicity mediated by interleukin-2. *Cancer Immunol. Immunother.*, **31**, 342–348.

57. Pleisca, O. J., Smith, A. H., and Greenwick, K. (1975). Subversion of the immune system by tumour cells and the role of prostaglandins. *Proc. Natl. Acad. Sci.*, **72**, 1848–1851.

58. Droller, M. J., Schneider, M. H., and Perlmann, P. (1978). A possible role of prostaglandins in the inhibition of natural and antibody-dependant cell-mediated cytotoxicity against tumour cells. *Cell Immunol.*, **39**, 165–171.

59. Balch, C. M., Dougherty, P. A., Cloud, G. A., and Tilden, A. B. (1984). Prostaglandin E2 mediated suppression of cellular immunity in colon cancer patients. *Surgery*, **95**, 71–76.

60. Tilden, A. B. and Balch, C. M. (1981). Indomethacin enhancement of immunocompetence in melanoma patients. *Surgery*, **90**, 77–84.

61. Sedman, P. C., Ramsden, C. W., Brennan, T. G., Giles, G. R., and Guillou, P. J. (1988). Augmentation of lymphokine-activated killer cell activity in patients with gastointestinal cancer. *Br. J. Surg.*, **75**, 591–594.

62. Maxwell, W. J., Keating, J., Hogan, F. P., McDonald, G. S. A., and Keeling, P. W. N. (1988). Enhanced prostaglandin E2 production by tissue fixed macrophages from colonic tumours. *Gastroenterology*, **94**, A292.

63. Wanebo, H. J., Pace, R., Hargett, S., Katz, D., and Sando, J. (1986). Production and response to interleukin-2 in peripheral blood lymphocytes of cancer patients. *Cancer*, **57**, 656–662.

64. Itoh, K., Pellis, N. R., Balch, C. M. (1989). Monocyte-dependent, serum-borne suppressor of induction of lymphokine-activated killer cells in lymphocytes from melanoma patients. *Cancer Immuno. Imunother.*, **29**, 57–62.

65. Kamo, I. and Friedman, H. (1977). Immunosuppression and the role of suppressive factors in cancer. *Adv. Cancer Res.*, **25**, 271–321.

66. Ting, C. C., Hargrove, M. E., and Stephany, D. (1987). Generation of activated killer cells in tumor-bearing hosts. *Int. J. Cancer*, **39**, 232–236.

67. Shu, S., Chou, T., and Rosenberg, S. A. (1987). Generation from tumor-bearing mice of lymphocytes with *in vivo* therapeutic efficacy. *J. Immunol.*, **139**, 295.

68. Gregorian, S. K., and Battisto, J. R. (1990). Immunosuppression in murine renal cell carcinoma. I. Characterisation of extent, severity and sources. *Cancer Immunol. Immunother.*, **31**, 325–334.

69. Gregorian, S. K. and Battisto, J. R. (1990). Immunosuppression in murine renal cell carcinoma. II. Identification of responsible lymphoid cell phenotypes and examination of elimination of suppression. *Cancer Immunol. Immunother.*, **31**, 335–341.

70. Sondak, V. K., Wagner, P. D., Shu, S., and Chang, A. E. (1991). Suppressive

effects of visceral tumour on the generation of anti-tumour T-cells for adoptive immunotherapy. *Arch. Surg.*, **126**, 442–446.

71. Thomas, K. A. (1987). Fibroblast growth factors. *FASEB J*, **6**, 443–440.

72. Anzano, M. A., Rieman, D., Prichett, W., Bowen-Pope, D. F., and Greig, R. (1989). Growth factor production by human colon carcinoma cell lines. *Cancer Res.*, **49**, 2898–2904.

73. Childs, C. B., Proper, J. A., Tucker, R. F., and Moses, H. L. (1982). Serum contains a platelet-derived transforming gowth factor. *Proc. Natl. Acad. Sci. USA*, **79**, 5312–5314.

74. Assoian, R. K., Komoriya, A., Meyers, C. A., Miller, D. M., and Sporn, M. B. (1983). Transforming growth factor-beta in human platelets; identification of a major storage site, purification and characterization. *J. Biol. Chem.*, **258**, 7155–7162.

75. Sporn, M. B., Roberts, A. B., Wakefield, L. M., and Assoian, R. K. (1986). Transforming growth factor-$\beta$: Biologic function and chemical structure. *Science*, **233**, 532–539.

76. Knabbe, C., Lippman, M. E., Wakefield, L. E., Flanders, K. C., Kasid, A., Derynck, R. *et al.* (1987). Evidence that transforming growth factor-$\beta$ is a hormonally regulated negative growth factor in human breast cancer cells. *Cell*, **48**, 417–428.

77. Mule, J. J., Schwarz, S. L., Roberts, A. B., Sporn, M. B., and Rosenberg, S. A. (1988). Transforming growth factor-beta inhibits the *in vitro* generation of lymphokine-activated killer cells and cytotoxic T-cells. *Cancer Immunol. Immunother.*, **26**, 95–101.

78. Grimm, E. A., Crump, W. L., Durett, A., Hester, J. P., Lagoo-Deenadalayan, S., and Owen-Schlaub, L. B. (1988). TGF-beta inhibits the *in vitro* induction of lymphokine-activted killing activity. *Cancer Immunol. Immunother.*, **27**, 53–58.

79. Rook, A. H., Kehrl, J. H., Wakefield, L. M., Roberts, A. B., Sporn, M. B., Bulington, D. B. *et al.* (1986). Effects of transforming growth factor-beta on the functions of natural killer cells: depressed cytolytic activity and blunting of interferon responsiveness. *J. Immunol.*, **36**, 3916–3920.

80. Kehrl, J. H., Taylor, A. S., Delsing, G. S., Roberts, A. B., Sporn, M. B., and Fauci, A. (1989). Further studies of the role of transforming growth factor-beta in human B-cell function. *J. Immunol.*, **143**, 1868–1871.

81. Kehrl, J. H., Wakefield, L. M., Roberts, A. B., Jakowlel, S., Alvarez-Mon, M., and Derynck, R. (1986). The production of TGF-beta by human T-Lymphocytes and its potential role in the regulation of T-cell growth. *J. Exp. Med.*, **163**, 1037–1041.

82. Kuppner, M. C., Hamou, M.-F., Bodmer, S., Fontana, A., and de Tribolet, N. (1988). The glioblestoma-derived T-cell suppressor factor/transforming growth factor beta inhibits the generation of lymphokine-activated killer (LAK) cells. *Int. J. Cancer*, **42**, 562–567.

83. Torre-Amione, G., Beuchamp, R. D., Koeppen, H., Park, B. H., Schreiber, H., Moses, H. L. *et al.* (1990). A highly immunogenic tumor transfected with a murine transforming growth factor type $\beta$ cDNA escapes immune surveillance. *Immunol.*, **86**, 1486–1490.

84. Snyderman, R. and Cianciolo, G. J. (1984). Immunosuppressive activity of the retroviral envelope protein p15E and its possible relationship to neoplasia. *Immunol. Today*, **5**, 240–246.

85. Steffen, D. I. and Robinson, L. L. (1982). Endogenous retroviruses of mice and chickens. *Curr. Top. Microbiol. Immunol.*, **98**, 1–6.

86. Cianciolo, G. J., Lostrom, M. E., Tam, M., and Synderman, R. (1983). Murine malignant cells synthesise a 19,000-dalton protein that is physicochemically and antigenically related to the immunosuppressive retroviral protein, p15E. *J. Exp. Med.*, **158**, 885–893.

87. Harris, D. T., Cianciolo, G. J., Snyderman, R., Argov, S., and Koren, H. S. (1987). Inhibition of human natural killer cell activity by a synthetic peptide homologous to a conserved region in the retroviral protein p15E. *J. Immunol.*, **138**, 889–894.

88. Kizaki, T., Mitani, M., Gaic, G. J., Ogasawara, M., Good, R. A., and Day, N. K. (1991). Specific association of retroviral envelope protein p15E with human cell surfaces. *Immunol. Lett.*, **28**, 11–18.

89. Schmidt, D. M. and Snyderman, R. (1988). Retroviral protein P15E and tumorigenesis. *J. Immunol.*, **140**, 4035–4041.

90. Foulds, S., Wakefield, C. H., Giles, M., Gillespie, J., Dye, J. F., and Guillou, P. J. (1993). Expression of a suppresive P15-E related epitope in colorectal and gastric cancer. *Br. J. Cancer*. (In press.)

91. Remacle-Bonnet, M. M., Pommier, G. J., Luc, C., Rance, R. J., and Depieds, R. C. (1978). Nonspecific suppressivc and cytostatic activities mediated by human colonic carcinoma tissue or cultured cell extract. *J. Immunol.*, **121**, 44–49.

92. Roth, J. A., Chee, D. O., Morton, D. L., and Holmes, E. C. (1978). Inhibition of concanavalin-A mediated lymphocyte stimulation by extracts of lung carcinomas. *Proc. Am. Assoc. Cancer Res.*, **19**, 135–141.

93. Mohagbeghpour, N., Parhami, B., Dowlatshahi, K., Kadjehnouri, D., Elder, J. H., and Chisari, F. V. (1979). Immunotherapy properties of human esophageal tumour extract. *J. Immunol.*, **122**, 1350–1356.

94. Nelson, M., Nelson, D. S., Kuchroo, V. K., Spadbrow, P. B., and Jennings, P. A. (1987). Depression of cell-mediated immunity by tumour cell products: induction of resistance by immunotherapeutically active extracts of bovine ocular squamous cell carcinoma. *Cancer Immunol. Immunother.*, **24**, 231–236.

95. Roth, J. A., Grimm, E. A., Gupta, R. K., and Ames, R. S. (1982). Immuno-regulatory factors derived from human tumors. I. Immunologic and biochemical characterizations of factors that suppress lymphocyte proliferation and cytotoxic responses *in vitro*. *J. Immunol.*, **128**, 1922.

96. Roth, J. A., Osborne, B. A., and Ames, R. S. (1983). Immunoregulatory factors derived from human tumors. II. Partial prufication and further immuno-biochemical characterization of a human sarcoma-derived immunosuppressive factor expressing HLA-DR and immunoglobulin-related determinants., 303–308.

97. Medoff, J. R., Clack, V. D., and Roche, J. K. (1986). Characterization of an immunosuppressive factor from malignant asictes that resembles a factor induced *in vitro* by carcinoembryonic antigen. *J. Immunol.*, **137**, 2057–2064.

98. Werkmeister, J., Zbroja, R., McCarthy, W., and Hersey, P. (1980). Detection of an inhibitor of cell division in cultures of tumour cells with immunosuppressive activity *in vitro*. *Clin. Exp. Immunol.*, **40**, 168–170.

99. Whitehead, J. S. and Kim, Y. S. (1980). An inhibitor of lymphocyter proliferation produced by a human colonic adenocarcinoma cell line in culture. *Cancer Res.*, **40**, 29–35.

100. Hersey, P., Bindon, C., Czerniecki, M., Spurling, A., Wass, J., and McCarthy, W. H. (1983). Inhibition of interleukin 2 production by factors released from tumor cells. *J. Immunol.*, **131**, 2837–2842.

101. Farram, E., Nelson, M., Nelson, D. S., and Moon, D. K. (1982). Inhibition of cytokine production by a tumour cell product. *Immunology*, **46**, 603–612.

102. Putnam, J. B. and Roth, J. A. (1985). Identification and characterisation of a tumour derived immunosuppressive glycoprotein from murine melanoma K-1735. *Cancer Immunol. Immunother.*, **19**, 90–94.

103. Ebert, E. C., Roberts, A. I., O'Connell, S. M., Robertson, F. M., and Nagase, H. (1987). Characterization of an immunosuppressive factor derived from colon cancer cells. *J. Immunol.*, **38**, 2161–2168.

104. Pommier, G. J., Garrouste, F. L., Bettetini, D., Culouscou, J. M., and Remacle-Bonnet, M. M. (1987). *In vivo* delayed rejection of tumors and inhibition of delayed-type hypersensitivity by HT-29 human colonic adenocarcinoma cell line. *Cancer Immunol. Immunother.*, **24**, 225–230.

105. Muraki, J., Fischer, J., Addonizio, J. C., Nagamatsu, G. R., and Chiao, J. W. (1989). Immunosuppressive factor derived from renal cancer cells. *Urology*, **34**, 205–209.

106. Fujiwara, H. and Ellner, J. J. (1986). Spontaneous production of a suppressor factor by the human macrophage-like cell line U937. *J. Immunol.*, **136**, 181–185.

107. Fujiwara, H., Toossi, Z., Ohnishi, K., Edmonds, K., and Ellner, J. J. (1987). Spontaneous preduction of a suppressor factor by a human macrophage-like cell line U937. *J. Immunol.*, **138**, 197–203.

108. Sugimura, K., Ueda, Y., Takeda, K., Fukuda, S., Tsukahara, K., Habu, Y. *et al.* (1989). A cytokine, lymphocyte blastogenesis inhibitory factor (LBIF), arrests mitogen-stimulated T-lymphocytes at early G phase with no influence on interleukin 2 production and interleukin 2 receptor light chain expression. *Eur. J. Immunol.*, **19**, 1357–1364.

109. Sugimura, K., Ohno, T., Fukuda, S., Wada, Y., Kimura, T., and Azuma, I. (1990). Tumor gowth inhibitory activity of a lymphocyte blastogensis inhibitory factor. *Cancer Res.*, **50**, 345–349.

110. Serrano, R., Yiangou, Y., Solana, R., Sachs, J., and Pena, J. (1990). Isolation of a novel tumor protein that induces resistance to natural killer cell lysis. *J. Immunol.*, **145**, 3516–3523.

111. Somers, S. S., Dye, J. F., and Guillou, P. J. (1991). Comparison of transforming growth factor-beta and a human tumour derived suppressor factor. *Cancer Immunol. Immunother.*, **33**, 217–222.

112. Trinchieri, G. and Perussia, B. (1985). Immune Interferon: a pleiotropic lymphokine with multiple effects. *Immunol. Today*, **6**, 131–136.

113. Novelli, F., Giovarelli, M., Reber-Liske, R., Virgallita, G., Garotta, G., and Forni, G. (1991). Blockade of physiologically secreted IFN-γ inhibits human T-lymphocyte and natural killer cell activation. *J. Immunol.*, **147**, 1445–1452.

114. Farrar, W. L., Birchenall-Sparks, M. C., and Young, H. B. (1986). Interleukin 2 induction of interferon-γ mRNA synthesis. *J. Immunol.*, **137**, 3836–3840.

# 17

# Psychoneuroimmunology: a critical analysis of the implications for oncology in the twenty-first century

D.H. BOVBJERG

## 1  Introduction

The chain of reasoning implicit in much of the current thinking concerning the implications of psychoneuroimmunology for oncology (in what will be called here the 'conventional view') is the following: (1) there is evidence that some psychosocial factors affect the incidence and progression of some types of cancer; (2) there is evidence that some activities of the immune system affect the incidence and progression of some types of cancer; (3) there is evidence that some psychological factors affect some activities of the immune system; and, (4) therefore, psychological influences on the immune system may mediate the influence of psychological factors on cancer progression (1, 2). As direct studies of this last aspect (the 'mediational hypothesis') are scant, the 'conventional view' relies on the strength of evidence supporting each of the links in the chain. This evidence has been reviewed in depth in the previous chapters of this book.

In this brief chapter, three challenges are posed to this conventional view of the importance of psychoneuroimmunology to cancer. First, (in what will be called the 'weak link' view) the difficulties facing researchers in each of the three separate research literatures (that is psychooncology, tumour immunology, and psychoimmunology) underlying the mediational hypothesis will be outlined. Second, (in what will be called the 'chutzpah view') a case will be made for the links being weak *because* the chain is strong. That is, the evidence for the link between psychological factors and cancer, as well as for links between immune factors and cancer would be stronger if investigators in each of these areas had taken the mediational hypothesis into consideration when designing their research. Third, (in what will be called the 'wider view') a case will be made for psychological influences on the immune system being only a small part of the impact of psychoneuroimmunology on oncology in the twenty-first century.

## 2  The conventional view of the implications of psychoneuroimmunology for oncology

The 'conventional view' of psychoimmune mechanisms mediating the influence of psychological factors on cancer progression is schematically shown as in Figure 1.

The naive reader, having made it this far through the book, has surely been struck by the conceptual and methodological difficulties *within* each of three individual links making up this chain of reasoning (Figure 1, Points 1–3), and may perhaps have been boggled by the challenges facing researchers having the temerity to consider confronting the three-headed Hydra of the 'mediational hypothesis' (Figure 1, Point 4). For those readers who habitually

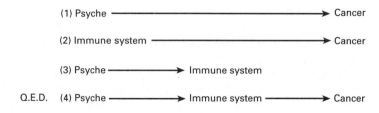

Figure 1

start their reading with a peek at the end to see how it comes out, or those who just skip to the end out of indolence and sloth, it may be helpful to briefly note some of the more pressing challenges to researchers within each of the three research literatures. It should be noted that these are selective (some might say idiosyncratic) overviews, and do not consider more specific methodological issues which are outlined in greater depth in previous chapters.

## 2.1 EVIDENCE FOR THE INFLUENCE OF VARIOUS PSYCHOSOCIAL FACTORS ON THE INCIDENCE AND PROGRESSION OF SOME TYPES OF CANCER

Putative psychosocial risk/protection factors are likely to interact with each other and with physical risk factors in ways that may differ from tumour to tumour, or from step to step in the natural history of a given tumour. Eysenck (Chapter 5) has noted the considerable evidence for physical and behavioural risk factors (for example smoking, drinking) interacting synergistically to contribute to the individual's risk of cancer, and emphasized the accumulating evidence for analogous synergies with psychosocial factors. For example, 'stress' or 'personality' may show a minimal relation to lung cancer when considered by itself, but when considered in conjunction with other individual risk factors (for example genetic predisposition, smoking), the increase in total risk due to stress may be profound. That is, individual risk factors have to be multiplied and not simply added to yield the total risk. Such interactive models are likely to be the norm for cancer researchers in the twenty-first century. One can foresee productive collaborations between psychologically oriented investigators and perceptive epidemiologists, working together to determine the causal connections in the complex web of risk factor interactions. Such research will of course, be hypothesis driven, avoiding the dangers of a fishing expedition through the data, focusing on particular, predicted interactions.

It is likely that changes in behaviour may make a contribution to the relationship of psychosocial risk factors to cancer in a way that is larger than putative psychobiological pathways (see Figure 2). Several of the authors of

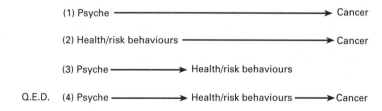

**Figure 2**

previous chapters (for example Classen *et al.*, Chapter 4; Richardson *et al.*, Chapter 8; Levenson *et al.*, Chapter 9) have noted the importance of considering the links between psychological factors (for example emotional distress) and a broad class of behavioural variables (health/risk behaviours) that have been found to positively and negatively affect the incidence and/or progression of many types of cancer. The effects of such variables (for example smoking) on cancer incidence may be profound. Indeed, cigarette smoking has been estimated to play a role in 30 per cent of all cases of cancer in the United States, providing perhaps the most dramatic example of the impact behavioural variables may have on cancer. Psychosocial variables may be related to dietary choices, screening behaviours, compliance with treatment, and so on, which may have a major impact on cancer incidence and progression. Changes in such behaviours patterns (which are independent of putative psychoimmune influences) could account for relationships between psychosocial factors and survival in both correlational and intervention studies (for example Fawzy *et al.*, Chapter 11). Lasting changes in behaviour are difficult to achieve however, suggesting the importance of continued basic research in this area. One can hope that the twenty-first century will see the development of effective interventions for risky behaviours, which would make a significant contribution to cancer prevention.

Another challenge to researchers exploring the putative effects of psychosocial variables on cancer is the clear effect of cancer and its treatment on psychosocial variables. Several of the authors of previous chapters (for example Classen *et al.*, Chapter 4; Richardson *et al.* Chapter 8; Fawzy *et al.*, Chapter 11) have noted that the diagnosis and treatment of cancer have profound psychological consequences (for example depression, anxiety). Indeed, the evidence for cancer and its treatment affecting psychological factors is stronger than the evidence for a causal relationship in the opposite direction. In studies with humans it is difficult to determine the direction of causality. Even in prospective studies conducted prior to diagnosis, it is difficult to rule out the possibility that patients have considerable information about their medical status. Moreover, the tumour itself can have psychological consequences (for example paraneoplastic syndromes), which may be the presenting symptoms. The arrow linking psychological factors and cancer in Figure 1 (Point 1) should thus point in both directions, indicating bidirectional causal relationships. Research with inbred strains of animals having well established genetic risks for cancer would greatly facilitate the prospective study of psychological influences. By the twenty-first century, such studies may provide a wealth of information about the role of psychological factors in the development of cancer.

## 2.2 EVIDENCE FOR THE INVOLVEMENT OF THE IMMUNE SYSTEM IN THE INCIDENCE AND PROGRESSION OF SOME TYPES OF CANCER

Putative immune defenses against cancer are multifactorial, mediated by both specific (for example cytotoxic T-cell activity) and non-specific mechanisms (for example natural killer cell activity) with extensive cytokine cross-talk, as reviewed by Dalgliesh and Souberbielle (Chapter 10). The relative contribution of these mechanisms may differ from tumour to tumour (even within an individual). A less well recognized contributor to the complexity of tumour immunity is the accumulating evidence that immune mechanisms can have a positive influence on tumour cells (for example by providing growth factors, or by suppressing immune effector cells). Tumour immunity is also a dynamic process of interactions between the developing tumour and the immune system, as neoplastic cells have multiple strategies for escaping immune control (Somers and Guillou, Chapter 16), and may exert suppressive influences on various immune functions. The arrow linking the immune system and cancer in Figure 1 (Point 2) should thus also point in both directions, indicating bidirectional causal relationships analogous to those seen between the psyche and cancer above.

## 2.3 EVIDENCE FOR THE INFLUENCE OF PSYCHOLOGICAL FACTORS ON SOME IMMUNE FUNCTIONS

Much of the research concerning the effects of psychological factors on the immune system has focused on the immunological consequences of 'stressors' of various kinds, as noted by Biondi and Kotzalidis (Chapter 1). The effect of other psychological variables on immune function has rarely been directly explored. Animal models, for example, have typically involved physical stressors which may affect the immune system via a role that is independent of putative psychologically induced mediators. For example, restraining an animal in a small tube results in increased body temperature that may affect immune parameters; electric shock may increase the animal's attempts to escape and the increased muscular activity may affect recirculation patterns of leukocytes, quite independent of any putative distress the animal may be experiencing. One can hope that researchers in the twenty-first century will routinely use stressors with a more obvious psychological component (for example loss of control, aversive social interactions, conditioned aversive responses).

Studies with humans are beginning to examine the links between psychological variables and alteration in immune function outside the context of mental illness (for example depression). Much remains to be learned about these. For example, if a stressor induces anger, does that have different

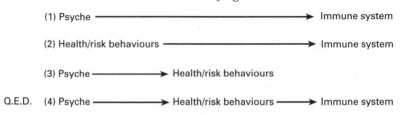

Figure 3

immunological consequences than if it induces anxiety? Are the effects specific to particular aspects of immune function? Use of experimental stressors under controlled conditions may help to provide the answers to such questions in the future.

As with research linking psychological variables with cancer, research linking psychological variables with alteration in immune function must be aware of the contribution of behavioural variables (for example changes in sleep) known to affect the immune system (see Figure 3).

Correlational studies of psychoimmune relations may be complicated under certain circumstances by the potential for immunological influences on psychological variables (for example see Biondi and Kotzalidis, Chapter 1). Administration of cytokines has been reported to have psychological consequences in humans and a variety of behavioural effects in animals. The psychological consequences of various forms of immune activity *in vivo* (for example production of cytokines) induced or altered by cancer or its treatment have yet to be explored. If such influences do prove to have an effect on psychological factors, the determination of the direction of causal relations between cancer, immune function, and psychological factors becomes even more challenging. In addition to the conventional view, one can propose a 'contrary view' that relationships between psychological factors and cancer may be mediated in part by the effects of cancer and its treatment on the immune system (see Figure 4).

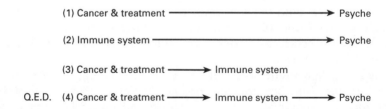

Figure 4

## 3 The chutzpah view of the implications of psychoneuro-immunology for oncology

If one does not accept the evidence supporting the view that psychological factors influence cancer, or the evidence supporting the immunological influences on cancer, is one forced to dismiss the possibility that psychological influences on immune function may affect the incidence or progression of cancer? Possibly not. The failure to consider the influences of psychological factors on immune function may have compromised much of the previous literature in each of these areas. For example, researchers investigating the influence of immune variables on the progression of cancer rarely indicate in their published studies the circumstances under which blood was collected for immune assessments. Was it collected in the clinic as patients awaited a diagnostic test, or after they had received the bad news? Although most investigators would not think of collecting blood at various times of day because they are aware that circadian effects on immune function could compromise their data, they are largely unaware of the potential effects of psychological variables. Unexamined psychological influences on immune function could thus obscure underlying links between immune function and cancer. On the other hand, researchers investigating the influence of psychological variables on cancer rarely consider the immunological literature, the psychoimmune literature, or the psychological measures to be used when selecting patients for a given study. For example, immunological effects are better established for some cancers than others (for example virally induced tumours) and are better established at some stages in the natural history of cancer than others (for example when tumour burden is lower). Psychological investigations of patients selected on that basis may be more likely to reveal significant effects of psychological factors on cancer.

## 4 The wider view of the implications of psychoneuro-immunology for oncology

As outlined above, both the conventional view and the chutzpah view focus on the mediational role of *psychological* influences on immune function in cancer. From this perspective, the neuroendocrine links between the brain and immune system (for example Bellinger *et al.*, Chapter 2) have been viewed as mediating psycho-immune links (see Figure 5).

Little attention has been paid to neuroendocrine effects on the immune system that may occur independent of psychological factors. Although psychological influences on immune function may be mediated by some of these

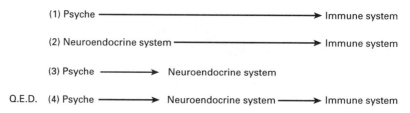

**Figure 5**

pathways, there is likely to be considerable regulatory activity taking place without the involvement of the psyche. As with neural regulation of other physiological systems (for example the cardiovascular system) there are likely to be regulatory loops that can function without psychological input or conscious awareness. As Bellinger and colleagues (Chapter 2) amply illustrate, an increasing number of both efferent and afferent pathways linking the brain and the immune system have now been identified. A few of these are shown in Figure 6.

There are numerous potential pathways for efferent output from the central nervous system to the immune system, including autonomic innervation of lymphoid organs as well as classical neuroendocrine responses. There are also a myriad of potential pathways for afferent input from the immune system to the brain, including a wide range of cytokines and neuropeptides produced by the leukocytes in response to antigenic stimulation. Direct evidence that any of these pathways are involved in *regulation* of immune function is scant. The secretion of interleukin-1 (IL-1) by monocytes may provide one rare example of a feedback control mechanism involving the neuroendocrine system. Increased levels of IL-1 in the bloodstream, can trigger increased level of ACTH secretion, which in turn triggers increased corticosteroid levels, which in turn reduces the production of IL-1. Evidence for feedforward regulation of the immune system by the brain is provided by studies demonstrating that immune function can be modulated by classical conditioning (3). Considerable research remains to be done to determine the extent and specificity of such neural regulation of immune function. When and where does the brain become involved? How do neural regulatory loops interact with regulatory loops within the immune system? Hopefully, the twenty-first century will see the answers to such questions.

The autonomic regulatory component of psycho*neuro*immunology, may prove to make a more profound contribution to oncology in the future than the psychological component. Greater understanding of the connections between brain and immune system is likely to reveal a plethora of novel strategies for the enhancement of immune defences against cancer (see Plotnikoff and Faith, Chapter 15).

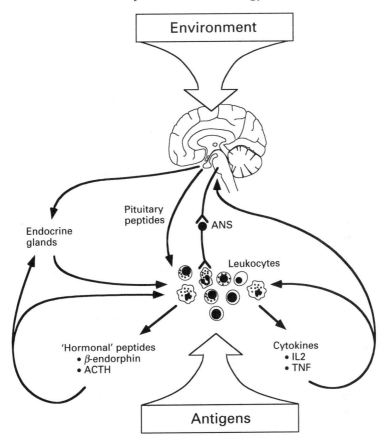

Figure 6

## 5   Summary and conclusions

The potential implications of psychoneuroimmunology for oncology have only just begun to be appreciated. Greater understanding of psychological and neuroendocrine influences on immune function may make a major contribution to our understanding and treatment of cancer, or contribute very little. The jury is still out, awaiting the results of research to come.

# 6 References

1. Bovbjerg, D. H. (1989). Psychoneuroimmunology and cancer. In *Handbook of Psychooncology*, (ed. J. C. Holland and J. H. Rowland), pp. 727–734. Oxford University Press, New York.
2. Bovbjerg, D. H. (1991). Psychoneuroimmunology—implications for oncology? *Cancer*, **67**, 828–832.
3. Bovbjerg, D. H. and Ader, R. (1986). The central nervous system and learning: Feedforward regulation of immune responses. In *Pituitary Function and Immunity*, (ed. I. Berczi) pp. 252–259. CRC Press, Boca Raton, FL.

# Index